PLANTS FROM TEMPERATE ZONE USED IN HOMOEOPATHIC MEDICINE

Botanical, Ecological &
Pharmacognostic features

José Waizel-Bucay*

Formerly
Escuela Nacional de Medicina &
Homeopatía
Instituto Politécnico Nacional
Mexico City
MEXICO

*B. Sc., M. Sc., Dr. Sc., Senior Researcher

PLANTS FROM TEMPERATE ZONE USED IN HOMOEOPATHIC MEDICINE

Botanical, Ecological & Pharmacognostic features

José Waizel-Bucay

First Edition: 2019

Copyright © José Waizel-Bucay, 2016.

ISBN: 9781698578422

Independently published

All rights reserved.

The entire content of this book is copyrighted and no part whatsoever may be copied and used -privately, for educational purposes, publishing or for commercial application- without the written permission of the author.

Dedicatory

To my wife, my children, granddaughters and daughter-in-law, for all what they mean to me. Also I want to leave public testimony of appreciation, remembrance and tribute to the memory of many traditional healers and physicians formed in universities, which ungratefully were unregistered and therefore not remembered by the history of the world, but contributed anonymously, to the discovery and research of several remedies that are now in common use. Likewise, my sincere appreciation to those at all times —even at the cost of their lives-, devoted or dedicated their lives to try to restore health or mitigate the suffering of their brothers -men-, regardless of their race, religion or the color of their skin and with or without economic remuneration. Similarly I pay tribute to the blessed memory of my parents: Teresa and Alberto, grandfather Mair, and to my brother-in-law David, for the legacy they have left us.

Table of Contents

Acknowledgements..
Preface...

CHAPTER I. Introduction....................................... 1
I.1. Major groups of plants in the world...............2
I.2. Plants & Homeopathy....................................3
I.3. Plant metabolites & chemical composition... 4
CHAPTER II. The World's Climate Classification.. 7
II.1. The Köppen's Classification...........................8
II.2. Temperate Climate... 9
II.3. The Temperate Zones..................................10
CHAPTER III. The plants of temperate zones used in Homeopathy...13
III.1. Format Design of the Checklist and Description of the Elements of the Text............13
III.2. Temperate plant remedies used by Homoeophatic Therapy.......................................17
CHAPTER IV. Illustrations of some plants mentioned in the book...307
CHAPTER V. References....................................316
CHAPTER VI. Index of Homeopathic Remedies
....325
CHAPTER VII. About the Author..................347

Acknowledgments

The author wishes to make public recognition to authorities from the Instituto Politécnico Nacional, Mexico (IPN) the support given. It also wishes to express its gratitude to: Drs. Sc.; Miss Nury Pérez-Hernández and Dr. Juan S. Salas-Benito, for their remarks into the English translation to the introductory book's chapter, as well as to MD, & M. Sc. Marco Polo Franco-Hernández his collaboration for the digital format of the remedie's monographs. And to all my companions from the Escuela Nacional de Medicina y Homeopatía (in Mexico City) for their friendship over many years. I do not forgot and will appreciate forever the teachings of all my teachers throughout my life.

Preface

Plants, animals, minerals and chemical substances are used for the preparation of the homeopathic drugs, – also known as "remedies"-. The largest number of materials comes from the plant kingdom. The number of the employed species varies depending on the Pharmacopoeia or Materia Medica revised, and fluctuates between 390 and 1.000 or more. More than a seventh of our planet surface area is considered temperate.

The purpose of this work is to allow the reader to know quickly and in a summarized form, different aspects of the plants that are used by homeopathy (that grow wild or cultivated) in temperate world zones for the remedies elaboration, such as: their common and scientific names (includes the synonyms), botanical family. Their geographic distribution, and form life, the part of the plant used and if they are prepared from fresh or dried form material and some bibliographical references for further information.

CHAPTER I. Introduction

Since ancient times, humans have found plants to be a useful resource for satisfying several of their needs, not only the most basic one for food but also, among others, for obtaining relief from illness and disease. There have never been a people or culture that has not left oral or written testimony regarding its use of plants for this latter purpose, or that has not searched the surrounding flora for possible remedies for disease. Since Paleolithic times update, the search has continued without interruption, first, based only on intuition and trial-and-error, and later, by observing the similarities between the shapes of some of the fruits, seeds and flowers and the nature of the disease or the shape of the affected organ. At present, the exploration of flora continues in an empirical manner, keeping popular wisdom and conviction, knowing that a big proportion, over 75%, of flora still remains unexplored (Waizel & Waizel, 2009).

I.1. Major groups of plants in the world

DIVISION	GROUP	Species number
Spermatophytes or Phanerogams (plants with flowers and will reproduced by seeds)	Angiosperms / Dicotyledons (Magnoliophyta)	199,350
	Angiosperms / Monocotyledons or Liliopsida (Palms, grasses, etc.)	59,300
	Gymnosperms or Pinophyta (Conifers, cycads, Gnetales and Gingkoales)	980
Cryptogams (plants that reproduced by spores)	Ferns & allies (Pteridophyta)	13,025
	Mosses & Hepatics (Bryophyta)	19,900
	Algae	27,000
Fungi*	Mushrooms	70,000
TOTAL		**389,525**

Table 1. Major groups of world plants*
Adapted from: Llorente-Bousquets y Ocegueda (2008).

*Although they are listed as a separate group, in this work are deemed algae and fungi as part of the plant Kingdom's (Plantae).

I.2. Plants & Homeopathy

Homeopathy is a medical therapy discovered and test in a modern form by the physician Samuel C. Hahnemann, -born in Meissen, Germany in 1755 and died in Paris in 1843-. To prepare its medicines (also known as homeopathic remedies), this medical doctrine make use of raw materials obtained from complete plants and animals or some of their parts or secretions, as well as minerals and isolated and purified organic or inorganic chemicals. The major source of materials comes from the plant kingdom. The number of the employed species varies depending on the Pharmacopoeia or Materia Medica revised, and fluctuates between 390 and 1.000 or more. The first figure was obtained from the review of the species mentioned in the "Comisión Editora de la Farmacopea Homeopática de los Estados Unidos Mexicanos", (1988), and in the "American Institute of Homeopathy (1979) or [The Homeopathic Pharmacopoeia of the United States of America], as others books as: Guajardo (1988); Guermonprez; Pinkas & Torck (1989), and additional bibliographic sources that are mentioned in the chapters related to references.

In a previous paper (Waizel, 2005), I presented the plants that inhabit in arid zones and are used in Homeopathy. In this book, I reviewed those that grow in the temperate zones, so considered by the climatic Aristotle's as well as Köppen's classifications, which are also used as homeopathic remedies.

I.3. The plant metabolites and their chemical composition

Plants manufacture a great number of organic substances essential for their subsistence called primary metabolites, as well as other several types of compounds in smaller amount and concentration, known as secondary metabolites. Among the first group, sugars or carbohydrates, fatty acids, fats, amino acids, proteins and vitamins are basically found; while among the second group the main components included are: alcohols, alkaloids, antibiotics, balsams, carotenoids, coumarines, essential or volatile oils, flavonoids, glycosides, glycosides, gums, ketones, lactones, mucilages, organic acids, pectines, phenols, phytosterols, phytotoxins, quinones, resins, saponins, steroids, tannins, terpenes (terpenoids), and several others with an assorted biological activity. Therefore the plants are used as drugs or medicaments for humans or in the veterinary medicine (phytomedicines), either directly or after undergoing some chemical laboratory processes (Rotblatt & Ziment, 2002).

The chemical composition (qualitative and/or quantitative) of plants is variable; it depends on the botanic family and species, and on the chemical race to which the plant belongs; also may be individual variations between equal specie (Filipowicz, 2006). This variability can also be affected by ecological conditions of the growing habitat such as soil type and composition, altitude above the sea level, climate, and water availability (ecotypes or ecological races). In some cases, the properties of the plant can be affected even for the hour of the day or the year season of collection, or the phenological conditions of the plant, as well as age and ripeness of the organism.

Furthermore when a plant is subject to farming, the production (and thus the concentration) of any selected metabolites such as alkaloids, may be accelerated or increased, in comparison with the production under natural conditions (Waizel, 1979).

Therefore, some of the secondary metabolites may increase or decrease their concentration as a response to some environmental abiotic, stressing agents such as low or high temperature, lack or excess of available moisture, salinity, high insolation, etc., which among other issues are the matter of study of ecophysiology.

For all the above reasons, it is not unusual to find variations in the "quality" of different lots of the raw materials employed to manufacture phytopharmaceuticals, in accordance with their source (site and country of origin). In a similar way, for the manufacture of homeopathic remedies, there is a preference to use materials coming from the country where the plant was assayed and employed for the first time.

Therefore, it is possible that a given species shows ecological differentiation and that its composition varies depending on the habitat where it develops and consequently its chemical constituents are going to vary depending on the place of growth (tropical, temperate or arid zone).

CHAPTER II. The World's Climate Classification

One of the first attempts to climate classification was performed by the ancient Greek scholar Aristotle. He hypothesized that the earth was divided into three types of climatic zones, each one characterized by its distance from the equator. Though we actually know that Aristotle's theory was extremely oversimplified, it unfortunately persists at present days.

Based on the consideration that the area near the equator was too hot to be inhabited, Aristotle dubbed the region comprised between the Tropic of Cancer at 23.5° North, passing over the equator, latitude 0°, to the Tropic of Capricorn 23.5° South, as the "Torrid Zone." Despite Aristotle's beliefs, great civilizations flourished in the Torrid Zone, in Latin America, India, and Southeast Asia.

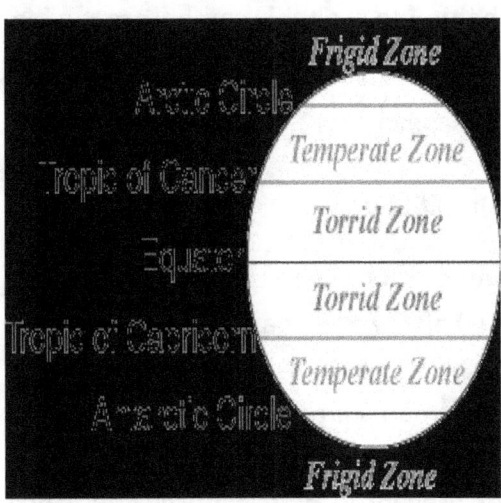

Fig. 1. The world climatic classification (Rosenberg, 1999).

Aristotle reasoned that the area to the North of the Arctic Circle (66.5° North) and to the South of the Antarctic Circle (66.5° South) were permanently frozen. He called this uninhabitable zone as the "Frigid Zone." But now we know that the areas to the North of the Arctic Circle are indeed habitable. For instance, the world's largest Asian city to the north of the Arctic Circle, Murmansk, Russia, is home to almost half a million people. Because of to the months lacking of sunlight, it is true that the city residents live under artificial light, but nevertheless the city actually lies in the Frigid Zone.

The only area that Aristotle believed fit for habitation and able to support the flourishing of human civilization was the "Temperate Zone." The two Temperate Zones were suggested to lie between the Tropics and the Arctic and Antarctic Circles. Aristotle's belief that the Temperate Zone was the most habitable probably came from the fact that it was the zone where he dwelt.

II.1. The Köppen's classification

Since Aristotle's time, others have attempted to classify the regions of the earth over climatic basis. The most successful classification probably was the system developed by the German climatologist and amateur botanist Wladimir Köppen co-authored with his student Rudolph Geiger and presented as a wall map in 1928. They assigned capital letters to design the zones as follows: A (tropical, tropical rainy); B (subtropical, dry climate); C (temperate); D (cold, snow, or boreal); E (polar or snow) and F (everlasting ice). The criteria to define the climatic zones are the measurements of temperature and precipitation (Sachs, 2000).

Those groups were further subdivided as a function of the rain regime and environmental temperatures and were also notated by a letter, using this time small case letters that together with capital letters specify the climatic variety of a particular area within each major category. So, for instance, a Csa type climate means one with temperate, dry hot summers and moist mild winters, so known as "Mediterranean climate".

Köppen's multiple-category classification system has been slightly modified since his final classification in 1936, but it is still the most frequently used and widely accepted as the authoritative map of the world climates up to this time (Rosenberg, 1999, 2005).

II.2. Temperate climate

"Temperate climate" is something of a misnomer. Tropical, Oceanic and Mediterranean climates undergo a moderate weather change along the year but some regions within the temperate climate zone, experience distinct changes across the four seasons. In a great area of eastern North America, from the Ohio Valley in the United States of America to the southern shores of Hudson Bay in Canada, the "temperate" climate can involve episodes of both arctic and tropical weather in the same year. Such changes are greater the further the area is from the influence of large water bodies, and decrease in the areas where oceans and other large water bodies exert a more strong influence over the climate. A constant common factor of the world's temperate zones is the climatic variability; these regions have all four seasons distinctly marked, while those in the tropical zone have only two seasons (summer "wet" and winter "dry") (Rosenberg, 2005).

D'Ambrosio (2008), classified the temperate climate in 4 subtypes: Mediterranean, chinese, oceanic, and continental.

II.3. The Temperate zones

In the temperate zones the three large groups of plants (herbs, shrubs and trees) are commonly found, the trees can either keep their leaves or not, depending on the season of the year, and are: the evergreen that keep their foliage through two or more consecutive seasons, in opposition to which lose their leaves every year as the cold season approaches, and are commonly called deciduous.

More than a seventh of our planet surface area is considered temperate. The temperate zones are regions that only a few people regard as rich in vegetal diversity. This appreciation is not correct because even if those areas are not as rich in diversity as a tropical rain forest, the people living there have inherited from immemorial times, and they have the knowledge of how to use the resources that nature has put on their hands for their own benefit. From several of those resources, the man has obtained, in addition of food, several other products as wood (timber), resins, essential or volatile oils (perfumes), etc. Likewise, a number of ancient cultures have employed the plants of temperate zones as a therapeutic resource.

There are two stripes located further to the north and south of the subtropics. In those zones the sun always stays in the sky to the South (North Temperate Zone) or to the North (South Temperate Zone). Summers are quite hot, but winters carry freezing temperatures in both the air and the soil. In order to survive there, the organisms must be able to tolerate frost and freeze processes; therefore it is not surprising that as the latitude increases, the diversity of organism's decreases.

A major part of Europe is located in the temperate zone and only its southern regions belong to the subtropical zone. For that reason the most typical forest growing almost through all Europe are deciduous trees and only in the very northern part of the continent the taiga and tundra do occur.

Because of its size, Asia includes practically all the climatic zones, e.g., from tundra and taiga through the temperate zone to subtropical and tropical regions. The largest portion of this continent shows an arid character, with deforested territories and only in the most humid regions of Eastern Asia broad-leaved forests with numerous species of plants can be found. The south-eastern part of Asia, e.g., the so-called Indo-Malaysian region, is located in the rainfall virgin forest zone. Only the Northern part and a little portion of the Southwest Africa is considered temperate or subtropical.

The temperate zone covers a good part of North America and tundra and taiga may be found only at the north of that region. In the middle latitudes of the eastern half of North America broad-leaved and mixed forest predominate, while in the west there are extensive prairies.

South America is located in the tropical region, and a temperate zone is only found in its utmost southern part. The Australian territory is partially tropical and partially temperate (Ross, 1994; ZOO, 1998).

Considering that a number of plants that inhabit the temperate zones of the globe are used for medical purposes, it should not be a surprise that Homeopathy uses them.

Chapter III. The plants of temperate zones used in homeopathy

We present below, more than 700 plants that grow wild or cultivated in several regions of the temperate zones of the world, including those growing within the farming fields, e.g., those known as "undergrowth", "weeds" or "arvensis", as well as the so called "ruderal" that grow at the roadsides, on the garbage surface, or construction wastes or abandoned fields, and that are used for preparing medicaments in homeopathic therapeutics. The list shows the species alphabetically ordered according to the name of the remedy, its scientific name and respective family, the common name(s) (mainly in English and French), their life's form, the part of the plant used for the preparation of the remedy, also if the plant is used in its dried or fresh form, as well as its geographical distribution.

III.1. Format Design of the checklist and description of the elements of the text

Homeopathic Remedy Name: These names were taken from the consulted references and reviewed -between others-, from Bharatan et al. (2002).

Scientific Name(s) / [Botanical Family]: The scientific names presented comprises the species name, and the complete plant or abbreviated taxon author's name, e.g., Linn. or (L.) refer to Carl Linnaeus. In some cases, after the "=" symbol the relevant scientific synonyms are added. Note: This information is not updated in all cases. Occasionally, two or more names of Botanical families are quoted for a same plant or species, which means that she can be placed in one or more families interchangeably.

The scientific names were reviewed as far as possible from Bharatan et al. (formerly mentioned) and from the following Internet Taxonomic Data Bases:

The Missouri Botanical Garden's VAST (VAScular Tropicos). <http://mobot.mobot.org/cgi-bin/search_vast>

The International Plant Names Index (IPNI). <http://www.ipni.org/index.html>

The GRIN Taxonomy, GRIN-Global Species Data. <https://npgsweb.ars-grin.gov/gringlobal/taxon/taxonomysearch.aspx>

The Integrated Taxonomic Information System (ITIS). <https://www.itis.gov>

USDA, ARS, National Genetic Resources Program. Germplasm Resources Laboratory. <http://plants.usda.gov/index.html>

There are other categories infraespecifics; i.e.: subsp. = subspecie, a lower taxonomic rank than species; var. = variety, a taxonomic rank below subspecies and above form; x = hybrid between 2 different species, or varieties, etc.

Sometimes two or more family's names are cited for a plant, it means that will be placed indistinctly in one or more families. About the current denomination of the Botanical families: Asteraceae, Compositae; Labiatae = Lamiaceae; Gramineae = Poaceae; Cruciferae = Brassicaceae; Leguminosae = Fabaceae; Umbelliferae = Apiaceae, being the second name the present-day.

Common Name(s): the common names are mentioned in different languages or just in English. The square brackets "[ ]" indicate the language. In the case of the Chinese, Japanese or Russian, are transcribed.

Life form: epiphytes: air-borne plants that form symbiotic relationships with host plants.

Fungi: includes microorganisms such as yeasts and molds, as well as the more familiar mushrooms.

Herbs: small, fragile plants lacking woody stems, which can be annual, biennial or perennial (e.g., grasses).

Lianas: woody plants that take the form of vines supported on tree and shrubs.

Shrubs: woody perennials having several stems branching from a base near the soil surface.

Trees: large woody perennial plants having an upright single trunk, branching into a crown.

Weed: low-lying broad-leaved plants.

Part(s) Used: show the vegetable part or organ employed in the remedy manufacture, and in some cases, if are used starting from Fresh or Dried material.

Geographic distribution: It indicates the main regional area that's inhabited by a particular specie, and may not properly represent the total globe geographical distribution of the specie, e.g., North America, South Europa, USA = United States of America.

Cosmopolitan: means an organism found in most parts of the world.

Naturalized: Indicate a plant adapted or acclimated to a new environment or introduced and established as if native.

Reference(s): As mentioned in abbreviated form. There are cited complete in the References chapter, for instance: American Institute of Homeopathy, 1979; Bharatan et al. 2002; Remedia/at, 2010; Tiwari et al. 2013; n.d. = no publication date.

III.2. Temperate plant remedies used by Homoeophatic therapy

Abies canadensis

Scientific Name(s) / [Botanical Family]: *Abies canadensis* Mill. = *Abies canadensis* (L.) Michx. = *Picea canadensis* (Mill.) Britton, Sterns & Poggenb. = *Picea canadensis* (Mill.) Link = *Picea glauca* (Moench) Voss = *Pinus canadensis* L. = *Tsuga canadensis* (L.) Carrièrre. [Pinaceae].

Common Name(s): Tuya del Canada [Spanish]. Alberta white spruce, American white spruce, Black Hills spruce, Canadian spruce, hemlock spruce, porsild spruce, weastern white spruce, white spruce [English]. Épinette blanche, pruche du Canada, sapin du Canada [French].

Life form: Tree. **Part(s) Used:** Bark, leaf, shoot, bud / Fresh. **Geographic distribution:** North America.

Reference(s): Bharatan *et al.* 2002; Remedia/at, 2010; Tiwari *et al.* 2013; American Institute of Homeopathy, 1979.

Abies nigra

Scientific Name(s) / [Botanical Family]: *Abies mariana* Mill. = *Abies nigra* Du Roi = *Abies nigra* (Aiton) Poir. = *Picea mariana* (Mill.) Britton, Sterns & Poggenb. = *Picea nigra* (Aiton) Link. = *Pinus nigra* Arnold [Pinaceae].

Common Name(s): Black or double spruce [English]. Sapin noir [French].

Life form: Tree. **Part(s) Used:** Root resin / **Geographic distribution:** North America.

Reference(s): Bharatan *et al.* 2002; Tiwari *et al.* 2013; American Institute of Homeopathy, 1979.

Abrotanum

Scientific Name(s) / [Botanical Family]: *Artemisia abrotanum* L. [Asteraceae, Compositae].
Common Name(s): Abrótano, abrótano macho, boja, hierba lombriguera, incienso [Spanish]. Herb royal, lady's love, old-man womwood, southern wormwood [English]. Armoise aurone, aurone mâle, citronelle, citronelle aurone [French].
Life form: Herb. **Part(s) Used:** Leaf, Stem / Fresh. **Geographic distribution:** South Europe.
Reference(s): Clarke, 2008; Fuentes, 1996; Gotfredsen, 2009.

Abrus

Scientific Name(s) / [Botanical Family]: *Abrus precatorius* L. = *Abrus abrus* (L.) W. Wight = *Glycine abrus* L. [Fabaceae, Leguminosae].
Common Name(s): Árbol del rosario, bejuco de peonia, jequiriti, paternostera, regaliz americano [Spanish]. Grain d'église, graine diable, herbe de diable, jéquirity [French]. Bead tree, coral-beadplant, crab's-eye, Indian-licorice, jequirity, jequirity-bean, licorice-vine, love-bean, lucky-bean, minnie-minnies, prayer-beads, precatory, red-beadvine, rosary-pea, weatherplant [English]. Arvoreiro, assacú mirim, carolina miúda [Portuguese].
Life form: Tree. **Part(s) Used:** Fruit mature or seeds / Dried.
Geographic distribution: Temperate & tropical-Asia.
Reference(s): Bharatan *et al.* 2002; Clarke, 2008; Dorta Soares, n.d.; Fuentes, 1996; Gotfredsen, 2009; American Institute of Homeopathy, 1979.

Absinthium

Scientific Name(s) / [Botanical Family]: *Artemisia absinthium* L. [Asteraceae, Compositae].
Common Name(s): Absintio, ajenjo, ajenjo mayor, ajorizo,

artemisia amarga, hierba santa, incienso [Spanish]. Absinthe, armoise absinthe, armoise amère, armoise amčre [French]. Absinth, absinthe wormwood, absinthium, common wormwood, wormwood [English]. Absinto, aluina, erva dos vermes, losna [Portuguese].
Life form: Shrub. **Part(s) Used:** Aerial part in bloom, leaf, root / Fresh.
Geographic distribution: North Africa. West Asia. Siberia. Sovietic Central Asia. India. Europe. etc., naturalized in several places. Cosmopolitan.
Reference(s): Allen, 2006-2010; Bharatan *et al.* 2002; Clarke, 2008; Dorta Soares, n.d.; Fuentes, 1996; Gotfredsen, 2009; Guermonprez *et al.* 1989; Plants for a future, 2009; Tiwari *et al.* 2013.

Acanthus mollis

Scientific Name(s) / [Botanical Family]: *Acanthus mollis* L. = *Acanthus spinulosus* Host [Acanthaceae].
Common Name(s): Acanto, ala de ángel, alas de ángel, carnerona, hierba gigante [Spanish]. Acanthe, acanthe molle [French]. Bear's breech, common cow parsnip, cow parsley, hogweed, masterwort [English]. Acanto, erva gigante [Portuguese].
Life form: Herb. **Part(s) Used:** Complete plant / fresh, complete plant in bloom / fresh. **Geographic distribution:** Europe. Cosmopolitan. Cultivated.
Reference(s): Allen, 2006-2010; Dorta Soares, n.d.; Gotfredsen, 2009; American Institute of Homeopathy, 1979; Zandvoort, 2006.

Achyrantes calea

Scientific Name(s) / [Botanical Family]: *Iresine celosioides* L. = *Iresine celosia* L. = *Iresine diffusa* H. & B. = *Iresine calea* (Ibañez)

Standl. = *Achyranthes calea* Ibañez [Amaranthaceae].
Common Name(s): Hierba del tabardillo (typhus), hierba de la calentura (fever), tlatlancuaya [Spanish]. Erva da febre, erva do tifo [Portuguese].
Life form: Herb. **Part(s) Used:** Complete plant / Fresh / Dried. Stem & leaf collected before bloom / Fresh. **Geographic distribution:** Mexico. Central & South America.
Reference(s): Bharatan *et al.* 2002; Dorta Soares, n.d.; American Institute of Homeopathy, 1979.

Aconitum anthora

Scientific Name(s) / [Botanical Family]: *Aconitum anthora* L. [Ranunculaceae].
Common Name(s): Anthore, Acónito amarillo [Spanish]. Aconit anthore, Aconit anti-thora [French]. Pyrenees monkshood, yellow monkshood [English].
Life form: Herb. **Part(s) Used:** Complete plant / fresh, root and complete plant in bloom. **Geographic distribution:** Temperate-Asia. Europe.
Reference(s): Bharatan *et al.* 2002; Dorta Soares, n.d.

Aconitum cammarum

Scientific Name(s) / [Botanical Family]: *Aconitum x cammarum* L. [probably are a hibrid between *Aconitum variegatum* x *Aconitum napellus*]. This remedy name also includes: *Aconitum neomontanum* Willd. = *Aconitum intermedium* DC. = *Aconitum stoerckianum* Reich. [Ranunculaceae].
Common Name(s): Monkshood [English].
Life form: Herb. **Part(s) Used:** Root, rhizome / **Geographic distribution:** Europe & cultivated.
Reference(s): Allen, 2006-2010; Bolte *et al.* 1997; Clarke, 2008; Dorta Soares, n.d.

Aconitum e radice

Scientific Name(s) / [Botanical Family]: *Aconitum napellus* L. = *Aconitum neomontanum* Wulfen [Ranunculaceae].
Common Name(s): Acónito, acónito común, aconitum napellus, anapelo, matalobos, nabillo del diablo, napelo [Spanish]. Aconit napel [French]. Monkshood, common aconite, bear's-foot, blue rocket, priest´s pintle [English]. Acónito, capacete de Júpter, capuz de frade [Portuguese].
Life form: Herb. **Part(s) Used:** Complete plant in bloom / Fresh / Dried. **Geographic distribution:** WestEurope, Siberia-Himalaya, cultivated.
Reference(s): Bharatan *et al.* 2002; Dorta Soares, n.d.; Gotfredsen, 2009; Plants for a future, 2009; American Institute of Homeopathy, 1979.

Aconitum ferox

Scientific Name(s) / [Botanical Family]: *Aconitum ferox* Wallich ex Ser. = *Aconitum virosum* Don. *Delphinium ferox* Baill. [Ranunculaceae].
Common Name(s): Acónito de la india, acónito de Nepal [Spanish]. Aconitum feroxe, aconit blanc [French]. Ativisha, bisch, bikh, Indian aconite, moonkshood, Nepalese aconite [English]. Acônito da Índia [Portuguese].
Life form: Herb. **Part(s) Used:** Root, rhizome / Fresh, mature seeds / Dried. **Geographic distribution:** Asia (Bhutan, Himalaya, India, Nepal).
Reference(s): Allen, 2006-2010; Bolte *et al.* 1997; Dorta Soares, n.d.; Gotfredsen, 2009; Müntz, n.d.; Tiwari *et al.* 2013.

Aconitum lycoctonum

Scientific Name(s) / [Botanical Family]: *Aconitum lycoctonum* L. = *Aconitum* excelsum Rchb. = *Aconitum septentrionale* Koelle = *Aconitum vulparia* Reichb. This remedies's name also include

Aconitum telyphonum Reich. [Ranunculaceae].
Common Name(s): Aconit blanc, Aconit tue-loup [French]. Badgersbane, great yellow wolfsbane, wolfbane, yellow aconite [English].
Life form: Herb. **Part(s) Used:** Complete plant / Fresh.
Geographic distribution: Temperate-Asia. Europe.
Reference(s): Allen, 2006-2010; Bharatan *et al.* 2002; Bolte *et al.* 1997; Clarke, 2008; Dorta Soares, n.d.; Gotfredsen, 2009; Tiwari *et al.* 2013.

Aconitum napellus see also *Aconitum e radice*

Aconitum napellus

Scientific Name(s) / [Botanical Family]: *Aconitum napellus* L. [Ranunculaceae].
Common Name(s): Acónito, acónito común, capucha del monje, napelo [Spanish]. Aconit napel, Casque de Jupiter [French]. Common aconite, European monkshood, helmet-flower, monkshood, priest´s pintle, Venus'chariot, wolfsbane [English].
Life form: Herb. **Part(s) Used:** Complete plant, Flower / Fresh.
Geographic distribution: West & Central Europe (Siberia). Central Asia. Himalaya, cultivated.
Reference(s): Bolte *et al.* 1997; Clarke, 2008; Comisión Editora de la Farmacopea Homeopática de los Estados Unidos Mexicanos, 1988; Dorta Soares, n.d.; Gotfredsen, 2009; Tiwari *et al.* 2013.

Aconitum septentrionale see Aconitum lycoctonum

Acorus calamus

Scientific Name(s) / [Botanical Family]: *Acorus calamus* L. = *Acorus aromaticus* Lam. = *Acorus vulgaris* Simk. [Acoraceae, Araceae].

Common Name(s): Acoro aromático, cálamo aromático, cálamo verdadero, calamís [Spanish]. Acore, acore calame, acore odorant, acore roseau, acore vrai [French]. Acorus roseau, calamus, flagroot, myrtle-flag, sweet calamus, sweet-flag, sweetroot [English]. Ácoro verdadeiro, cálamo aromático [Portugués].
Life form: Herb. **Part(s) Used:** Root, rhizome / Dried. **Geographic distribution:** Europe, North America. Temperate-Asia & tropical. Naturalized in several places.
Reference(s): Dorta Soares, n.d.; Gotfredsen, 2009; Plants for a future, 2009.

Actaea racemosa see *Cimifuga racemosa*

Actaea spicata

Scientific Name(s) / [Botanical Family]: *Actaea spicata* L. = *Actaea christophoriana* Gouan = *Christophoriana spicata* (L.) Moench [Ranunculaceae].
Common Name(s): Barba de cabra, cristobalina, hierba de San Cristóbal [Spanish]. Actée in épi, herbe-de-Saint-Christophe [French]. Baneberry, bugbane, cohosh, herb Christopher, toadroot [English]. Erva de Sâo Cristovâo [Portuguese].
Life form: Herb. **Part(s) Used:** Root, rhizome / Fresh. **Geographic distribution:** North & Central Europe & Asia, North America.
Reference(s): Bolte *et al.* 1997; Dorta Soares, n.d.; Gotfredsen, 2009; Tiwari *et al.* 2013; American Institute of Homeopathy, 1979.

Actinidia chinensis e flores femineibus

Scientific Name(s) / [Botanical Family]: *Actinidia chinensis* Planchon = *Actinidia chinensis deliciosa* (A¡Error! Marcador no definido..Chev.) A.Chev. [Actinidiaceae].
Common Name(s): Mi hou tao, yang tao, zhong hua mi hou tao [Chinese]. Grosella china, kiwi [Spanish]. Actinidier de Chine,

actinidier à gros Fruits [French]. Chinese actinidia, chinese soft-hair kiwi, chinese goosebery, golden kiwi, kiwi, kiwi tree, yellow-fleshed actinidia [English].
Life form: Herb. **Part(s) Used:** Flower / Fresh. **Geographic distribution:** Temperate-Asia (China, Taiwan).
Reference(s): Remedia/at, 2010; Wang *et al.* 2010.

Adlumia fungosa

Scientific Name(s) / [Botanical Family]: *Adlumia fungosa* (Aiton) Greene ex Britton, Sterns & Poggenb. = *Adlumia cirrhosa* Rafinesque in DC. = *Bicuculla fungosa* (Aiton) Kuntze = *Fumaria fungosa* Aiton [Fumariaceae, Papaveraceae].
Common Name(s): Allegheny-vine, climbing-fumatory, mountain-fringe, woodfringe [English].
Life form: Herb. **Part(s) Used:** Aerial part / Fresh. **Geographic distribution:** Asia & Europe. North America (East & West Canada. North East, North, Central & Southeast United States of America). Siberia.
Reference(s): Bolte *et al.* 1997; Dorta Soares, n.d.; Müntz, n.d.; Tiwari *et al.* 2013.

Adonis vernalis

Scientific Name(s) / [Botanical Family]: *Adonis vernalis* L. = *Adonanthe* vernalis (L.) Spach [Ranunculaceae].
Common Name(s): Adonis primaveral, falso heléboro, ojo de faisán [Spanish]. Adonis du printemps, adonis [French]. False hellebore, ox-eye, pheasant´s eye, spring adonis, sweet vernal [English]. Olhos do diabo [Portuguese].
Life form: Herb. **Part(s) Used:** Complete plant / Fresh.
Geographic distribution: North Europe (France) & Asia. West United States of America.
Reference(s): Bolte *et al.* 1997; Clarke, 2008; Dorta Soares, n.d.; Gotfredsen, 2009; Tiwari *et al.* 2013; American Institute of

Homeopathy, 1979.

Adoxa
Scientific Name(s) / [Botanical Family]: *Adoxa moschatellina* L. = *Moschatellina tetragona* Moench = *Moschatellina fumariifolia* Bubani = *Moschatellina adoxa* All. = *Moscatella adoxa* Scop. [Adoxaceae, Caprifoliaceae].
Common Name(s): Moschatel/townhall clock, muskroot [English]. Adoxe moscatelle, moscatelline, moschatel [French]. Hierba del almizcle, moscatel, moscatelina [Spanish].
Life form: Herb. **Geographic distribution:** Europe (British Islands, Alpes), North America (United States of America).
Reference(s): Allen, 2006-2010; Bharatan *et al.* 2002; Bolte *et al.* 1997.

Aesculus glabra
Scientific Name(s) / [Botanical Family]: *Aesculus glabra* Willd. [Sapindaceae, Hippocastanaceae].
Common Name(s): Castaño de Asia [Spanish]. Marronnier de l'ohio, pavier de l'ohio, pavier glabre [French]. Fetid buckeye, Ohio buckeye, smooth-leaf ed horse chesnut, stinking buckeye [English]. Olho de Coelho [Portuguese].
Life form: Tree. **Part(s) Used:** Fruit, seeds / Fresh. **Geographic distribution:** North Asia. South Europe-England. North America (North East United States of America).
Reference(s): Clarke, 2008; Dorta Soares, n.d.; Gotfredsen, 2009; Tiwari *et al.* 2013; American Institute of Homeopathy, 1979.

Aesculus hippocastanum
Scientific Name(s) / [Botanical Family]: *Aesculus hippocastanum* L. [Sapindaceae, Hippocastanaceae].
Common Name(s): Castaño de India, castaño de Indias, castaño de Indias común [Spanish]. Marronnier, marronnier de l'Inde

[French]. Buckeye, common horse chestnut, conker, horse-chestnut, spanish chestnut, white chestnut [English]. Castanha da Índia [Portuguese].
Life form: Tree. **Part(s) Used:** Fruit, seeds / Fresh; young branches in bloom. **Geographic distribution:** India. Iran. North Turkey. Great Britain. France. United States of America.
Reference(s): Clarke, 2008; Dorta Soares, n.d.; Gotfredsen, 2009; Tiwari *et al.* 2013; American Institute of Homeopathy, 1979.

Aethusa
Scientific Name(s) / [Botanical Family]: *Aethusa cynapium* L. [Apiaceae, Umbelliferae].
Common Name(s): Apio de perro, cicuta Minor, cicuta of jardines, falso perejil, perejil de loco, perejil de perro [Spanish]. Ethuse, ethuse ciguë, petite ciguë [French]. Dog poison, dog parsley, fool's parsley, garden hemlock, lesser hemlock [English]. Cicuta dos jardins, cicuta pequena [Portuguese].
Life form: Herb. **Part(s) Used:** Complete plant / Fresh.
Geographic distribution: Europe, United States of America.
Reference(s): Bolte *et al.* 1997; Clarke, 2008; Dorta Soares, n.d.; Tiwari *et al.* 2013; American Institute of Homeopathy, 1979.

Agaricus
Scientific Name(s) / [Botanical Family]: *Amanita muscaria* (L.) Lam. = *Agaricus muscarius* L. = *Agaricus muscarius* Pers. [Amanitaceae].
Common Name(s): Falsa oronja, oronja venenosa, matamoscas [Spanish]. Amanite tue-mouche [French]. Fly agaric, fly amanita, fly mushroom [English]. Agárico mosqueado [Portuguese].
Life form: Fungi. **Part(s) Used:** Aerial part of the mushroom, or all without bark / Fresh. **Geographic distribution:** Asia. Europe. North America.
Reference(s): Bharatan *et al.* 2002; Dorta Soares, n.d.;

Gotfredsen, 2009; Guermonprez *et al.* 1989; Tiwari *et al.* 2013.

Agaricus citrina

Scientific Name(s) / [Botanical Family]: *Amanita citrina* (Schaeff.: Fr.) S. F. Gray. = *Agaricus citrinus* Schaeff.: Fr. [Amanitaceae].
Common Name(s): Amanita citrina [Spanish]. Amanite citrine [French]. Citron amanita, fals death cap [English].
Life form: Fungi. Plant **Part(s) Used:** Aerial part. **Geographic distribution:** Europe, North America.
Reference(s): Bharatan *et al.* 2002; Gotfredsen, 2009; Tiwari *et al.* 2013.

Agaricus emeticus

Scientific Name(s) / [Botanical Family]: *Russula emetica* (Schaeff.: Fr.) Gray = *Agaricus emeticus* Schaeff.: Fr. [Russulaceae].
Common Name(s): Seta [Spanish]. Russuke émétique [French]. The sickener, emetic russula, vomiting russula mushroom [English].
Life form: Fungi. **Part(s) Used:** Complete plant / Fresh. **Geographic distribution:** Northwest Europe. North America (United States of America, Mexico).
Reference(s): Allen, 2006-2010; Bharatan *et al.* 2002; Clarke, 2008; Tiwari *et al.* 2013.

Agaricus pantherina

Scientific Name(s) / [Botanical Family]: *Amanita pantherina* (DC.: Fr.) Krombh. = *Agaricus pantherinus* DC. [Amanitaceae].
Common Name(s): European panther, panther cap [English].
Life form: Fungi. **Part(s) Used:** Aerial part / Fresh. **Geographic distribution:** Europe, West Asia.
Reference(s): Bharatan *et al.* 2002; Tiwari *et al.* 2013.

Agaricus phalloides
Scientific Name(s) / [Botanical Family]: *Amanita phalloides* (Fr.: Fr.) Link = *Agaricus phalloides¡Error! Marcador no definido.* Fr. [Amanitaceae].
Common Name(s): Amanita bulbosa [Spanish]. Death cap, lethal death cap [English]. Cálice da Morte [Portuguese].
Life form: Fungi. **Part(s) Used:** Aerial part of the mushroom / Fresh. **Geographic distribution:** Australia. North America. North Europe.
Reference(s): Bharatan *et al.* 2002; Clarke, 2008; Dorta Soares, n.d.; Tiwari *et al.* 2013.

Agaricus procera
Scientific Name(s) / [Botanical Family]: *Macrolepiota procera* (Scop.: Fr.) Singer = *Lepiota procera* (Scop.: Fr.) Gray = *Agaricus procerus* Schaeff. [Agaricaceae].
Common Name(s): Hongo, seta de anillo [Spanish]. Coulenelle, cocherelle, Chevalier [French]. Parasol mushroom [English].
Life form: Fungi. **Part(s) Used:** Complete plant / **Geographic distribution:** Central Europe. Mexico.
Reference(s): Bharatan *et al.* 2002; Tiwari *et al.* 2013.

Agave americana
Scientific Name(s) / [Botanical Family]: *Agave americana* L. = *Agave americana* var. *expansa* (Jacobi) Gentry. *Agave expansa* Jacobi [Agavaceae, Amaryllidaceae].
Common Name(s): Acíbara, agave, maguey, maguey de lujo, pita [Spanish]. Agave d'Amérique, agave americaine [French]. Agave, american agave, american aloe, century plant, maguey [English]. Abecedária, agave, áloe americano, babosa brava [Portuguese].
Life form: Herb. **Part(s) Used:** Leaf, stem / Fresh; leaves collected in blooming time. **Geographic distribution:** North America & Mexico. Cultivated.

Reference(s): Clarke, 2008; Dorta Soares, n.d.; Gotfredsen, 2009; Tiwari *et al.* 2013; American Institute of Homeopathy, 1979.

Ageratina aromatica see *Eupatorium aromaticum*

Agnus castus
Scientific Name(s) / [Botanical Family]: *Vitex agnus-castus* L. [Verbenaceae].
Common Name(s): Agno casto, ajerobo, gatillo casto, hierba de la castidad, jorobo, sauzgatillo [Spanish]. Agneau-chaste, arbre chaste, gattilier [French]. Abraham's-bush, agnus castus, chaste berry, chaste tree, Hemp tree, lilac chastetree, monk's pepper [English]. Agno casto, árbore da castidade [Portuguese].
Life form: Shrub. **Part(s) Used:** Fruit, complete plant / Fresh / Dried. **Geographic distribution:** Mediterranean (South France-Greece) cultivated.
Reference(s): Bharatan *et al.* 2002; Dorta Soares, n.d.; François-Flores, 2007; Gotfredsen, 2009; Provings, 2008-2009; Tiwari *et al.* 2013; American Institute of Homeopathy, 1979.

Agraphis nutans
Scientific Name(s) / [Botanical Family]: *Scilla nutans* Sm. = *Agraphis nutans* Link. = *Hyacinthus nonscriptus* L. = *Hyacinthoides non-scriptus* L. Chouard ex Rothm. [Liliaceae].
Common Name(s): Auld man's bell, calverkeys, culverkeys, ring-o'-bells, jacinth, wild hyacinth, wood bells [English]. Endymion penché [French]. Campánula [Spanish].
Life form: Herb. **Part(s) Used:** Bulb / Dried; Complete plant / Fresh. **Geographic distribution:** West Europe. Great Britain. Mediterranean region.
Reference(s): Bharatan *et al.* 2002; Clarke, 2008; Dorta Soares, n.d.; Remedia/at, 2010; Tiwari *et al.* 2013.

Agrimonia

Scientific Name(s) / [Botanical Family]: *Agrimonia eupatoria* L. [Rosaceae].

Common Name(s): Agrimonia, amores pequeños, amoricos, hierba bacera, hierba de las heridas, hierba del podador, mermasangre, té del Norte [Spanish]. Aigremoine [French]. Agrimony, church steeples, cocklebur, european grovebur, philanthropos, sticklewort [English]. Erva de Sâo Guilherme, eupatoria dos gregos [Portuguese].

Life form: Herb. **Part(s) Used:** Aerial part in bloom / Dried.

Geographic distribution: Europe, Temperate-Asia.

Reference(s): Bharatan *et al.* 2002; Dorta Soares, n.d.; Fuentes, 1996; Gotfredsen, 2009; Müntz, n.d.

Agrostema githago

Scientific Name(s) / [Botanical Family]: *Agrostemma githago* L. = *Agrostemma githago* L. = *Githago segetum* Link = *Lychnis githago* (L.) Scop. = *Silene githago* E. H. L. Krause [Caryophyllaceae].

Common Name(s): Candelaria, clavellina, neguilla, negrilla, neguillón [Spanish]. Nielle des blés [French]. Agrostemma, cockle, corn-cockle, corn pink, githage, lychnis garbage [English]. Joio venenoso, nigela dos trigais [Portuguese].

Life form: Herb. **Part(s) Used:** seeds / Dried. **Geographic distribution:** Europe, Asia, Africa. Cosmopolitan.

Reference(s): Bharatan *et al.* 2002; Clarke, 2008; Dorta Soares, n.d.; Gotfredsen, 2009; Plants for a future, 2009; Tiwari *et al.* 2013; American Institute of Homeopathy, 1979.

Ailanthus glandulosus

Scientific Name(s) / [Botanical Family]: *Ailanthus glandulosa* Desfontaines = *Ailanthus altissima* (Mill.) Swingle = *Pongelion glandulosum* (Desf.) Pierre [Simaroubaceae].

Common Name(s): Ailanthus altissima, ailanto, árbol del cielo,

árbol del cielo chino, zumaque falso [Spanish]. Ailante, ailanthe glanduleux, arbre des dieux [French]. Ailanthus, ailanthus altissima, china-sumac, Chinese sumac, Chinese tree of heaven, copal tree, false varnish tree, paradise tree, stink tree, tree of heaven, tree of the gods, tree-of-heaven, varnish tree [English]. Ailanto, árvore do céu, árvore do paraiso [Portuguese].
Life form: Tree. **Part(s) Used:** Bark, Flower, bud, leaf / Fresh.
Geographic distribution: China, India, Pakistan, England.
Reference(s): Bolte *et al.* 1997; Dorta Soares, n.d.; Gotfredsen, 2009; American Institute of Homeopathy, 1979.

Ajuga reptans
Scientific Name(s) / [Botanical Family]: *Ajuga reptans* L. [Lamiaceae, Labiatae].
Common Name(s): Ajuga, ajuga reptans, blue bugle, bugle, bugle, bugleherb, bugleweed, carpet bugle, common bugle [English]. Consuelda media [Spanish]. Bugle rampante [French]. Búgula, erva de Sâo Leo [Portuguese].
Life form: Herb. **Part(s) Used:** Leaf, / Fresh. **Geographic distribution:** Europe, Southwest Asia & North Africa.
Reference(s): Bolte *et al.* 1997; Dorta Soares, n.d.; Gotfredsen, 2009; Plants for a future, 2009.

Aletris
Scientific Name(s) / [Botanical Family]: *Aletris farinosa* L. [Melanthiacaeae, Liliaceae, Nartheciaceae].
Common Name(s): Aletris [Spanish]. Aletris farineux [French]. Ague-grass, ague-root, aloe-root, bettie-grass, colic root, crown corn, mealy colicroot, star grass, unicorn root, white coolicroot [English]. Erva estrelada, raiz estrelada [Portuguese].
Life form: Herb. **Part(s) Used:** Flowers / Dried; Root / Fresh.
Geographic distribution: North America.
Reference(s): Bharatan *et al.* 2002; Dorta Soares, n.d.; Gotfredsen, 2009; Remedia/at, 2010; Tiwari *et al.* 2013;

American Institute of Homeopathy, 1979.

Alkekengi officinarum see *Physalis alkekengi*
Alfalfa
Scientific Name(s) / [Botanical Family]: *Medicago sativa* L. = *Medicago afghanica* Vassilcz. = *Medicago agropyretorum* Vassilcz = *Medicago coerula* Less. = *Medicago falcata* Lam. (and several scientific synonyms more) [Fabaceae, Leguminosae].
Common Name(s): Alfalfa, alfalfa silvestre, mielga, trébol [Spanish]. Luzerne, luzerne cultivée [French]. Alfalfa, buffalo grass, buffalo herb, chilean clover, cultivated lucern, lucerne, purple medic [English]. Alfalfa, luzerna [Portuguese].
Life form: Herb. **Part(s) Used:** Juice, complete plant / Fresh; dried leaves collected in bloom initiation. **Geographic distribution:** Temperate-Asia. Africa cultivated.
Reference(s): Dorta Soares, n.d.; Gotfredsen, 2009; Guermonprez *et al.* 1989; Tiwari *et al.* 2013; Vithoulkas, n.d.; American Institute of Homeopathy, 1979.

Allium cepa
Scientific Name(s) / [Botanical Family]: *Allium cepa* L. [Liliaceae, Alliaceae].
Common Name(s): Cebo, cebolla, cebolleta, chalote, thumps, xonácatl [Spanish]. Echalote, échalotte, oignon [French]. Bulb onion, Bermuda onion, common onion, onion, red onion, shallot, spanish onion [English]. Cebola [Portuguese].
Life form: Herb. **Part(s) Used:** Bulb mature, Complete plant / Fresh. **Geographic distribution:** Asia. Europe. Cultivated.
Reference(s): Dorta Soares, n.d.; Gotfredsen, 2009; Plants for a future, 2009; Tiwari *et al.* 2013; American Institute of Homeopathy, 1979.

Allium sativum
Scientific Name(s) / [Botanical Family]: *Allium sativa* L. = *Allium*

sativum L. var. *sativum* [Liliaceae, Alliaceae].
Common Name(s): Ajo [Spanish]. Ail, ail blanc, ail cultivé [French]. Cultivated garlic, garlic, poor man's teacle, rocambole, russian penicillin, serpent garlic, stinking rose [English]. Alho [Portuguese].
Life form: Herb. **Part(s) Used:** Bulb, Complete plant / Fresh.
Geographic distribution: Mediterranean. Cultivated in several places.
Reference(s): Dorta Soares, n.d.; Gotfredsen, 2009; Tiwari *et al.* 2013; American Institute of Homeopathy, 1979.

Allium ursinum
Scientific Name(s) / [Botanical Family]: *Allium ursinum* L. [Amaryllidaceae, Alliaceae, Liliaceae].
Common Name(s): Bear's garlic, broad-leaved garlic, buckrams, gypsy onion, hog garlic, ramsons, wild garlic, wood garlic [English]. Ail des bois, ail des ours [French].
Life form: Herb. **Part(s) Used:** Complete plant collected in bloom initiation / Fresh. **Geographic distribution:** Temperate-Asia Europe.
Reference(s): Dorta Soares, n.d.; Remedia/at, 2010; Tiwari *et al.* 2013.

Alnus
Scientific Name(s) / [Botanical Family]: *Alnus glutinosa* (L.) Gaertn. = *Alnus alnus* (L.) Britton = *Alnus vulgaris* Hill [Betulaceae].
Common Name(s): Black alder, common alder of Europe, European alder, swartels, tag alder [English]. Aulne glutineux [French].
Life form: Tree. **Part(s) Used:** Bark, bud / Fresh?. **Geographic distribution:** North Africa. Temperate-Asia. Europe. Naturalized in several places.
Reference(s): Bolte *et al.* 1997; Clarke, 2008.

Alnus

Scientific Name(s) / [Botanical Family]: *Alnus rubra* Bong. = *Alnus oregana* Nutt. [Betulaceae].
Common Name(s): Oregon alder, red alder, tag alder [English]. Aulne rouge [French].
Life form: Tree. **Part(s) Used:** Bark, bud / Fresh. **Geographic distribution:** North America (Alaska, Canada, North & Southwest United States of America).
Reference(s): Bolte *et al.* 1997; Clarke, 2008; Müntz, n.d.

Alnus serrulata

Scientific Name(s) / [Botanical Family]: *Alnus serrulata* (Aiton) Willd. = *Alnus noveboracensis* Britton = *Alnus rubra* Desf. ex Spach [Betulaceae].
Common Name(s): Common smooth, common alder, hazel alder, red alder, tag alder [English].
Life form: Tree. **Part(s) Used:** Bark & young branches / Fresh.
Geographic distribution: North America (East Canada, United States of America).
Reference(s): Bolte *et al.* 1997; Dorta Soares, n.d.; Tiwari *et al.* 2013; American Institute of Homeopathy, 1979.

Aloe

Scientific Name(s) / [Botanical Family]: *Aloe barbadensis* Mill. = *Aloe abyssinica* Lam. = *Aloe vera* (L.) Burm. f. = *Aloe vulgaris* Lam. [Liliaceae, Aloeaceae].
Common Name(s): Barbados aloe, Curaçao aloe, true aloe, medicinal aloe, star cactus, true aloe, west Indian aloe [English]. Aloès, alòes vulgaire [French]. Acibar, áloe, Flor del desierto, pitasábida, sábila, sávila [Spanish]. Áloe, azebre vegetal, babosa [Portuguese].
Life form: Herb. **Part(s) Used:** Leaf, leaves juice / Dried;
Geographic distribution: Asia, Macronesia, Spain. Cultivated.

Reference(s): Boericke, 1927, 1927b.; Dorta Soares, n.d.; Fuentes, 1996; American Institute of Homeopathy, 1979.

Alpinia officinarum
Scientific Name(s) / [Botanical Family]: *Alpinia officinarum* Hance = *Languas officinarum* Hance [Zingiberaceae].
Common Name(s): Chinese-ginger, galangal, lesser galanga, lesser galangal [English]. Galangal officinal, petit galanga [French]. Alpinia, galangal [Spanish]. Galinga [Portuguese].
Life form: Herb. **Part(s) Used:** Root, Rhizome/ Dried. **Geographic distribution:** Temperate-Asia (China).
Reference(s): Dorta Soares, n.d.; Fuentes, 1996; Provings, 2008-2009.

Althaea officinalis
Scientific Name(s) / [Botanical Family]: *Althaea officinalis* L. = *Althaea taurinensis* DC. [Malvaceae].
Common Name(s): Marsh-mallow, white-mallow [English]. Guimauve officinale, guimauve sauvage [French]. Malvavisco [Spanish]. Altéia, malva branca, malvaísco [Portuguese].
Life form: Herb. **Part(s) Used:** firewood before bloom / Dried; root / Fresh / Dried. **Geographic distribution:** Europe, Asia Minor. England. United States of America.
Reference(s): Dorta Soares, n.d.; American Institute of Homeopathy, 1979.

Ambrosia artemisiaefolia
Scientific Name(s) / [Botanical Family]: *Ambrosia artemisiaefolia* L. [Asteraceae, Compositae].
Common Name(s): Hogweed, rag weed, roman wormwood [English]. Ambroisie à feuilles d'armoise [French]. Altamisa, altemisa, ambrosia, artemisa, artemisia, camemba, hierba amargosa [Spanish]. Ambrosia americana, carprimeira, cravo da roça [Portuguese].

Life form: Herb. **Part(s) Used:** Flower, Bud / Fresh; Complete plant / Fresh. **Geographic distribution:** North America (Canada), Asia, Europe.
Reference(s): Clarke, 2008; Dorta Soares, n.d.; American Institute of Homeopathy, 1979.

Ampelopsis quincefolia
Scientific Name(s) / [Botanical Family]: *Ampelopsis quinquefolia* Michx. = *Parthenocissus quinquefolia* (L.) Planch. = *Vitis quinquefolia* (Michx.) Hemsl. = *Vitis quinquefolia* (Michx.) Lam. [Vitaceae].
Common Name(s): American ivy, false grape, five leaf, Virginia creeper, woodbine [English]. Vitis quinquefolia [French].
Life form: Liana. **Part(s) Used:** Bark / Fresh. **Geographic distribution:** North America (Canada, United States of America, Mexico). Central America (Guatemala). Naturalized in several places.
Reference(s): Tiwari *et al.* 2013; American Institute of Homeopathy, 1979; Zandvoort, 2006.

Amygdala amara see *Amygdalus dulcis*

Amygdalus dulcis
Scientific Name(s) / [Botanical Family]: *Prunus dulcis* (Mill.) D. A. Webb = *Prunus amygdalus* Batsch = *Amygdalus dulcis* Mill. = *Amygdalus communis* L. [Rosaceae].
Common Name(s): Almond, bitter almond, sweet almond [English]. Amandier, amandier commun [French]. Amendoeira, cerejeira [Portuguese]. Almendra dulce, almendro [Spanish].
Life form: Tree. Plant **Part(s) Used:** seeds / Dried; bark with flower / Fresh. **Geographic distribution:** South & West Asia. Europe (Mediterranean). Cultivated in Europe & Asia.
Reference(s): Bharatan *et al.* 2002; Dorta Soares, n.d.; Remedia/at, 2010; American Institute of Homeopathy, 1979.

Amygdalus persica

Scientific Name(s) / [Botanical Family]: *Prunus persica* (L.) Batsch. = *Prunus vulgaris* Mill. = *Persica vulgaris* Mill. = *Amygdalus persica* L. [Rosaceae].
Common Name(s): Common peach, peach pits, peach tree [English]. Pêcher, peacher [French]. Duraznero, durazno, melocotonero, melocotón, pérsico duraznero [Spanish].
Life form: Tree. **Part(s) Used:** Bark, Flower, leaf / **Geographic distribution:** Only cultivated.
Reference(s): Dorta Soares, n.d.; Remedia/at, 2010; Müntz, n.d.; Vithoulkas, n.d.; Zandvoort, 2006.

Anacardium orientale see *Semecarpus anacardium*

Anagallis arvensis.

Scientific Name(s) / [Botanical Family]: *Anagallis arvensis* L. [Primulaceae].
Common Name(s): Common pimpernel, scarlet pimpernel, weather-glass, red chickweed [English]. Buglosse des champs, Mouron des champs [French]. Anagálide, anagalis, coralilla, coralillo, hierba del pájaro, ixcuicuil, jabonera, murages, murajes, pimpinela escarlata, saponaria, tlalocoxóchitl [Spanish]. Bacuru, murriâo, pimpinela [Portuguese].
Life form: Herb. **Part(s) Used:** Complete plant / Fresh.
Geographic distribution: Europe. Asia. Africa. Europe. Cultivated.
Reference(s): Clarke, 2008; Dorta Soares, n.d.; Plants for a future, 2009; Tiwari *et al.* 2013; American Institute of Homeopathy, 1979.

Anantherum muricatum

Scientific Name(s) / [Botanical Family]: *Vetiveria zizanioides* (L.) Nash = *Phalaris zizanioides* L. = *Andropogon squarrosus* L. f. =

Andropogon muricatus Retz. = *Anantherum muricatum* (Retz.) P. Beauv. = *Chrysopogon zizanioides* (L.) Roberty [Gramineae, Poaceae].
Common Name(s): Cuscus grass, khus-khus, khus-khus grass, vetiver, vetiver grass chickweed [English]. Chiendent odorant, vetiver [French]. Patchuli-falso [Portuguese]. Zacate violeta [Spanish]. Capim de cheiro, cpim vetiver [Portuguese].
Life form: Herb. **Part(s) Used:** Complete plant, root, rhizome / Dried; plant without root / Dried. **Geographic distribution:** Extensively cultivated in tropical & subtropical regions.
Reference(s): Bharatan *et al.* 2002; Dorta Soares, n.d.

Anchusa officinalis
Scientific Name(s) / [Botanical Family]: *Anchusa officinalis* L. [Boraginaceae].
Common Name(s): Alkanet, bugloss, common alkanet, common bugloss, oxtongue, true bugloss chickweed [English]. Buglosse officinale [French]. Buglosa [Spanish].
Life form: Herb. **Part(s) Used:** Complete plant / **Geographic distribution:** Europe, West Asia.
Reference(s): Gotfredsen, 2009; Plants for a future, 2009.

Anemone nemorosa
Scientific Name(s) / [Botanical Family]: *Anemone nemorosa* Schang. = *Anemonoides nemorosa* (L.) Holub. [Ranunculaceae].
Common Name(s): Anémona of prados, nemorosa [Spanish]. Anémone sylvie [French]. European wood anemone, wood anemone, grove wind-flower chickweed [English]. Anêmola dos bosques, Silvia [Portuguese].
Life form: Herb. **Part(s) Used:** Leaf, Complete plant / Fresh. **Geographic distribution:** Europe. Boreal Asia. Boreal America.
Reference(s): Bolte *et al.* 1997; Dorta Soares, n.d.; Müntz, n.d.; Plants for a future, 2009.

Anethum

Scientific Name(s) / [Botanical Family]: *Anethum graveolens* L. = *Anethum sowa* Roxb. ex Fleming = *Peucedanum graveolens* (L.) Benth.& Hook. f. [Apiaceae, Umbelliferae].

Common Name(s): Dill, garden dill, indian dill, chickweed [English]. Shi luo [Chinese]. Aneth, aneth odorant, fenouil bâtard [French]. Ameto, anega, aneto, eneldo, falso anís, hinojo falso, hinojo hediondo [Spanish]. Aneto, endro [Portuguese].

Life form: Herb. **Part(s) Used:** Complete plant, leaf / Fresh.

Geographic distribution: South Europe (Mediterranean). Extensively cultivated.

Reference(s): Bolte *et al.* 1997; Dorta Soares, n.d.; Fuentes, 1996; Müntz, n.d.; Plants for a future, 2009.

Anisum stellatum

Scientific Name(s) / [Botanical Family]: *Illicium anisatum* L. = *Bandianifera anisata* Kuntze = *Illicium religiosum* Siebold & Zucc. [Illiciaceae].

Common Name(s): Bastard star anise, Japanese sacred anise tree, sacred anise tree, star anise [English]. Anise étoilé, anis du Japon [French]. Anís del Japón [Spanish].

Life form: Shrub. **Part(s) Used:** seeds / Dried. **Geographic distribution:** China, Japan.

Reference(s): Bharatan *et al.* 2002; Bolte *et al.* 1997; American Institute of Homeopathy, 1979.

Anthemis

Scientific Name(s) / [Botanical Family]: *Anthemis nobilis* L. = *Anthemis odorata* Lam. = *Chamaemelum nobile* (L.) All. = *Chamomilla nobilis* Godr. [Asteraceae, Compositae].

Common Name(s): English chamomile, garden chamomile, noble chamomile, Roman chamomile, Russian chamomile, camomille romaine [English]. Camomille noble, Camomille romaine [French]. Camomila de jardín, manzanilla, manzanilla

fina, manzanilla romana [Spanish].
Life form: Herb. **Part(s) Used:** Complete plant in bloom / Fresh; flower / Dried. **Geographic distribution:** Europe (England, France, Spain, Italy). United States of America.
Reference(s): Bharatan *et al.* 2002; Clarke, 2008; Dorta Soares, n.d.; Tiwari *et al.* 2013; American Institute of Homeopathy, 1979.

Anthoxanthum odoratum
Scientific Name(s) / [Botanical Family]: *Anthoxanthum odoratum* L. [Gramineae, Poaceae].
Common Name(s): Sweet vernal grass, ruchgras [English]. Flouve odorante [French]. Paleo odoroso, alesta olorosa, rama de olor [Spanish]. Feno de cheiro [Portuguese].
Life form: Herb. **Part(s) Used:** Complete plant / Fresh. **Geographic distribution:** Europe. North Africa & Asia. United States of America.
Reference(s): Bharatan *et al.* 2002; Dorta Soares, n.d.; Tiwari *et al.* 2013; American Institute of Homeopathy, 1979.

Apium graveolens
Scientific Name(s) / [Botanical Family]: *Apium graveolens* L. = *Carum graveolens* (L.) Koso-Pol. = *Celeri graveolens* (L.) Britton [Umbelliferae].
Common Name(s): Celery, celery-root, knob celery [English]. Ache des marais, célery à couper [French]. Apio [Spanish]. Aipo, aipo d'agua [Portuguese].
Life form: Herb. **Part(s) Used:** Complete plant / Fresh; seeds,fruit / Dried. **Geographic distribution:** Europe, Asia. cultivated, Cosmopolitan.
Reference(s): Clarke, 2008; Dorta Soares, n.d.; Tiwari *et al.* 2013.

Apocynum androsaemifolium
Scientific Name(s) / [Botanical Family]: *Apocynum*

androsaemifolium L. = *Cynopaema androsaemifolium* (L.) Lunell [Apocynaceae].
Common Name(s): Spreading dogbane [English]. Variété de chanvre du Canada [French]. Mata-câo, raiz amarga [Portuguese].
Life form: Herb. **Part(s) Used:** Root, rhizome / Fresh. **Geographic distribution:** North America (Canada, East United States of America).
Reference(s): Clarke, 2008; Dorta Soares, n.d.; Tiwari *et al*. 2013; American Institute of Homeopathy, 1979.

Apocynum cannabinum
Scientific Name(s) / [Botanical Family]: *Apocynum cannabinum* L. = *Apocynum pubescens* R. Br. = *Apocynum hypericifolium* Aiton = *Cynopaema cannabinum* Lunell [Apocynaceae].
Common Name(s): Cáñamo del Canada [Spanish]. Dogs'bane, Indian (American) hemp [English]. Chanvre du Canada [French]. Cânhamo americano [Portuguese].
Life form: Herb. **Part(s) Used:** Complete plant, root / Fresh.
Geographic distribution: North America (Canada. East United States of America).
Reference(s): Bharatan *et al*. 2002; Clarke, 2008; Dorta Soares, n.d.; Tiwari *et al*. 2013.

Aquilegia vulgaris
Scientific Name(s) / [Botanical Family]: *Aquilegia vulgaris* L. [Ranunculaceae].
Common Name(s): Aguileña, muela de San Cristóbal, palomas [Spanish]. Columbine, garden columbine, capon´s feather, culver key, european columbine, europeann crowfoot, granny's-bonnet [English]. Ancholie vulgaire [French]. Columbina, erva pombinha [Portuguese].
Life form: Herb. **Part(s) Used:** Complete plant in bloom / Fresh.
Geographic distribution: Central & South Europe. Temperate-

Asia (China). North Africa. Naturalized in several places.
Reference(s): Bharatan *et al.* 2002; Bolte *et al.* 1997; Clarke, 2008; Dorta Soares, n.d.; Müntz, n.d.; Plants for a future, 2009.

Aragallus lambertii see *Oxytropis lambertii*

Aralia
Scientific Name(s) / [Botanical Family]: *Aralia nudicaulis* L. = *Aralia edulis* Siebold & Zucc. = *Aralia nudicaulis* Blume, non L. = *Aralia nutans* Franch. & Sav. = *Aralia schmidtii* Pojark. = *Dimorphanthus edulis* (Siebold & Zucc.) Miq. [Araliaceae].
Common Name(s): Japanese-asparagus, Japanese spikenard, spikenard, wild sarsaparilla [English]. Aralie à feuilles cordées, aralie à tige nue, aralie du Japon [French]. Aralia del Japan, aralia pequeña [Spanish].
Life form: Herb. **Part(s) Used:** Root / Fresh?. **Geographic distribution:** North America (Canada-United States of America). Reference: Plants for a future, 2009.

Aralia hispida
Scientific Name(s) / [Botanical Family]: *Aralia hispida* Vent. [Araliaceae].
Common Name(s): Bristly-sarsaparilla, bristly-spikenard, dwarf-elder, wild elder [English]. Aralie hispide [French].
Life form: Herb. **Part(s) Used:** Root? / Fresh?. **Geographic distribution:** North America (Canada-United States of America). Reference: Bharatan *et al.* 2002.

Aralia racemosa
Scientific Name(s) / [Botanical Family]: *Aralia racemosa* L. [Araliaceae].
Common Name(s): American spikenard, aralia, berry-bearing aralia, life-of-man, petty morrel, small spikenard [English]. Aralie à grappes [French]. Arália de cachos, salsaparilha brava

[Portuguese].
Life form: Herb. **Part(s) Used:** Root / Fresh; Dried leaves collected during bloom time. **Geographic distribution:** North America (Canada-Mexico).
Reference(s): Bharatan *et al.* 2002; Dorta Soares, n.d.; Guermonprez *et al.* 1989; Müntz, n.d.; Tiwari *et al.* 2013; American Institute of Homeopathy, 1979.

Arbutus andrachne
Scientific Name(s) / [Botanical Family]: *Arbutus andrachne* L. [Ericaceae].
Common Name(s): Eastern strawberry tree, Greak strawberry tree, Greecen madrone [English]. Arbousier de Candie [French]. Frutilla de Levante, madroño de Greece, madroño de Chipre [Spanish].
Life form: Shrub. **Part(s) Used:** Buds / **Geographic distribution:** Europe (Mediterranean). Minor Asia.
Reference(s): Bharatan *et al.* 2002; Boericke, 1927, 1927b.; Clarke, 2008; Müntz, n.d.; Vithoulkas, n.d.

Arbutus menziesii
Scientific Name(s) / [Botanical Family]: *Arbutus menziesii* Pursh = *Arbutus procera* Douglas. non Sol. [Ericaceae].
Common Name(s): Pacific Madrone [English]. Madroña, madroño [Spanish].
Life form: Shrub. **Part(s) Used:** leaf / Fresh. **Geographic distribution:** North America (British Columbian West Coast to Central California).
Reference(s): Bharatan *et al.* 2002; Müntz, n.d.

Argemone mexicana
Scientific Name(s) / [Botanical Family]: *Argemone mexicana* L. = *Argemone grandiflora* Sweet = *Argemone mucronata* Dum.-Cours. = *Argemone sexualis* Stokes = *Argemone versicolor* Salisb.

= *Echtrus trivialis* Lour. = *Echtrus mexicanus* (L.) Nieuwl = *Papaver mexicanum* (L.) E. H. L. Krause [Papaveraceae].
Common Name(s): Mexican prickly poppy, Prickly poppy, yellow-flower Mexican poppy, yellow-thistle [English]. Argémone du Mexique [French]. Cardo santo, cardo santo de Yucatán, chicalote, chicalotl, chichillotl, xalé [Spanish]. Cardo santo, papoula do Mexico [Portuguese].
Life form: Herb. **Part(s) Used:** Complete plant bloom beginig / Fresh. **Geographic distribution:** North America (Mexico). Central America. Cultivated.
Reference(s): Bharatan *et al.* 2002; Bolte *et al.* 1997; Dorta Soares, n.d.; USA,1979.

Argemone ochroleuca
Scientific Name(s) / [Botanical Family]: *Argemone ochroleuca* Sweet = *Argemone mexicana* var. *ochroleuca* Reiche [Papaveraceae].
Common Name(s): Creasted prickle poppy [English]. Chicalote, chicalotl [Spanish].
Life form: Herb. **Part(s) Used:** Complete plant / Fresh. **Geographic distribution:** North America & Mexico. Cultivated Cosmopolitan.
Reference(s): De Legarreta, 1961; American Institute of Homeopathy, 1979.

Argemone pleicantha
Scientific Name(s) / [Botanical Family]: *Argemone pleiacantha* Greene [Papaveraceae].
Common Name(s): Bluestern or crested or southwesten prickly poppy [English].
Life form: Herb. **Part(s) Used:** Complete plant? / **Geographic distribution:** North America (South Central & Southwest United States of America).
Reference: Bolte *et al.* 1997.

Aristolochia clematitis

Scientific Name(s) / [Botanical Family]: *Aristolochia clematitis* L. [Aristolochiaceae].
Common Name(s): Asarabacca, birthwort, birthroot, long birtworth [English]. Aristoloche clématite [French]. Aristoloquia, jarrinha da Europe [Portuguese].
Life form: Liana. **Part(s) Used:** Aerial part / Fresh. **Geographic distribution:** Temperate-Asia. Europe. Cultivated.
Reference(s): Bharatan *et al.* 2002; Bolte *et al.* 1997; Dorta Soares, n.d.; American Institute of Homeopathy, 1979.

Arnica montana

Scientific Name(s) / [Botanical Family]: *Arnica montana* L. = *Arnica helvetica* Loudon = *Arnica petiolata* Schur = *Arnica plantaginisfolia* Gilib. = *Chrysanthemum latifolium* (DC.) Baksay = *Doronicum arnica* Desf. = *Doronicum arnica* Garsault = *Doronicum montanum* Lam. = *Doronicum oppositifolium* Lam. = *Senecio arnica* E.H.L. Krause [Asteraceae, Compositae].
Common Name(s): Arnica, arnica, arnikablomst, Almindelig guldblomme, Bjerg-guldblomme, Bjergvolverlej, Gammelmand, Volverlejblomst [Danish]. Valkruid, valkruid sort, wolverlei [Dutch]. Arnica, Celtic nard, cure all, European arnica, fallherb, golden-fleece, lambskin, leopard's bane, mountain arnica, mountain daisy, mountain-tobacco, sneezewort, tumblers, wolf's bane [English]. Arniko monta [Esperanto]. Arnikki, etelänarnikki, telänarnikki [Finnish]. Arnica des montagnes, arnique, bétoine des montagnes, doronic des Vosges, herbe aux prêcheurs, panacée des chutes, quinquina des pauvres, souci des Alpes, tabac des Savoyards, tabac des Vosges [French]. Arnika, berg-wohlverleih, echte arnica [German]. Sungorsiusaq [Greenlanders]. Árnika, hegyi árnika [Hungarian]. Fjallagullblóm [Icelandic]. Arnica [Italian]. Kalninė arnika [Lithuanian]. Solblom, Gullblom, Hestesoleie, Jonsokblom, Slåtteblom, Slåttermann,

Snusblad, Tobakksblom [Norwegian]. Arnika, arnika górska, arnica pospolita, pomornik [Polish]. Arnica vulgar, arnica-da-montanha, betónica-dos-saboianos, cravo-dos-Alpes, dórico-da-Alemanha, panaceia-das-queda, quina-dos-pobres, tabaco-dos-saboianos, tanchagem-dos-Alpes, tabaco-dos-Vosgos [Portuguese]. Арника горная [Russian]. Arnika horská, brdnja, navadna arnika [Slovene]. Arnika, hästfibbla, hästfibla, slåttergubbe [Sweeden]. Árnica, arnica, Arnicón, arnika, árnika, dorónico de Alemania, estabaco, esternudera, estornudadera, flor de tabaco, herba capital, hèrba capital, herba cheirenta, herba da papeira, herba de buitre, herba de les caigudes, hierba de las caídas, hierba santa, tabac de muntanya, tabac de pastor, tabaco, tabaco borde, tabaco de la montaña, tabaco de montanya, tabaco de montaña, tabaco de monte, tabaco del diablo, talpa, talpica, usin-belar, yerba de las caidas, zebadilla, [Spanish, includes: Aragonese, Asturian, Castillian, Catalan, Euskera, Galician, Valencian]. Hästfibbla, Slåttergubbe [Swedish]. Altın Çiçek, arnika, Öküzgözüotu [Turkish]. Арніка гірська [Ukraine].
Life form: Herb. **Part(s) Used:** Complete plant / Fresh.
Geographic distribution: Europe, North de Asia. Russia. Northwest United States of America.
Reference(s): Bharatan *et al.* 2002; Dorta Soares, n.d.; Gotfredsen, 2009; Greuter, (2006) ; American Institute of Homeopathy, 1979; USDA, 2013.

Artemisia abrotanum
Scientific Name(s) / [Botanical Family]: *Artemisia abrotanum* L. = *Artemisia* paniculata Lam. = *Artemisia procera* Willd. [Asteraceae, Compositae].
Common Name(s): Lady's love, old man, southern-wood [English]. Aurõne mãle [French]. Abrotano, artemísia dos jardins [Portuguese].
Life form: Shrub. **Part(s) Used:** Leaf, Aerial part in bloom / Fresh.

Geographic distribution: South & Central Europe. Temperate-Asia.
Reference(s): Allen, 2006-2010; Bharatan *et al.* 2002; Dorta Soares, n.d.; Guermonprez *et al.* 1989; Tiwari *et al.* 2013; American Institute of Homeopathy, 1979.

Artemisia absinthum see *Absinthum*

Artemisia dracunculus
Scientific Name(s) / [Botanical Family]: *Artemisia dracunculus* L. [Asteraceae, Compositae].
Common Name(s): French tarragon, silky wormwood, tarragon [English]. Estragon [French]. Dragon, estragon, estragão [Portuguese]. Dragoncillo, estragón [Spanish].
Life form: Herb. **Part(s) Used:** Root? / Dried?. **Geographic distribution:** Temperate-Asia Europe. North America (Canada, United States of America, Mexico). Extensively cultivated.
Reference(s): Bolte *et al.* 1997; Rowe, 2006.

Artemisia vulgaris
Scientific Name(s) / [Botanical Family]: *Artemisia vulgaris* L. = *Artemisia heterophylla* Nutt. = *Artemisia superba* Pamp. [Asteraceae, Compositae].
Common Name(s): Common wormwood, felon herb, mugwort, St. John's plant, wegwood, wild wormwood [English]. Armoise citronnelle, armoise commune, armoise vulgaire [French]. Artemisia, hierba de San Juan, sisim [Spanish]. Artemigem, artemísia verdadeira, Flor de Diana [Portuguese].
Life form: Shrub. **Part(s) Used:** Root, rhizome / Fresh. Complete plant. **Geographic distribution:** Europe. United States of America.
Reference(s): Allen, 2006-2010; Bharatan *et al.* 2002; Dorta Soares, n.d.; Guermonprez *et al.* 1989; Tiwari *et al.* 2013; American Institute of Homeopathy, 1979.

Arum dracontium
Scientific Name(s) / [Botanical Family]: *Arisaema dracontium* (L.) Schott = *Muricauda dracontium* (L.) Small [Araceae].
Common Name(s): Arisčme dragon, Dragon root, green dragon [English]. Dragâo verde, serpentaria [Portuguese].
Life form: Herb. **Part(s) Used:** Root, rhizome / Fresh. **Geographic distribution:** North America (United States of America).
Reference(s): Bharatan *et al.* 2002; Dorta Soares, n.d.; Tiwari *et al.* 2013; American Institute of Homeopathy, 1979.

Arum maculatum
Scientific Name(s) / [Botanical Family]: *Arum maculatum* L. = *Arum vulgare* Lam. [Araceae].
Common Name(s): Adam-and-Eve, common arum, cuckoo pint, lords-and-ladies [English]. Pied-de-veau [French]. Aro muchacho, culebrera [Spanish]. Arum vulgar [Portuguese].
Life form: Herb. **Part(s) Used:** Root / Fresh; tuber / Fresh. **Geographic distribution:** West Asia. Europe.
Reference(s): Bharatan *et al.* 2002; Dorta Soares, n.d.; Plants for a future, 2009; Tiwari *et al.* 2013; American Institute of Homeopathy, 1979.

Arum triphyllum
Scientific Name(s) / [Botanical Family]: *Arum triphyllum* L. = *Arisaema triphyllum* (L.) Schott [Araceae].
Common Name(s): Bog onion, Canada turnip, Indian turnip, Dragon's root [English]. Arum à trois feuilles, navet indien [French].
Life form: Herb. **Part(s) Used:** Root / Fresh. **Geographic distribution:** United States of America. Canada.
Reference(s): Bharatan *et al.* 2002; Guermonprez *et al.* 1989; Tiwari *et al.* 2013; American Institute of Homeopathy, 1979.

Asarum canadense

Scientific Name(s) / [Botanical Family]: *Asarum canadense* L. = *Asarum acuminatum* (Ashe) Bickn. = *Asarum latifolium* Salisb. = *Asarum reflexum* Bickn. [Aristolochiaceae].

Common Name(s): American wild ginger, asaro, Canada Indian or wild snake root, Canadian or Kidney-leaf ed asarabacca, Canada ginger, wild ginger [English]. Asaret du Canada, serpentaire du Canada [French]. Asaro, serpentaria [Spanish]. Gengibre bravo, gengibre da Índia [Portuguese].

Life form: Herb. **Part(s) Used:** Root, rhizome / Fresh; Dried leaves collected during bloom. **Geographic distribution:** North America (East & West Canada. North East, North, Central & Southeast United States of America).

Reference(s): Bharatan *et al.* 2002; Dorta Soares, n.d.; Tiwari *et al.* 2013; American Institute of Homeopathy, 1979.

Asarum europaeum

Scientific Name(s) / [Botanical Family]: *Asarum europaeum* L. [Aristolochiaceae]. **Common Name(s):** Asarabacca, European snake-root hazelwort, Fole´s foot, wild [English]. Asaret, asaret d'Europe [French]. Asarum, orelha de homen [Portuguese].

Life form: Herb. **Part(s) Used:** Complete plant root included / Fresh. **Geographic distribution:** West Asia Siberia, Europe.

Reference(s): Bharatan *et al.* 2002; Clarke, 2008; Dorta Soares, n.d.; American Institute of Homeopathy, 1979.

Asclepias cornuti

Scientific Name(s) / [Botanical Family]: *Asclepias cornuti* Decne = *Asclepias apocinum* Gaterau = *Asclepias capitellata* Raf. = *Asclepias eliptica* Raf. = *Asclepias fragans* Raf. = *Asclepias grandifolia* Bertoloni = *Asclepias intermedia* Vail = *Asclepias kansana* Vail = *Asclepias pubescens* Moench = *Asclepias pubigera* Dumort. = *Asclepias serica* Raf. = *Asclepias syriaca* L. [Asclepiadaceae].

Common Name(s): Solimán vegetal [Spanish]. Common milkweed, milk plant, silkweed, wild cotton [English]. Ascelpiade a la Soie, herbe à la ouate [French].
Life form: Shrub. **Part(s) Used:** Subterraneous parts / Fresh.
Geographic distribution: North America (East & Southeast United States of America).
Reference(s): Bharatan *et al.* 2002; Bolte *et al.* 1997; Remedia/at, 2010; Tiwari *et al.* 2013.

Asclepias incarnata
Scientific Name(s) / [Botanical Family]: *Asclepias incarnata* L. [Asclepiadaceae].
Common Name(s): Flesh-colored asclepias or swallow-wort, rose-colored or swamp silkweed, swamp milkweed [English]. Algodoncillo, señorita, soldadillo [Spanish].
Life form: Herb. **Part(s) Used:** Root / Fresh. **Geographic distribution:** Boreal America (Canada, United States of America).
Reference(s): Bharatan *et al.* 2002; Bolte *et al.* 1997; Tiwari *et al.* 2013; American Institute of Homeopathy, 1979.

Asclepias syriaca
Scientific Name(s) / [Botanical Family]: *Asclepias syriaca* L. = *Asclepias cornuti* Decne = *Asclepias intermedia* Vall. = *Asclepias kansana* Vall. [Asclepiadaceae].
Common Name(s): Broadleaf milkweed, common milkweed, silkweed, milkweed, Virginian swallow-wort [English]. Herber la ouate [French]. Algodoncillo, asclepias [Spanish].
Life form: Herb.
Part(s) Used: Subterraneous parts / Dried.
Geographic distribution: Siria, Europe, North America (East & West Canada. North East, North, Central & Southeast United States of America).
Reference(s): Allen, 2006-2010; Bharatan *et al.* 2002; Bolte *et al.* 1997; Müntz, n.d.

Asclepias syriaca see *Asclepias cornuti*

Asclepias tuberosa
Scientific Name(s) / [Botanical Family]: *Asclepias tuberosa* L. [Asclepiadaceae].
Common Name(s): Butterfly milkweed, butterfly weed, Canada root, colic root, flux Root, Indian posy, orange apocynum, pleurisy-root [English]. Asclepiade tubereuse [French]. Raíz de la pleuresía [Spanish].
Life form: Herb. **Part(s) Used:** Root / Fresh. **Geographic distribution:** North America (United States of America & North Mexico).
Reference(s): Bharatan *et al.* 2002; Clarke, 2008; Tiwari *et al.* 2013; American Institute of Homeopathy, 1979.

Asimina triloba
Scientific Name(s) / [Botanical Family]: *Asimina triloba* (L.) Dunal = *Annona triloba* (L.) Dunal = *Orchidocarpum arietinum* Michx. = *Porcelia triloba* (L.) Pers. = *Uvaria triloba* (L.) Torr. & Gray [Annonaceae].
Common Name(s): American custard-apple, common pawpaw, cherimoya, papaw, fetid-shrub, wild banana [English]. Asminier [French]. Asimina [Spanish].
Life form: Tree. **Part(s) Used:** seeds / Fresh; Leaves / fresh. **Geographic distribution:** North America (East Canada & United States of America).
Reference(s): Bharatan *et al.* 2002; Dorta Soares, n.d.; Tiwari *et al.* 2013; American Institute of Homeopathy, 1979.

Asparagus officinalis
Scientific Name(s) / [Botanical Family]: *Asparagus officinalis* L. [Liliaceae].
Common Name(s): Asparagus, garden asparagus, sperage,

spearage [English]. Asperge [French]. Esparraguera, espárrago [Spanish].
Life form: Herb. **Part(s) Used:** Bud / Fresh. **Geographic distribution:** Asia. Great Britain. Europe. Cultivated Cosmopolitan.
Reference(s): Dorta Soares, n.d.; Müntz, n.d.; Tiwari *et al.* 2013; American Institute of Homeopathy, 1979.

Assa-foetida
Scientific Name(s) / [Botanical Family]: *Ferula assa-foetida* L. = *Ferula foetida* (Bunge) Regel [Apiaceae, Umbelliferae].
Common Name(s): Asafetida, asafoetida, assa-foetida, devil's-dung [English]. Férule persique [French]. Asafétida [Spanish]. Asa fétida [Portuguese].
Life form: Herb. **Part(s) Used:** Goma o resin which emanates when punching or chopping the Root / Dried. **Geographic distribution:** West Asia (Iran, Afganistan). Naturalized in Asia temperate.
Reference(s): Bolte *et al.* 1997; Dorta Soares, n.d.; Rowe, 2006; Tiwari *et al.* 2013.

Astragallus lamberti
Scientific Name(s) / [Botanical Family]: *Astragalus lambertii* (Pursh) Spreng = *Oxytropis hookeriana* Nutt. = *Oxytropis plattensis* Nutt. = *Spiesia lamberti* (Pursh) Kuntze [Fabaceae, Leguminosae].
Common Name(s): Colorado loco vetch, Lambert's crazyweed, lambert's locoweed, Lamberet loco, locoweed, purple locoweed, stemless loco, white woollyloco, whitepoint locoweed [English].
Life form: Herb. **Part(s) Used:** Complete plant?. / Fresh.
Geographic distribution: North America (West Canada, North Central, Northwest, South Central & Southwest United States of America. North Mexico).

Reference: Bharatan *et al.* 2002.

Astragalus campestris see *Astragallus lamberti*

Astragalus exscapus
Scientific Name(s) / [Botanical Family]: *Astragalus exscapus* L. = *Astragalus exscapus* var. *transsilvanicus* (Barth ex Schur) Gams = *Astragalus exscapus* subsp. *transsilvanicus* = *Astragalus transsilvanicus* Barth ex Schur [Fabaceae, Leguminosae].
Common Name(s): Milkvetch, tragant [English]. Astragale sans tige [French].
Life form: Herb. **Part(s) Used:** Complete plant, Flower / Fresh.
Geographic distribution: Temperate-Asia (West Asia), Europe (Central, East & Southeast).
Reference(s): Bharatan *et al.* 2002; Bolte *et al.* 1997; Müntz, n.d.

Astragalus menziesii
Scientific Name(s) / [Botanical Family]: *Astragalus nuttallii* (Torr. & A. Gray) J. T. Howell = *Astragalus menziesii* A. Gray = *Astragalus nuttallii* var. *nuttallii* = *Erigeron asteroides* Roxb. = *Phaca nuttallii* Torr. & A. Gray [Fabaceae, Leguminosae].
Common Name(s): Nuttall's milkvetch [English].
Life form: Herb. **Part(s) Used:** Leaf / Fresh. **Geographic distribution:** California (Southwest United States of America).
Reference(s): Allen, 2006-2010; Bharatan *et al.* 2002.

Astragalus mollisimus
Scientific Name(s) / [Botanical Family]: *Astragalus mollisimus* Torr. = *Astragalus argillophilus* Cory = *Astragalus earlei* Greene ex Rydb. = *Astragalus thompsoniae* S. Watson = *Astragalus mollissimus* var. *thompsoniae* [Fabaceae, Leguminosae].
Common Name(s): Crazyweed, loco, locoplant, purple locoweed, milkvetch, wolly locoweed, woolly milk vetch [English].
Life form: Herb. **Part(s) Used:** Complete plant / Fresh.

Geographic distribution: North America (United States of America, Mexico).
Reference(s): Boericke, 1927, 1927b.; Bolte *et al.* 1997; Vithoulkas, n.d.; Zandvoort, 2006.

Athamanta oreoselinum
Scientific Name(s) / [Botanical Family]: *Athamanta oreoselinum* L. = *Athamanta oreoselinum* Huds. = *Peucedanum oreoselinum* (L.) Moench [Umbelliferae].
Common Name(s): Galbanum, mountain parsley, speddwell [English].
Life form: Herb. **Part(s) Used:** Complete plant / Fresh.
Geographic distribution: Central Europe, (Germany, Caucasus).
Reference(s): Allen, 2006-2010; Bharatan *et al.* 2002; Dorta Soares, n.d.; American Institute of Homeopathy, 1979.

Avena sativa
Scientific Name(s) / [Botanical Family]: *Avena sativa* L. = *Avena byzantina* K. Koch = *Avena byzantina* var. *anopla* Mordv. = *Avena diffusa* var. *segetalis* Vavilov = *Avena diffusa* var. *volgensis* Vavilov = *Avena orientalis* Schreb = *Avena volgensis* (Vavilov) Nevski [Gramineae, Poaceae].
Common Name(s): Common oats, oat, red oat, side oat [English]. Avoine [French]. Avena, avena común, avena roja [Spanish]. Aveia, aveia branca [Portuguese].
Life form: Herb. **Part(s) Used:** seeds or / and Aerial parts in bloom / Fresh; seeds / Dried; Fruit / Fresh. **Geographic distribution:** cultivated Cosmopolitan.
Reference(s): Bharatan *et al.* 2002; Dorta Soares, n.d.; American Institute of Homeopathy, 1979.

Baptisia confusa

Scientific Name(s) / [Botanical Family]: *Baptisia australis* (L.) R. Br. = *Baptisia confusa* G. Don. = *Baptisia minor* Lehm. = *Sophora australis* L. [Fabaceae, Leguminosae].

Common Name(s): Baptisia, blue false indigo, blue wild indigo [English].

Life form: Herb. **Part(s) Used:** Root, Subterraneous parts / Fresh?. **Geographic distribution:** North America (Canada, United States of America of America).

Reference(s): Bharatan *et al.* 2002; Bolte *et al.* 1997; Tiwari *et al.* 2013.

Baptisia tinctoria

Scientific Name(s) / [Botanical Family]: *Baptisia tinctoria* (L.) Vent. = *Sophora tinctoria* L. = *Podalyria tinctoria* L = [Fabaceae, Leguminosae].

Common Name(s): Horselfly weed, indigo broom, rattleweed, wild indigo [English]. Baptisia tinctoria [French]. Índigo silvestre, índigo salvaje [Spanish]. Índigo salvagem [Portuguese].

Life form: Shrub. **Part(s) Used:** Root, Subterraneous parts / Fresh-Dried. **Geographic distribution:** East North America (Canada-United States of America of America).

Reference(s): Bharatan *et al.* 2002; Bolte *et al.* 1997; Clarke, 2008; Dorta Soares, n.d.; Guermonprez *et al.* 1989; Müntz, n.d.; Plants for a future, 2009; Remedia/at, 2010; Tiwari *et al.* 2013.

Belladona

Scientific Name(s) / [Botanical Family]: *Atropa belladona* L. = *Atropa bella-dona* L. = *Belladona baccifera* Lam. = *Belladona trichotoma* Scop. [Solanaceae].

Common Name(s): Belladonna, deadly nightshade, dwale

[English]. Belladone [French]. Belladona [Spanish]. Beladona, tabaco bastardo [Portuguese]. Xdzunyal [Other languages].
Life form: Herb. **Part(s) Used:** Complete plant / Fresh.
Geographic distribution: Europe. North America, cultivated.
Reference(s): Bharatan *et al.* 2002; Bolte *et al.* 1997; Dorta Soares, n.d.; Fuentes, 1996; Tiwari *et al.* 2013; American Institute of Homeopathy, 1979.

Bellis perennis
Scientific Name(s) / [Botanical Family]: *Bellis perennis* L. [Asteraceae, Compositae].
Common Name(s): Daisy, English daisy, garden daisy [English]. Pâquerette vivace [French]. Vellorita [Spanish]. Bela margarida, bobina [Portuguese].
Life form: Herb. **Part(s) Used:** Complete plant / Fresh. Complete plant in bloom / Fresh. **Geographic distribution:** Libya, West Asia, Caucasus, Europe. Great Britain.
Reference(s): Bharatan *et al.* 2002; Dorta Soares, n.d.; Tiwari *et al.* 2013; American Institute of Homeopathy, 1979.

Benzoin
Scientific Name(s) / [Botanical Family]: *Lindera benzoin* (L.) Blume [Lauraceae].
Common Name(s): American spicebush, feverbush, benjaminbush, wild allspice [English]. Laurier faux-benjoin [French].
Life form: Tree. **Part(s) Used:** Branch. **Geographic distribution:** East & North United States of America of America (Maine-Ontario; Kansas, Texas & Florida).
Reference(s): Allen, 2006-2010; Bharatan *et al.* 2002; Bolte *et al.* 1997; Tiwari *et al.* 2013; American Institute of Homeopathy, 1979.

Berberis
Scientific Name(s) / [Botanical Family]: *Berberis vulgaris* L.

[Berberidaceae].
Common Name(s): Barberry [English]. Epinette-vinette [French]. Agracejo [Spanish]. Berberis, uva espim [Portuguese].
Life form: Shrub. **Part(s) Used:** Bark or stem or / and de root / Dried; Root / Fresh-Dried. **Geographic distribution:** Temperate-Asia. Europe.
Reference(s): Allen, 2006-2010; Dorta Soares, n.d.; Tiwari *et al.* 2013.

Berberis aquifolium
Scientific Name(s) / [Botanical Family]: *Berberis aquifolium* Pursh = *Berberis diversifolia* (Sweet) Steud = *Mahonia aquifolium* (Pursh) Nutt. = *Mahonia diversifolia* Sweet [Berberidaceae].
Common Name(s): Blue barberry, holly barberry, holly mahonia, mahonie, Oregon grape, mountain Grape, trailing mahonia, holly-leaf ed [English]. Mahonia faux-houx [French]. Mahonia, uva do monte [Portuguese].
Life form: Shrub. **Part(s) Used:** Root-bark, root / Fresh; bark / Dried; Dried leaves collected before bloom. **Geographic distribution:** North America (West Canada, Northwest & Southwest United States of America of America). Naturalized in East Canada, Europe & New Zealand.
Reference(s): Bharatan *et al.* 2002; Dorta Soares, n.d.; Guermonprez *et al.* 1989; Plants for a future, 2009; Tiwari *et al.* 2013.

Berberis vulgaris
Scientific Name(s) / [Botanical Family]: *Berberis vulgaris* L. = *Berberis jacquinii* Hort. ex K. Koch = *Berberis sanguinea* Hort. ex K. Koch [Berberidaceae].
Common Name(s): Barberry, european barberry, beet, jaundice-berry, piprage, pipperidge tree [English]. Agracejo, espino cambrón [Spanish]. Berbéris vulgaire, vinettier [French].
Life form: Shrub. **Part(s) Used:** Bark, Aerial & subterraneous

parts / Dried; Root / Fresh-Dried.
Geographic distribution: Europe-North Asia. New England. United States of America of America. Cultivated.
Reference(s): Bolte *et al.* 1997; Bharatan *et al.* 2002; Dorta Soares, n.d.; Müntz, n.d.; Tiwari *et al.* 2013; American Institute of Homeopathy, 1979.

Betula alba
Scientific Name(s) / [Botanical Family]: *Betula alba* Ehrh. = *Betula alba* L. = *Betula czerepanovii* N. I. Orlova = *Betula pubescens* Ehrh. subsp. *tortuosa* (Ledeb.) Nyman = *Betula pubescens* Ehrh. subsp. *czerepanovii* (N. I. Orlova) Hämet-Ahti [Betulaceae].
Common Name(s): Birch, downy or silver birch, tar of birchwood, white birch [English]. Bouleau blanc [French]. Bétula, vidoeiro branco [Portuguese].
Life form: Tree. **Part(s) Used:** Branches bark / Fresh / Dried. Young leaves / Fresh. **Geographic distribution:** Asia (Caucasus, Siberia). Europe. North America (Subarctic America. Greenland).
Reference(s): Bharatan *et al.* 2002; Bolte *et al.* 1997; Dorta Soares, n.d.; Müntz, n.d.; American Institute of Homeopathy, 1979.

Blumea balsamifera
Scientific Name(s) / [Botanical Family]: *Blumea balsamifera* (L.) DC. = *Conyza balsamifera* L. = *Placus balsamifer* (L.) Baill. [Asteraceae, Compositae].
Common Name(s): Blumea camphor, Ngai camphor, ngai camphorshrub, ngai camphortree, sambong, sembung [English]. Camphrier [French]. Kakarondra [India]. Sembung [Indo].
Life form: Shrub. **Part(s) Used:** Leaf. **Geographic distribution:** Temperate-Asia (China).
Reference(s): Anonymous, 2008; Bharatan *et al.* 2002; Bolte *et al.* 1997.

Blumea odorata see Blumea balsamifera

Boerhavia diffusa
Scientific Name(s) / [Botanical Family]: *Boerhavia diffusa* L. = *Boerhavia diffusa* Engelm. & A. Gray = *Boerhavia paniculata* Lam. = *Boerhavia paniculata* Rich. = *Boerhavia repens* L. = *Boerhavia repens* Rojas = *Boerhavia repens* Sievers = *Boerhavia viscosa* Ehrenb. ex Schweinf. = *Boerhavia viscosa* Fresen. = *Boerhavia viscosa* Lag. & Rodr. [Nyctaginaceae].
Common Name(s): Punarnava, red spiderling, spreading hogweed [English]. Huang xi xin [Chinese]. Ipecacuanha de Cayenne [French]. Hierba de cabro, mochi, mata de pavo [Spanish].
Life form: Herb. **Part(s) Used:** Root. **Geographic distribution:** Africa, Temperate-Asia, Tropical-Asia. United States of America of America. Central America. South America. Southwest Pacific. Cosmopolitan.
Reference(s): Bharatan *et al.* 2002; Tiwari *et al.* 2013.

Boletus see *Lariciformes officinalis*

Borago officinalis
Scientific Name(s) / [Botanical Family]: *Borago officinalis* L. [Boraginaceae].
Common Name(s): Beebread, beeplant, borage, star-flower [English]. Bourrache [French]. Boragem [Portuguese]. Borraja [Spanish]. Borragem [Portuguese].
Life form: Herb. **Part(s) Used:** Flower / Fresh / Dried. Leaf / Fresh. **Geographic distribution:** Africa. Orient (Temperate-Asia), Europe (Mediterranean) cultivated.
Reference(s): Bharatan *et al.* 2002; Dorta Soares, n.d.; Tiwari *et al.* 2013.

Bougainvillea

Scientific Name(s) / [Botanical Family]: *Bougainvillea glabra* Choisy = *Bougainvillea spectabilis* var. *glabra* (Choisy) Hook. [Nyctaginaceae].
Common Name(s): Paper flower [English]. Azalia de guía, bugambilia [Spanish].
Life form: Liana, Shrub. **Part(s) Used:** Flower. **Geographic distribution:** cultivated.
Reference(s): Bharatan *et al.* 2002; Bolte *et al.* 1997; Müntz, n.d.

Bovista

Scientific Name(s) / [Botanical Family]: *Calvatia gigantea* (Batsch = Pers.) Lloyd. = *Langermannia gigantea* (Batsch.) Rotsk.; *Lycoperdon gigantea* Batsch. Pers. = *Lycoperdon bovista* (L.) Fr. = *Bovista gigantea* Bull. [Lycoperdaceae, Agaricaceae].
Common Name(s): Giant puf-ball [English]. Tête de mort, vesse de loup géante [French]. Cuesco grande de lobo [Spanish].
Life form: Fungi. **Part(s) Used:** "Fruit" or "seed's purse" / Dried.; complete mushroom collected in autumn time. **Geographic distribution:** Asia-Minor. Europe, North America.
Reference(s): Dorta Soares, n.d.; Müntz, n.d.; Tiwari *et al.* 2013.

Branca ursina

Scientific Name(s) / [Botanical Family]: *Heracleum sphondylium* L. = *Heracleum lanatum* Michx. = *Heracleum maximum* W. Bartram = *Heracleum montanum* Schleich. ex Gaudin = *Heracleum palmatum* Baumg. = *Heracleum sibiricum* L. = *Heracleum ternatum* Velen. = *Heracleum transsilvanicum* Schur (each synonymous has their respective subspecies) [Apiaceae, Umbelliferae].
Common Name(s): Cow-parsnip, hogweed, meadow-parsnip [English]. Branc-ursine [French]. Ursina [Spanish]. Bunda de urso [Portuguese].
Life form: Herb. **Part(s) Used:** Complete plant / Fresh collected

in bloom. North Africa, Temperate-Asia. Europe. Naturalized in other regions.
Reference(s): Allen, 2006-2010; Bharatan *et al.* 2002; Bolte *et al.* 1997; Comisión Editora de la Farmacopea Homeopática de los Estados Unidos Mexicanos, 1988; Dorta Soares, n.d.; Remedia/at, 2010; Tiwari *et al.* 2013; American Institute of Homeopathy, 1979.

Brassica napus
Scientific Name(s) / [Botanical Family]: *Brassica napus* L. [with many forms (f), subspecies (subsp.) or / and variedades (var.)]. = *Brassica campestris* f. *annua* [Brassicaceae, Cruciferae].
Common Name(s): Bargeman's cabbage, Bergman's cabbage, bird rape, birdseeds, repe [English]. Chou oléifère [French]. Col, colza, nabo comestible, nabo de verano [Spanish].
Life form: Herb. **Part(s) Used:** Complete plant / Fresh.
Geographic distribution: cultivated.
Reference(s): Allen, 2006-2010; Bharatan *et al.* 2002; Müntz, n.d.

Brassica oleracea
Scientific Name(s) / [Botanical Family]: *Brassica oleracea* L. (with different varieties (var.), for example: *Brassica oleracea* var. *botrytis*). [Brassicaceae, Cruciferae].
Common Name(s): Cabbage [English]. Chou pommé [French]. Berza, col, coliFlower, col enana, col de Milán, nabo, repollo, [Spanish]. Repolho, repolho branco [Portuguese].
Life form: Herb. **Part(s) Used:** Complete plant / Fresh.
Geographic distribution: Europe. Extensively cultivated in other regions.
Reference(s): Bharatan *et al.* 2002; Dorta Soares, n.d.; Tiwari *et al.* 2013; Zandvoort, 2006.

Brucea

Scientific Name(s) / [Botanical Family]: *Brucea antidysenterica* J. F. Mill. = *Brucea antidysenterica* Lam. [Rutaceae, Simaroubaceae].
Common Name(s): Brucea [English]. Angustura falsa [Portuguese]. Mrikawandu [Other languages].
Life form: Tree. **Part(s) Used:** Bark. **Geographic distribution:** Africa Oriental, Tanganyika.
Reference(s): Bharatan *et al.* 2002; Dorta Soares, n.d.; Zandvoort, 2006.

Bryonia

Scientific Name(s) / [Botanical Family]: *Bryonia alba* L. = *Bryonia aspera* Bauh. = *Bryonia monoeca* Krause ex Sturm = *Bryonia nigra* Dum. = *Bryonia nigra* Gilib. = *Bryonia vulgaris* Gueldenst. ex Ledeb [Cucurbitaceae].
Common Name(s): Bastard turnip, black-berried bryony, devil's turnip, european white bryony, parsnip turnip, snakeweed, white bryony, wild hops [English]. Bryone blanche, navet du diable, vigne blanche [French]. Brionia blanca, nueza blanca [Spanish]. Nabo do diabo, vinha branca [Portuguese].
Life form: Liana. **Part(s) Used:** Subterraneous parts / Fresh.
Geographic distribution: Temperate-Asia. Central, East & Southeast Europe.
Reference(s): Bharatan *et al.* 2002; Dorta Soares, n.d.; Tiwari *et al.* 2013; Zandvoort, 2006.

Bryonia

Scientific Name(s) / [Botanical Family]: *Bryonia cretica* L. [Cucurbitaceae].
Common Name(s): Aegean bryony [English]. Bryone [French]. Brionia cretica [Spanish].
Life form: Liana. **Part(s) Used:** Root / Fresh. **Geographic distribution:** Africa. Temperate-Asia. Central, East & Southeast Europe.

Reference(s): Bharatan *et al.* 2002; Guermonprez *et al.* 1989; Plants for a future, 2009; Tiwari *et al.* 2013; American Institute of Homeopathy, 1979.

Bunias orientalis

Scientific Name(s) / [Botanical Family]: *Bunias orientalis* L. [Brassicaceae, Cruciferae].

Common Name(s): Hill mustard, Turkish rocket, wartycabbage [English]. Bunias d'Orient, fausse roquette d'Orient [French]. Cascellore [Italian].

Life form: Herb. **Part(s) Used:** Leaf. **Geographic distribution:** Temperate-Asia. Central, East & Southeast Europe. Naturalized in Great Britain.

Reference: Remedia/at, 2010.

Buxus

Scientific Name(s) / [Botanical Family]: *Buxus sempervirens* L. [Buxaceae].

Common Name(s): Box, boxtree, boxwood, boxwood tree, Caucasian boxwood, common box, common boxwood, European box, French boxwood, Persian boxwood, Turkish boxwood [English]. Buis toujours vert [French]. Buxo [Portuguese].

Life form: Tree. **Part(s) Used:** Branch & leaf / Fresh; Tillers (buds) & leaves. **Geographic distribution:** North Africa, Temperate-Asia (East-Asia, Caucasus). Europe (North, Central, Southeast & Southwest). Naturalized in several places.

Reference(s): Bharatan *et al.* 2002; Dorta Soares, n.d.; Remedia/at, 2010; Zandvoort, 2006.

Cainca (cahinca)

Scientific Name(s) / [Botanical Family]: *Chiococca alba* (L.) Hitchc. = *Chiococca racemosa* L. = *Lonicera alba* L. [Rubiaceae].

Common Name(s): Bejuco de berac, buenda, canica, perlilla, ti branda [Spanish]. Jasmin-bois, liane des sorciers [French]. David's milkberry, David's root, Davis root, milkberry, snowberry, West Indian Snowberry [English]. Cahinca, caninana, casinga [Portuguese].

Life form: Herb. **Part(s) Used:** Root bark, root / Dried.

Geographic distribution: North America (South United States of America of America, Mexico). Central & South America.

Reference(s): Allen, 2006-2010; Bharatan *et al.* 2002; Dorta Soares, n.d.; Plants for a future, 2009.

Cajuputum

Scientific Name(s) / [Botanical Family]: *Melaleuca cajuputi* Powell = *Melaleuca cajuputi* Roxb. = *Melaleuca cuninghami* Schau. = *Melaleuca leucadendra* (L.) L. = *Melaleuca leucadendron* L. = *Melaleuca minor* Sm. = *Melaleuca saligna* Bl. [Myrtaceae].

Common Name(s): Cajaput, cajeput, cajuput, Kajeputbaum, swamp teatree, White tea tree [English]. Cajuputier [French]. Árvore branca, árvore do óleo, cajeputi, cajuputum [Portuguese].

Life form: Tree. **Part(s) Used:** Oil obtained from the distillation of recent leaves & buds. **Geographic distribution:** Tropical Asia. Australia. Cultivated in Asia.

Reference(s): Allen, 2006-2010; Bharatan *et al.* 2002; Dorta Soares, n.d.; Tiwari *et al.* 2013.

Calabar

Scientific Name(s) / [Botanical Family]: *Physostigma*

venenosum Balf. [Fabaceae, Leguminosae].
Common Name(s): Eserina, haba del Calabar, nuez de Eseré [Spanish]. Fève de Calabar [French]. Calabar bean, ordeal-bean [English]. Eserê, fava de calabar [Portuguese].
Life form: Herb. Plant **Part(s) Used:** Seeds / Dried; complete plant.
Geographic distribution: West Africa.
Reference(s): Bharatan *et al.* 2002; Dorta Soares, n.d.; Müntz, n.d.

Caladium seguinum

Scientific Name(s) / [Botanical Family]: *Dieffenbachia seguine* [Jacq.]. Schott [Araceae].
Common Name(s): Amoena, aro seguino, caña muda, caña silenciosa, cochinilla, hierba de la noche [Spanish]. Arum des Antilles, canne à gratter [French]. American arum, dumb cane, dumbplant, mother-in-law-plant, poison arum [English]. Aninga-pára, cana de imbê [Portuguese].
Life form: Herb. **Part(s) Used:** Leaf, stem / Fresh; Complete plant / Dried; rhizome recently collected with leaves. **Geographic distribution:** North, Central & South America. Cultivated as ornamental plant in several world's regions.
Reference(s): Dorta Soares, n.d.; Remedia/at, 2010; Tiwari *et al.* 2013.

Calea

Scientific Name(s) / [Botanical Family]: *Calea ternifolia* Kunth = *Calea zacatechichi* Schltdl. [Asteraceae, Compositae].
Common Name(s): Ahuapantli, chichicxiuitl, hoja madre, sacachichic, sacatechichi, yerba amarga, zacachichi, zacate amargo, zacatechichi [Spanish]. Bitter-grass, dog's-grass, Mexican calea [English]. Capim de cachorro [Portuguese].
Life form: Herb. **Part(s) Used:** Complete plant / Fresh.
Geographic distribution: North America (North & Central

Mexico). Central America.
Reference(s): Bharatan *et al.* 2002; Dorta Soares, n.d.; Remedia/at, 2010.

Calendula

Scientific Name(s) / [Botanical Family]: *Calendula officinalis* L. [Asteraceae, Compositae].
Common Name(s): Caléndula, copetuda, mercadela, reinita, virreina [Spanish]. Souci des jardins, souci officinal [French]. Calendula, garden marigold, marigold, pot-marigold, ruddles, Scotch-marigold [English]. Bem me quer, calêndula [Portuguese].
Life form: Herb. **Part(s) Used:** Aerial part or complete plant in bloom / Fresh. **Geographic distribution:** Europe (Mediterranean). Cultivated & naturalized in temperate areas.
Reference(s): Bharatan *et al.* 2002; Dorta Soares, n.d.; Tiwari *et al.* 2013.

Calendula arvensis

Scientific Name(s) / [Botanical Family]: *Calendula arvensis* L. = *Calendula aegyptiaca* Pers. = *Calendula gracilis* DC. = *Calendula micrantha* Tineo & Guss. = *Calendula persica* C. A. Mey. [Asteraceae, Compositae].
Common Name(s): Caléndula, caléndula campestre, caléndula silvestre, flamenquilla, Flor de cada mes, Flor de muerto, hierba del podador, maravilla, maravilla of campos, maravilla del campo Maravilla silvestre [Spanish]. Souci des champs [French]. Field marigold, marigold, wild marigold [English].
Life form: Herb. **Part(s) Used:** Aerial part in bloom. **Geographic distribution:** Temperate-Asia Europe. Extensively naturalized in several places.
Reference(s): Allen, 2006-2010; Bharatan *et al.* 2002; Bolte *et al.* 1997; Fuentes, 1996; Guermonprez *et al.* 1989; Remedia/at,

2010; American Institute of Homeopathy, 1979.

Calla aethiopica

Scientific Name(s) / [Botanical Family]: *Calla aethiopica* L. = *Zantedeschia aethiopica* (L.) Spreng. [Araceae].
Common Name(s): Cala, cartucho [Spanish]. Calla, florist calla [French]. Altar-lily, arum-lily, calla-lily, common calla, common calla-lily, pig-lily, trumpet-lily [English].
Life form: Herb. **Part(s) Used:** Leaf / Fresh. **Geographic distribution:** South Africa. Australia. New Zealand.
Reference(s): Boericke, 1927, 1927b.; Dorta Soares, n.d.; Gotfredsen, 2009; Plants for a future, 2009; Remedia/at, 2010.

Calotropis

Scientific Name(s) / [Botanical Family]: *Asclepias gigantea* (L.) Willd = *Asclepias gigantea* Willd. = *Calotropis gigantea* (L.) W. T. Aiton = *Calotropis gigantea* (Dryand.) Aiton = *Calotropis gigantea* (L.) R. Br. [Apocynaceae, Asclepiadaceae].
Common Name(s): Algodón de seda, lechoso [Spanish]. Arbre à soie, mercure végétal, mudar [French]. Akanda, bowstring-hemp, crownplant, giant-milkweed, madar. [English]. Bombardeira, ciúme, Flor de seda, madar [Portuguese].
Life form: Herb. **Part(s) Used:** Bark, bark root / Dried; Complete plant / Fresh. **Geographic distribution:** Temperate-Asia (Iran, China). Cultivated & naturalized in several countries.
Reference(s): Dorta Soares, n.d.; Remedia/at, 2010; Tiwari *et al.* 2013.

Caltha palustris

Scientific Name(s) / [Botanical Family]: *Caltha palustris* L. = *Caltha arctica* R. Br. = *Caltha cornuta* Schott, Nyman & Kotschy = *Caltha laeta* Schott, Nyman & Kotschy = *Caltha longirostris* Beck = *Caltha minor* Mill. = *Caltha polypetala* Hochst. ex Lorent

[Ranunculaceae].
Common Name(s): Aro palustre, hierba centella, centella de agua, calta, cala de agua [Spanish]. Caltha des marais, populage des marais, populage, souci d'eau [French]. Common marsh marigold, cowflock, cowslip, kingcup, marsh marigold, mayflower, meadow-bright, yellow marsh marigold [English]. Calta, malmequer dos brejos [Portuguese].
Life form: Herb. **Part(s) Used:** Complete plant / Fresh. Complete plant in bloom. **Geographic distribution:** Temperate-Asia, Tropical-Asia, Europe, North America (Canada-United States of America of America), also cultivated.
Reference(s): Bharatan *et al.* 2002; Dorta Soares, n.d.; Tiwari *et al.* 2013.

Calystegia sepium
Scientific Name(s) / [Botanical Family]: *Convolvulus sepium* L. = *Calystegia sepium* (L.) R. Br. = *Volvulus sepium* (L.) Junger [Convolvulaceae].
Common Name(s): Campañilla blanca, corregula mayor, correhuela mayor, campanilla blanca, hiedra campana, hierba campana [Spanish]. Liseron des haies, liseron des prés, veillée [French]. Bearbind, bindweed, greater binweed, hedge bindweed, wild morning-glory [English].
Life form: Herb. **Part(s) Used:** Root. **Geographic distribution:** North hemisphere.
Reference(s): Bharatan *et al.* 2002; Bolte *et al.* 1997; American Institute of Homeopathy, 1979.

Camphora
Scientific Name(s) / [Botanical Family]: *Cinnamomum camphora* (L.) J. Presl = *Laurus camphora* L. [Lauraceae].
Common Name(s): Kanferboom [African]. Alcanfor, alcanfor del Japón, alcanforero [Spanish]. Arbre à camhre, camphre, camphrier [French]. Camphor, camphor tree, Formosa camphor,

formosan wood, gum camphor, hon-sho, Japanese camphor, laurel camphor, tree camphor [English]. Canfora [Italian]. Kuso-no-ki [Japanese]. Ŕrvore-da-camphora [Portuguese].
Life form: Tree. **Part(s) Used:** Wood. **Geographic distribution:** Temperate-Asia (China. East de Asia. Japan. Taiwan). Naturalized in South Europe, South Africa & United States of America of America.
Reference(s): Seror, 2000; Tiwari *et al.* 2013.

Canchalagua

Scientific Name(s) / [Botanical Family]: *Centaurium minus* Moench = *Centaurium minus* Auct. = *Centaurium littorale* (Turner) Gilmour = *Centaurium erythraea* Rafn. = *Erythraea centaurium* (L.) Persoon [Gentianaceae].
Common Name(s): Centáurea Minor [Spanish]. Petite centaurée [French]. Centaury gentian, centaury, common centaury, European centaury, pink centauro, red centaury, sea century, kustarun [English].
Life form: Herb. **Part(s) Used:** Flower. **Geographic distribution:** Europe, Southwest Asia (Bosnia, Estocolmo, etc.). North America, Australia.
Reference(s): Allen, 2006-2010; Bharatan *et al.* 2002; Bolte *et al.* 1997; Fuentes, 1996; Tiwari *et al.* 2013.

Cannabis indica

Scientific Name(s) / [Botanical Family]: *Cannabis indica* Lam. = *Cannabis sativa* L. subsp. *indica* (Lam.) E. Small & Cronquist = *Cannabis sativa* var. *indica* Lam. = *Cannabis chinensis* Delile [Cannabaceae].
Common Name(s): Hashish, [Árabe. Cáñamo, doña Juanita, Juanita, grifa, mariguana, marihuana, marijuana [Spanish]. Chanvre d'Inde, chanvre indien [French]. Ganja, gallow-grass, grass, indian hemp, hemp, marijuana, neck-weed, pot, reed-root, soft-true hemp [English]. [English]. Cânhamo, diamba, dirijo, maconha

[Portuguese].
Life form: Herb. **Part(s) Used:** Female plant in bloom / Fresh / Dried. Terminal buds in plant bloom; flower's bud / Fresh.
Geographic distribution: Extensively cultivated & naturalized. Plant use prohibited by law.
Reference(s): Bharatan *et al.* 2002; Bolte *et al.* 1997; Dorta Soares, n.d.; Plants for a future, 2009; Tiwari *et al.* 2013.

Cannabis sativa see *Cannabis indica*

Capsicum
Scientific Name(s) / [Botanical Family]: *Capsicum annuum* L. (with several varieties), = *Capsicum cerasiforme* Mill. = *Capsicum conoides* Mill. = *Capsicum cordiforme* Mill. = *Capsicum frutescens* L. (with several varieties), = *Capsicum grossum* L. = *Capsicum hispidum* Dunal var. *glabriusculum* Dunal = *Capsicum minimum* Blanco = *Capsicum petenense* Standl. [Solanaceae].
Common Name(s): Ají, charapilla, chile, chile chocolate, chile picante, chile piquín, chiltepín, pimiento [Spanish]. Piment annuel, piment de Cayenne, piment des jardins, piment rouge, poivre de Guienee [French]. African pepper, bell pepper, capsicum, cayenne pepper, cherry peppe, chili, chilli, chilly pepper, cone pepper, green pod pepper, hot chili pepper, red pepper, sweet pepper [English]. Pimentâo [Portuguese].
Life form: Herb. **Part(s) Used:** Fruit mature / Dried; complete plant fruit with seeds / Dried. **Geographic distribution:** cultivated. North America (South, South Central & Southwest United States of America of America. Mexico.) Central America. West South America.
Reference(s): Bharatan *et al.* 2002; Bolte *et al.* 1997; Dorta Soares, n.d., Fuentes, 1996; Tiwari *et al.* 2013; American Institute of Homeopathy, 1979.

Capsicum frutescens see *Capsicum*

Carduus benedictus

Scientific Name(s) / [Botanical Family]: *Cnicus benedictus* L. = *Carduus benedictus* L. = *Carduus arvensis* (L.) E. Robson = *Centaurea benedicta* (L.) L. = *Centaurea benedicutus* (L.) L. = *Carbeni benedicta* (L.) Benth. = *Cirsium segetum* Bunge = *Cirsium setosum* (Willd.) Besser ex Middle Bieb. = *Cnicus arvensis* (L.) Roth = *Serratula arvensis* L. = *Serratula setosa* Willd. = *Carduus benedictus* [Mattioli], (this is a name before-Linnaeus) [Asteraceae, Compositae].

Common Name(s): Cardo bendito, cardo benedictino, cardo-santo [Portugués, Spanish]. Centaurée bénie, chardon béni, chardon bénit, cnicaut béni, safran sauvage. [French]. Bitter thistle, blessed thistle, cardin, cnicus, holy thistle, lady's thistle, sacred thistle, spotted thistle, St. Benedicts thistle [English]. Cardo-bendito, cardo santo [Portuguese].

Life form: Herb. **Part(s) Used:** Complete plant / Fresh.
Geographic distribution: North Africa, Asia-temperate, Europe (Southeast & Southwest), United States of America of America (East & West). Naturalized in several regions of the world.
Reference(s): Dorta Soares, n.d., American Institute of Homeopathy, 1979.

Carduus marianus

Scientific Name(s) / [Botanical Family]: *Carduus marianus* L. = *Silybum marianum* (L.) Gaertn. [Asteraceae].
Common Name(s): Cardo de María, cardo lechero, cardo mariano [Spanish]. Chardon-Marie, silybe de Marie [French]. Blessed milk thistle, bull thistle, gundagai thistle, holy thistle, lady's thistle, milk thistle, variegated artichocke [English]. Cardo-leiteiro, cardo de Santa Maria, cardo santo [Portuguese].
Life form: Herb. **Part(s) Used:** Fruit mature / Dried; mature seeds / Dried; root, seeds, complete plant. **Geographic distribution:**

Europe (England, Italy), North Africa & West Asia. Cultivated & naturalized in several regions of the world.
Reference(s): Allen, 2006-2010; Bharatan *et al.* 2002; Dorta Soares, n.d., Fuentes, 1996; Gotfredsen, 2009; Tiwari *et al.* 2013.

Carissa schimperi

Scientific Name(s) / [Botanical Family]: *Carissa schimperi* A.DC. = *Acokanthera schimperi* (A. DC.) Oliv. = *Acokanthera schimperi* (A. DC.) Benth. & Hook. f. ex Schweinf. [Apocynaceae].
Common Name(s): Arrow-poison tree, common poison bush, quabain, wabayo [English].
Life form: Herb. **Part(s) Used:** Leaf. **Geographic distribution:** Temperate-Asia. East Africa (Abisinia).
Reference(s): Bharatan *et al.* 2002; Comisión Editora de la Farmacopea Homeopática de los Estados Unidos Mexicanos, 1988; Plants for a future, 2009; Remedia/at, 2010.

Carpinus betulus

Scientific Name(s) / [Botanical Family]: *Carpinus betulus* L. = *Carpinus betulus* L. form *pendula* (H. Massé) G. Kirchn. = *Carpinus caucasica* Grossh. [Betulaceae, Corylaceae].
Common Name(s): Abedulillo, carpe, charmilla, haya blanca, haya de espalleres, hojaranzo [Spanish]. Charme, Charme faux bouleau [French]. Common hornbeam, european hornbeam, hornbeam, hornbeam, white beech [English].
Life form: Tree. **Part(s) Used:** Bark, Leaf. **Geographic distribution:** West Asia, Caucasus, Europe. United States of America of America.
Reference(s): Bharatan *et al.* 2002; Bolte *et al.* 1997.

Carya alba

Scientific Name(s) / [Botanical Family]: *Carya tomentosa* (Poir.) Nutt. = *Carya tomentosa* (Lam.) Nutt. = *Carya ovata* (Miller) C.

Koch = *Juglans tomentosa* Poir. = *Carya alba* (L.) K. Koch = *Carya alba* (Mill.) K. Koch. [Juglandaceae].
Common Name(s): Caria blanca [Spanish]. Carya blanc, caryer blanc, caryer ovale, hickory véritable [French]. Big-Bud hickory, little shellbark hickory, scaly-barked hickory, shagbark hickory, mockernut hickory, shellbark, or shagbark hickory, upland hickory, white-heart hickory [English]. Nogueira americana [Portuguese].
Life form: Tree. **Part(s) Used:** Fruit, mature seeds / Dried.
Geographic distribution: United States of America of America (North East, North Central, South & South Central).
Reference(s): Bolte *et al.* 1997; Dorta Soares, n.d.

Cascara sagrada

Scientific Name(s) / [Botanical Family]: *Rhamnus purshiana* DC. = *Rhamnus alnifolia* Pursh. = *Frangula purshiana* (DC.) J. G. Cooper [Rhamnaceae].
Common Name(s): Cáscara sagrada [Spanish]. Ècorce sacrée, cascara [French]. Bark buckthorn, cascara sagrada, chittambark, western buckthorn [English].
Life form: Shrub, Tree. **Part(s) Used:** Bark, collected in bloom / Dried. **Geographic distribution:** North America (Canada, Northwest & Southwest, United States of America of America).
Reference(s): Allen, 2006-2010; Bharatan *et al.* 2002; Bolte *et al.* 1997; Clarke, 2008; Dorta Soares, n.d.; American Institute of Homeopathy, 1979.

Castanea sativa

Scientific Name(s) / [Botanical Family]: *Castanea sativa* Mill. = *Castanea vulgaris* Lam. = *Castanea vesca* Gaertn = *Castanea vesca* Bunge = *Fagus castanea* L. = *Fagus procera* Salisb. [Fagaceae].
Common Name(s): Castaña, castaño común, castaño regoldo,

marrón, marrón comestible, regoldo [Spanish]. Châtaignier commun [French]. Chestnut, chesnut tree, sweet chestnut, Spanish chestnut, European chestnut [English]. Castanheira, castanheira da Europe [Portuguese].
Life form: Tree. **Part(s) Used:** Leaf / Fresh; leaves collected in summer. **Geographic distribution:** North America (United States of America of America). North Africa. Temperate-Asia. Europe (Central & Southeast Europe). Cultivated in several regions of the world.
Reference(s): Allen, 2006-2010; Bolte *et al.* 1997; Bharatan *et al.* 2002; Clarke, 2008; Dorta Soares, n.d.; Remedia/at, 2010; Tiwari *et al.* 2013; American Institute of Homeopathy, 1979.

Castanea vesca see *Castanea sativa* or also *Vesca*

Catalpa

Scientific Name(s) / [Botanical Family]: *Catalpa bignonioides* Walter = *Catalpa catalpa* (L.) Karst. = *Catalpa syringifolia* Sims. = *Bignonia triloba* T. Freeman & Custis [Bignoniaceae].
Common Name(s): Arbre aux haricots, catalpa commun, catalpa de caroline, catalpa [French]. Catawba, cigartree; common catalpa, Indian-bean, smoking-bean, southern catalpa [English].
Life form: Tree. **Part(s) Used:** Bark; root / Fresh. **Geographic distribution:** North America (Southeast United States of America of America). Japan. Naturalized in several parts of South Europe & in North America (Canada & the United States of America of America). Also cultivated.
Reference(s): Allen, 2006-2010; Bolte *et al.* 1997; Bharatan *et al.* 2002; Dorta Soares, n.d.

Cataria nepeta see *Nepeta cataria*

Caulophyllum

Scientific Name(s) / [Botanical Family]: *Caulophyllum*

thalictroides (L.) Michx. = *Leontice thalictroides* L. [Berberidaceae].

Common Name(s): Cohosh bleu [French]. Squaw root, blueberry root, leontice, pappoose root, blue cohosh [English]. Leontice [Portuguese].

Life form: Herb. **Part(s) Used:** Subterranean parts / Fresh / Dried. branche's inner bark collected in bloom. **Geographic distribution:** North America (East & West Canada. North East, North, Central & Southeast United States of America of America).

Reference(s): Bharatan *et al.* 2002; Dorta Soares, n.d.; Tiwari *et al.* 2013.

Ceanothus

Scientific Name(s) / [Botanical Family]: *Ceanothus americanus* L. = *Ceanothus intermedius* Pursh [Rhamnaceae].

Common Name(s): Thé de Jersey [French]. New Jersey-tea ceanothus, mountainsweet, New Jersey-tea, red-root, wild snowball [English]. Ceanoto, chá de Nova Jersey [Portuguese].

Life form: Shrub. **Part(s) Used:** Leaf / Fresh / Dried. Leaves collected before bloom / Dried. **Geographic distribution:** North America (East Canada. North East, North Central, South Central & Southeast United States of America of America). Also cultivated.

Reference(s): Allen, 2006-2010; Bharatan *et al.* 2002; Bolte *et al.* 1997; Cowperthwaite, 2008; Dorta Soares, n.d.; Tiwari *et al.* 2013.

Ceanothus thyrsiflorus

Scientific Name(s) / [Botanical Family]: *Ceanothus thyrsiflorus* Eschsch. [Rhamnaceae].

Common Name(s): Blueblossum, bluebrush, California-lilac [English].

Life form: Shrub. **Part(s) Used:** Leaf? / Fresh. **Geographic distribution:** North America (Northwest & Southwest United States of America of America). Also cultivated.
Reference(s): Bharatan *et al.* 2002; Bolte *et al.* 1997; Clarke, 2008.

Celtis

Scientific Name(s) / [Botanical Family]: *Celtis occidentalis* L. = *Celtis cordata* Pers. = *Celtis audibertiana* Spach = *Celtis crassifolia* Lam. = *Celtis occidentalis* var. *crassifolia* (Lam.) A. Gray = *Celtis pumila* Pursh [Cannabaceae, Celtidaceae, Ulmaceae].
Common Name(s): Vals witstinkhout [African]. Palo blanco [Spanish]. American hackberry, hackberry, nettletree, northern hackberry, sugarberry [English].
Life form: Shrub, Tree. **Part(s) Used:** Bark. **Geographic distribution:** North America (East & West Canada), North East, North Central, Northwest, South Central & Southeast United States of America). Naturalized in Australia & cultivated in other places.
Reference(s): Remedia/at, 2010.

Centaurea tagana

Scientific Name(s) / [Botanical Family]: *Centaurea tagana* Brot. = *Centaurea tagana* Willd. [Asteraceae, Compositae].
Common Name(s): Centaurea entera, centaurea mayor, centaurea portuguesa [Spanish]. Knapweed [English].
Life form: Herb. **Part(s) Used:** Root. **Geographic distribution:** Introduced around the world.
Reference(s): Allen, 2006-2010; Bharatan *et al.* 2002.

Centaurium umbellatum

Scientific Name(s) / [Botanical Family]: *Centaurium umbellatum*

Gilib. = *Centaurium erythraea* Rafn. = *Centaurium minus* auct. = *Erythraea centaurium* auct. [Gentianaceae].

Common Name(s): Centaury, common centaury, European centaury [English]. Centaura Minor, escobilla [Spanish].

Life form: Herb. **Part(s) Used:** Complete plant. **Geographic distribution:** Temperate-Asia. Europe. Cultivated & naturalized in several world's places.

Reference(s): Allen, 2006-2010; Bharatan *et al.* 2002; Zandvoort, 2006.

Cephalanthus

Scientific Name(s) / [Botanical Family]: *Cephalanthus occidentalis* L. [Rubiaceae].

Common Name(s): Bejuquillo [Spanish]. Bois bouton, céphalante [French]. Button-willow, buttonbush, common buttonbush, crane willow, honey-bells [English].

Life form: Shrub. **Part(s) Used:** Branch-bark / Fresh. Root-bark / Fresh. **Geographic distribution:** North America (East Canada. North East, North Central, Southeast & South Central, United States of America. Mexico). Also cultivated.

Reference(s): Bharatan *et al.* 2002; Zandvoort, 2006.

Cetraria

Scientific Name(s) / [Botanical Family]: *Cetraria islandica* (L.) Ach. [Parmeliaceae].

Common Name(s): Líquen de Islandia [Spanish]. Cetrarie d'Islande, lichen d'islande, mousse d'islande [French]. Iceland moss, island cetraria lichen, moss Icelandic [English]. Líquen Islândico, musgo amargo, musgo islândico [Portuguese].

Life form: Herb. **Part(s) Used:** Complete plant / Fresh / Dried. **Geographic distribution:** Islandia, Europe, North America (Canada to Alaska, United States of America).

Reference(s): Allen, 2006-2010; Bharatan *et al.* 2002; Bolte *et al.*

1997; Dorta Soares, n.d.; Tiwari *et al.* 2013.

Chamomilla

Scientific Name(s) / [Botanical Family]: *Matricaria chamomilla* L. = *Matricaria recutita* L. = *Chamomilla recutita* (L.) Rauschert = *Anthemis vulgaris* L. ex Steud. [Asteraceae, Compositae].
Common Name(s): Camomila, gguía-gueza, manzanico, manzanilla, manzanilla alemana, queza [Spanish]. Camomille vraie [French]. Blue chamomile, chamomile, common chamomile, German chamomile, Hungarian chamomile, matricaria, scented chamomile, scented mayweed, sweet false chamomile, true chamomile, wild chamomile [English].
Life form: Herb. **Part(s) Used:** Complete plant / Fresh.
Geographic distribution: Asia-temperate, Europe. Extensively world cultivated & naturalized.
Reference(s): Bharatan *et al.* 2002; Clarke, 2008; Dorta Soares, n.d.; Tiwari *et al.* 2013.

Chelidonium

Scientific Name(s) / [Botanical Family]: *Chelidonium majus* L. = *Chelidonium haematodes* Moench [Papaveraceae].
Common Name(s): Celandine, greater celandine, nipplewort, swallowwort, tellerwort, wollow-wort [English]. Grande chélidoine [French]. Amapola amrilla, calidonia, celidonia, celidonia mayor, celidueña, golondrinera, hierba de berros, hierba de la glolondrina extranjera, hierba de las golondrinas, hierba verrugera [Spanish]. Celidonia, ceruda, erva andorinha [Portuguese].
Life form: Herb. **Part(s) Used:** Complete plant in or before bloom / Fresh; Dried leaves collected in bloom. **Geographic distribution:** Temperate-Asia. Europe. Cultivated & naturalized in several places of temperate regions.
Reference(s): Bharatan *et al.* 2002; Fuentes, 1996; Gotfredsen,

2009; Dorta Soares, n.d.; Plants for a future, 2009; Tiwari *et al.* 2013.

Chenopodium ambrosioides

Scientific Name(s) / [Botanical Family]: *Chenopodium graveolens* Willd. = *Chenopodium ambrosioides* var. *graveolens* (Willd.) Speg. = *Chenopodium anthelminticum* L. = *Chenopodium incisum* Poir. = *Ambrina* ambrosoides Spach = *Dysphania graveolens* (Willd.) Mosyakin & Clemants = *Teloxys graveolens* (Willd.) W. A. Weber [Chenopodiaceae, Amaranthaceae, Dysphaniaceae].

Common Name(s): Apazote, epazote, epazote morado, epazotl, hierba hormiguera, ipazote, pazote [Spanish]. Ambroisie du Mexique, chénopode fausse ambroisie, thé du Mexique [French]. American wormseeds, epazote foetid goosefoot, wormseeds oil, mexican tea [English]. Ambrosia, ambrosia do Mexico, anserina vermífuga [Portuguese].

Life form: Herb. **Part(s) Used:** Complete plant / Fresh. Complete plant in bloom. **Geographic distribution:** America central, North America (Mexico), South America. Naturalized in several places of temperate regions.

Reference(s): Allen, 2006-2010; Bharatan *et al.* 2002; Bolte *et al.* 1997; Dorta Soares, n.d.; Tiwari *et al.* 2013; American Institute of Homeopathy, 1979.

Chenopodium vulvaria

Scientific Name(s) / [Botanical Family]: *Chenopodium vulvaria* L. [Chenopodiaceae, Amaranthaceae].

Common Name(s): Abadejo podrido, ageao hagea hedionda, cenizo hediondo, hediondilla, hierba sardinera, meaperros, vulvaria [Spanish]. Chénopode puant, L'anserine fétide [French]. Arrach, stinking goosefoot, vulvaria [English].

Life form: Herb. **Part(s) Used:** Complete plant / Fresh.

Geographic distribution: Temperate-Asia. Europe. Naturalized in several places.
Reference(s): Bharatan *et al.* 2002; Dorta Soares, n.d.; Fuentes, 1996; Guermonprez *et al.* 1989.

Chimaphila

Scientific Name(s) / [Botanical Family]: *Chimaphila umbellata* (L.) W. P. C. Barton = *Chimaphila umbellata* (L.) Nutt. = *Chimaphila acuta* Rydb. = *Chimaphila occidentalis* Rydb. = *Chimaphila corymbosa* Pursh. = *Pyrola umbellata* L. = *Pyrola corymbosa* (Pursh) Bertol. [Ericaceae, Pyrolaceae].
Common Name(s): Chimafila [Spanish]. Chimaphile ombellée, pyrole in ombelle [French]. Bitter wintergreen, common wintergreen, false wintergreen, ground holly, king's cure, pipsissewa, prince's pine, prince's pine, rheumatism weed, umbellate wintergreen [English].
Life form: Shrub. **Part(s) Used:** Complete plant / Fresh. Complete plant in bloom / Fresh. **Geographic distribution:** Temperate-Asia. Europe. North America (East Canada. North East, North, Central & Southeast United States of America. Mexico).
Reference(s): Allen, 2006-2010; Bharatan *et al.* 2002; Dorta Soares, n.d.; Gotfredsen, 2009; Tiwari *et al.* 2013.

Chionanthus

Scientific Name(s) / [Botanical Family]: *Chionanthus virginica* L. = *Chionanthus virginicus* L. [Oleaceae].
Common Name(s): Árbol de nieve, cionanto de Virginia [Spanish]. Arbre à fleurs de neige, arbre à franges, arbre de neige [French]. Fringe tree, old-man's-beard, poison-ash, snow-flower, white fringetree [English]. Árvore da orla, árvore de neva, fresno florido [Portuguese].
Life form: Shrub. **Part(s) Used:** Bark, bark Root / Fresh.

Geographic distribution: United States of America (North East, North Central, Southeast & South Central), also cultivated.
Reference(s): Allen, 2006-2010; Bharatan *et al.* 2002; Dorta Soares, n.d.

Chrysanthemum

Scientific Name(s) / [Botanical Family]: *Chrysanthemum leucanthemum* L. = *Leucanthemum vulgare* Lam. [Compositae, Asteraceae].
Common Name(s): Bin ju [Chinese]. Margarita colombiana, margarita mayor [Spanish]. Grande camomille, Grandemarguerite, leucanthéme commun, leucanthéme vulgaire [French]. Dog daisy, margriet, marguerite daisy, moon daisy, oxeye daisy, white daisy, whiteweed, yellow daisy [English].
Life form: Herb. **Part(s) Used:** Flower. **Geographic distribution:** Temperate-Asia. Europe. Canada. United States of America. Cultivated & naturalized in several places & considered as weed.
Reference(s): Allen, 2006-2010; Anshutz, 2008; Bharatan *et al.* 2002.

Cichorium

Scientific Name(s) / [Botanical Family]: *Cichorium intybus* L. [Compositae, Asteraceae].
Common Name(s): Achicoria amarga, achicoria de Bruselas, achicoria de café, achicoria de Root, ahuirón, almeron, almirón, chirivía [Spanish]. Chicorée, chicorée de Bruxelles, endive witloof [French]. Belgium endive, chicory, coffee chicory, french endive, succory, wild or blue succory, wild or blue chiccory, wild endive, witloof [English]. Adicchio [Italian]. Almeirâo, chicórea verdadeira, chicória [Portuguese].
Life form: Herb. **Part(s) Used:** Complete plant in bloom. Root / Dried; Root / Fresh. **Geographic distribution:** Temperate-Asia.

Europe. Extensively naturalized & cultivated in several places.
Reference(s): Bharatan *et al.* 2002; Bolte *et al.* 1997; Dorta Soares, n.d.; Tiwari *et al.* 2013.

Cicuta maculata

Scientific Name(s) / [Botanical Family]: *Cicuta maculata* L. = *Cicuta bolanderi* S. Watson = *Cicuta maculata* var. *bolanderi* = *Cicuta curtissii* J. M. Coult. & Rose = *Cicuta maculata* var. *maculata* = *Cicuta mexicana* Coult. & Rose = *Cicuta maculata* var. *maculata* = *Cicuta occidentalis* Greene = *Cicuta maculata* var. *angustifolia* [Apiaceae, Umbelliferae].
Common Name(s): Beaver poison, children's-bane, muskrat-weed, musquash-root, spotted cowbane, spotted water-hemlock, water-hemlock [English]. Cicuta americana, cicuta grande [Portuguese].
Life form: Herb. **Part(s) Used:** Root / Fresh; root collected in summer. **Geographic distribution:** North America (Canada, United States of America, Mexico).
Reference(s): Allen, 2006-2010; Bharatan *et al.* 2002; Dorta Soares, n.d.; Tiwari *et al.* 2013.

Cimifuga racemosa

Scientific Name(s) / [Botanical Family]: *Cimifuga racemosa* (L.) Nutt = *Cimicifuga racemosa* (L.) Nutt. = *Actaea monogyna* Walter = *Actaea racemosa* L. = *Macrotys actaeoides* Rafin. = *Macrotys racemosa* Eat. [Ranunculaceae].
Common Name(s): Sauco, serpentaria [Spanish]. Actée à grappes, actée à grappes noires, cimicaire, cimicaire à grappes [French]. Black bugbane, black cohosh, black snake root, rattle root, squaw root, snake root, bugbane, deerweed, rattlesnake root [English]. Erva de são cristovão [Portuguese].
Life form: Herb. **Part(s) Used:** Root, rhizome / Fresh; Leaves collected in bloom / Dried. **Geographic distribution:** North

America (Canada, Georgia, West United States of America). Also cultivated in Asia, Europe.
Reference(s): Allen, 2006-2010; Bharatan *et al.* 2002; Dorta Soares, n.d.; Gotfredsen, 2009; Tiwari *et al.* 2013; American Institute of Homeopathy, 1979.

Cina

Scientific Name(s) / [Botanical Family]: *Artemisia contra* Wild. = *Artemisia cina* O. Berg = *Artemisia maritima* L. = *Seriphidium maritimum* (L.) Poljakov = *Seriphidium cinum* (O. Berg.) Poljakov [Asteraceae, Compositae].
Common Name(s): Tomillo blanco [Spanish]. Armoise de Judée, cina, semen contra, semencine [French]. Chamomille-leaved artemisia, cina, levant wormseeds, levant wormwood, santonica wormwood, wormseeds [English]. Barbotina, cina, santonica [Portuguese].
Life form: Herb, Shrub. **Part(s) Used:** Flower / Dried; inflorescences collected before bloom / Dried. **Geographic distribution:** East Asia (China, Russia, Turkestan).
Reference(s): Allen, 2006-2010; Bharatan *et al.* 2002; Bolte *et al.* 1997; Clarke, 2008; Dorta Soares, n.d.; Gotfredsen, 2009; Tiwari *et al.* 2013; American Institute of Homeopathy, 1979.

Cineraria

Scientific Name(s) / [Botanical Family]: *Cineraria maritima* L. = *Senecio cineraria* DC. = *Senecio bicolor* (Willd.) Tod [Compositae, Asteraceae].
Common Name(s): Cineraria gris [Spanish]. Cineraria, dusty miller, senecio, silver dust, silver ragwort [English]. Cineraria gris [Spanish]. Cinerária [Portuguese].
Life form: Herb. **Part(s) Used:** Complete plant / Fresh. Complete plant collected before inflorescences opened / Fresh. **Geographic distribution:** Temperate-Asia. Central America.

Europe (Mediterranean). Cultivated & naturalized in several places.

Reference(s): Bharatan *et al.* 2002; Dorta Soares, n.d.; Guermonprez *et al.* 1989; Plants for a future, 2009; Rowe, 2006; Tiwari *et al.* 2013; American Institute of Homeopathy, 1979.

Cirsium arvense

Scientific Name(s) / [Botanical Family]: *Cirsium arvense* (L.) Scop. = *Cardus arvensis* (L.) Robson. [Compositae, Asteraceae].

Common Name(s): Cardo blanco, cardo cundidor, cardo hemorroidal, cardo oloroso, cardo rastrero [Spanish]. Chardon des champs, chardon du Canada, cirse des champs [French]. Boar thistle, California thistle, Canadian thistle, corn thistle, creeping thistle, field thistle, perennial thistle, prickly thistle, way thistle [English]. Cardo Canadense [Portuguese].

Life form: Herb. **Part(s) Used:** Complete plant / Fresh.

Geographic distribution: Asia-temperate, Caucasus, Sovietic Central Asia. Europe. Naturalized in Africa, Australia, North & South America.

Reference(s): Bharatan *et al.* 2002; Dorta Soares, n.d.; Remedia/at, 2010.

Cistus

Scientific Name(s) / [Botanical Family]: *Cistus canadensis* L. = *Crocanthemum canadense* (L.) Britton = *Halimium candanense* (L.) Grosser = *Helianthemum canadense* (L.) Michx. [Cistaceae].

Common Name(s): Heliantemo del Canada [Spanish]. Ciste du Canada [French]. Canada frostweed, Canada sun-rose, frostweed, frostwort, longbranch frostweed [English]. Sargaço [Portuguese].

Life form: Herb. **Part(s) Used:** Complete plant / Fresh. Leaves collected before bloom / Dried. **Geographic distribution:** North America (Canada. North East, North, Central & Southeast United

States of America).
Reference(s): Bharatan *et al.* 2002; Dorta Soares, n.d.; Tiwari *et al.* 2013.

Citrus aurantium

Scientific Name(s) / [Botanical Family]: *Citrus x aurantium* L. = *Citrus vulgaris* Risso = *Citrus sinensis* Pers. [Rutaceae].

Common Name(s): Azahar, naranja, naranja amarga, naranja agria, naranjero agrio, naranjo, naranjo agrio, naranjo amargo, naranjo dulce [Spanish]. Bigaradier, orange amer, orange amère, orange doux [French]. Bigarade orange, bigrade, bitter, bitter orange, chinese bitter orange, immature orange fruit latin, neroli, orange, petitgrain, seville, seville orange, sour orange [English]. Laranja azeda [Portuguese].

Life form: Tree. **Part(s) Used:** Fruit bark / Fresh. **Geographic distribution:** cultivated in several places.

Reference(s): Bharatan *et al.* 2002; Dorta Soares, n.d.; Remedia/at, 2010; Tiwari *et al.* 2013.

Citrus decumana

Scientific Name(s) / [Botanical Family]: *Citrus maxima* (Rumph. ex Burm.) Merr. = *Citrus maxima* (Burm.) Merr = *Aurantium maximum* Rumph. ex Burm. = *Citrus aurantium* var. *decumana* L. = *Citrus decumana* (L.) L. = *Citrus decumana* Murr. [Rutaceae].

Common Name(s): Cidro, pampelmusa, pomelo, toronja [Spanish]. Pamplemousse doux des Antilles, chadec [French]. Chinese grapefruit, forbidden fruit, jabong, paradise apple, pomelo, pompelmoose, shaddock [English].

Life form: Tree. **Part(s) Used:** Fruit / Fresh. **Geographic distribution:** cultivated.

Reference(s): Bharatan *et al.* 2002; Remedia/at, 2010.

Citrus limonum

Scientific Name(s) / [Botanical Family]: *Citrus acida* Roxb. = *Citrus x limon* (L.) Osbeck. = *Citrus limon* (L.) Burman f = *Citrus limonum* Risso = *Citrus medica* L. var. *limon* L. = *Citrus medica* L. var. *medica* [Rutaceae].

Common Name(s): Fo shou gan, xiang yuan [Chinese]. Cidro, limón, limón de carne, limón de confitar, limonero [Spanish]. Cédrat, cédrat digité, cédratier, citronnier [French]. Citron, Buddha's-Hand, lemon, lemon tree, limon [English]. Cidra, cidreira [Portuguese].

Life form: Tree. **Part(s) Used:** Fruit / Fresh. **Geographic distribution:** Extensively cultivated.

Reference: Bharatan *et al.* 2002.

Citrus sinensis see *Citrus aurantium*

Citrus vulgaris see *Citrus aurantium*

Claviceps purpurea

Scientific Name(s) / [Botanical Family]: *Claviceps purpurea* (Fr.) Tul. & C. Tul. [Clavicipitaceae].

Common Name(s): Cornatillo, cornezuelo, cornezuelo del centeno, espolón del centeno, moro de centeno, tizón de centeno [Spanish]. Ergot de seigle [French]. Claviceps, clavus, ergot, ergot of rye, holy fire, mutterkorn, rye ergot, secale cornutum, siegle cornu, smit of rye, wheat ergot [English].

Life form: Fungi. **Part(s) Used:** "Fruit", sporangium. **Geographic distribution:** Extensively naturalized in several places.

Reference(s): Bharatan *et al.* 2002; Dorta Soares, n.d.; Gotfredsen, 2009; Tiwari *et al.* 2013.

Clematis

Scientific Name(s) / [Botanical Family]: *Clematis erecta* (L.) All. = *Clematis recta* L. [Ranunculaceae].

Common Name(s): Centoria, clematis, enredadera baja, flámula de Júpiter [Spanish]. Clematite droite [French]. Erect clematis, flammula jovis, ground clematis, ground virginsbower, upright Virgin's bower, Virgin's bower [English]. Arvoredo da Virgínia, congoca [Portuguese].
Life form: Herb. **Part(s) Used:** Leaf & stem. **Geographic distribution:** Asia-temperate, South Europe. Naturalized in several places.
Reference(s): Bharatan *et al.* 2002; Dorta Soares, n.d.; Guermonprez *et al.* 1989; Remedia/at, 2010; Tiwari *et al.* 2013.

Clematis

Scientific Name(s) / [Botanical Family]: *Clematis hirsutissima* Pursh = *Clematis arizonica* A. Heller = *Clematis scottii* Porter = *Coriflora hirsutissima* (Pursh) W. A. Weber [Ranunculaceae].
Common Name(s): Douglas'clematis, Scott's clematis [English].
Life form: Herb. **Part(s) Used:** Complete plant / Fresh.
Geographic distribution: North Central, Northwest, South Central & Southwest United States of America.
Reference(s): Allen, 2006-2010; Bharatan *et al.* 2002; Bolte *et al.* 1997; Gotfredsen, 2009; American Institute of Homeopathy, 1979.

Clematis erecta see *Clematis*

Clematis vitalba

Scientific Name(s) / [Botanical Family]: *Clematis vitalba* L. [Ranunculaceae].
Common Name(s): Abrazadera, ajan, barba de Dios, bedigueres, betiguerras, cabello de ángel, clemátide, hierba of pordioseros, muermera, vidarra, virgaza [Spanish]. Clématite, clématite blanche, clématite vigne blance, herbe aux gueux [French]. Evergreen clematis, old man's beard, traveller's joy, Virgin's bower, white Virgin's bowe, wild clematis [English]. Barba de

velho, vinha brava [Portuguese].
Life form: Herb. **Part(s) Used:** Leaf & stem / Fresh; Leaves collected during the bloom / Dried. **Geographic distribution:** North Africa. Temperate-Asia. Europe. Naturalized in Australia, New Zealand & United States of America, also cultivated.
Reference(s): Bharatan *et al.* 2002; Gotfredsen, 2009; Dorta Soares, n.d.

Cocculus indicus

Scientific Name(s) / [Botanical Family]: *Anamirta cocculus* (L.) Wight & Arn. = *Anamirta paniculata* Colebr. = *Cocculus indicus* Pharm. ex Wehmer = *Cocculus indicus* Royle = *Menispermum cocculus* L. [Menispermaceae].
Common Name(s): Cockles, fishberry, indian berry, indian cockle, levant nut [English]. Coque du Levant [French]. Coca del Levante, neguilla [Spanish]. Coca do Levante [Portuguese].
Life form: Tree. **Part(s) Used:** Mature fruits, seeds / Dried.
Geographic distribution: Europe. Boreal Asia (India).
Reference(s): Bolte *et al.* 1997; Bharatan *et al.* 2002; Dorta Soares, n.d.; Gotfredsen, 2009; Tiwari *et al.* 2013.

Cochlearia armoracia

Scientific Name(s) / [Botanical Family]: *Armoracia lapathifolia* Usteri = *Armoracia rusticana* Gaertn. Mey. & ScHerb. = *Armoracia armoracia* (L.) Cockerell = *Cochlearia rusticana* Lam. = *Cochlearia armoracia* L. = *Crucifera armoracia* (L.) E. H.L. Krause = *Nasturtium armoracia* (L.) Fr. = *Rorippa armoracia* (L.) Hitchc. [Brassicaceae, Cruciferae].
Common Name(s): Jaramago, mostaza romana, rábano de caballo, rábano picante, rábano rusticano [Spanish]. Cranson, moutard des capucins, moutarde des allemands, raifort cran [French]. Horseradish, red cole [English]. Rábano-picante, raiz-forte [Portuguese].

Life form: Herb. **Part(s) Used:** Root, rhizome / Fresh. **Geographic distribution:** East Europe. Russia. United States of America. Extensively cultivated & naturalized in several places.
Reference(s): Bharatan *et al.* 2002; Boericke, 1927, 1927b.; Bolte *et al.* 1997; Dorta Soares, n.d.; Gotfredsen, 2009; Tiwari *et al.* 2013.

Colchicum

Scientific Name(s) / [Botanical Family]: *Colchicum autumnale* L. = *Colchicum commune* Neck. [Colchicaceae, Liliaceae].
Common Name(s): Autumn-crocus, colchicum, meadow-saffron [English]. Cólchico [Spanish]. Açafrâo bastardo, colchico, narciso do outono [Portuguese].
Life form: Herb. **Part(s) Used:** Bulb, root / Fresh. **Geographic distribution:** Europe. Cultivated in several places.
Reference(s): Bharatan *et al.* 2002; Dorta Soares, n.d.; Tiwari *et al.* 2013; American Institute of Homeopathy, 1979.

Colocynthis

Scientific Name(s) / [Botanical Family]: *Citrullus colocynthis* (L.) Schrad. = *Colocynthis vulgaris* Schrad. = *Cucumis colocynthis* L. [Cucurbitaceae].
Common Name(s): Alhandal, calabacilla salvaje, coloquíntida, hiel de la tierra, manzana amarga, tuera, tuero [Spanish]. Coloquinte [French]. Bitter apple, bitter cucumber, colocynth, vine-of-Sodom, wild gourd [English].
Life form: Herb. **Part(s) Used:** Fruit / Fresh. **Geographic distribution:** India. Ceylon. Saudi Arabian. Japan. Extensive cultivated in Africa & Asia.
Reference(s): Bharatan *et al.* 2002; Clarke, 2008; Fuentes, 1996; Tiwari *et al.* 2013 , American Institute of Homeopathy, 1979.

Conium

Scientific Name(s) / [Botanical Family]: *Conium maculatum* L. = *Coriandrum cicuta* Crantz = *Cicuta major* Lam. [Apiaceae, Umbelliferae].

Common Name(s): Cañaleja, cañafierro, cañafleja, cicuta, cicuta mayor. Cicuta manchada, encaje cimarrón, panalillo, perejil de chucho, perejil de monte, zanahoria silvestre [Spanish]. Ciguë tachée, cigue, grande ciguë [French]. Carrot-fern, deadly hemlocj, fool's-parsley, hemlock, herb Bennet, poison-hemlock, spotted-hemlock, spotted-parsley [English]. Cicuta da Europe [Portuguese].

Life form: Herb. **Part(s) Used:** Complete plant collected during the bloom, flowers / Fresh. **Geographic distribution:** North & North East Africa. Temperate-Asia. Tropical Asia. Europe. Naturalized & cultivated in several places.

Reference(s): Bharatan *et al*. 2002; Dorta Soares, n.d.; Fuentes, 1996; Gotfredsen, 2009; Guermonprez *et al*. 1989; Rowe, 2006; Tiwari *et al*. 2013; American Institute of Homeopathy, 1979.

Convolvulus stans see also *Ipomoea stans*

Convolvulus stans

Scientific Name(s) / [Botanical Family]: *Calystegia spithamaea* (L.) Pursh. subsp. *stans* (Michx.) Brummitt. = *Convolvulus stans* Michx. [Convolvulaceae].

Common Name(s): Espanta lobos, espanta vaqueros, limpia tunas, pegajosa, tanibata, tumba jinetes [Spanish]. Low false bindweed [English].

Life form: Herb. **Part(s) Used:** Flower?. **Geographic distribution:** East United States of America.

Reference(s): Allen, 2006-2010; Bharatan *et al*. 2002; Gotfredsen, 2009; Remedia/at, 2010.

Coriaria ruscifolia

Scientific Name(s) / [Botanical Family]: *Coriaria ruscifolia* L. = *Coriaria microphylla* Poir = *Coriaria thymifolia* H. & B. ex Willd. [Coriariaceae].

Common Name(s): Borrego, chanchi, helecho de tierra, mio mio, shanshi [Spanish]. Redoul? [French].

Life form: Shrub. **Part(s) Used:** Fruit / Dried. **Geographic distribution:** Europe. North America (Mexico). Central & South America. Naturalized in several places.

Reference(s): Bharatan *et al.* 2002; Dorta Soares, n.d.

Corn-smut

Scientific Name(s) / [Botanical Family]: *Ustilago maydis* (DC.) Corda = *Ustilago zeae* (Beckm.) Unger [Ustilaginaceae].

Common Name(s): Cuitalcoche, huitlacoche, carbón del maíz [Spanish]. Boil, blister smut of corn, corn-smut, maize smut, tizon ustilago [English]. Ergot do milho, mofo do milho [Portuguese].

Life form: Fungi (It is a parasitic fungus corn & closely related species). **Part(s) Used:** Complete plant mushroom, mature spores, sporangium. **Geographic distribution:** America also it's distributed around the world in where the corn is grown.

Reference(s): Bharatan *et al.* 2002; Dorta Soares, n.d.

Corydalis

Scientific Name(s) / [Botanical Family]: *Dicentra canadensis* (Goldie) Walp. = *Corydalis formosa* (Hawort) Pursh = *Corydalis canadensis* Goldie [Fumariaceae, Papaveraceae].

Common Name(s): Dicentre du Canada, coeurs-saignants [French]. Bleeding-heart, squirrel corn, stagger weed, Turkey corn, wild turkey pea [English].

Life form: Herb. **Part(s) Used:** Root, rhizome / Fresh / Dried.

Geographic distribution: North America (Canada, East United States of America). China.
Reference(s): Bharatan *et al.* 2002; Dorta Soares, n.d.; Fuentes, 1996.

Corydalis cava

Scientific Name(s) / [Botanical Family]: *Corydalis cava* (L.) Schweigger & Koerte = *Corydalis tuberosa* DC. = *Corydalis bulbosa* L. = *Fumaria bulbosa* var. *cava* L. [Fumariaceae, Papaveraceae].
Common Name(s): Violeta bulbosa [Spanish]. Corydale à tubercule creux, corydale creux [French]. Bird-in-a-bush, bulbous corydalis, hollowroot-birthwort, hollowroot-larkspur, hollowroot, Turkey corn [English].
Life form: Herb. **Part(s) Used:** Tuber?. **Geographic distribution:** Temperate-Asia (West Asia, Caucasus). Europe, also cultivated.
Reference(s): Bharatan *et al.* 2002; Boericke, 1927, 1927b.; Bolte *et al.* 1997; Clarke, 2008.

Corylus avellana

Scientific Name(s) / [Botanical Family]: *Corylus avellana* L. = *Corylus colchica* Albov = *Corylus imeretica* Kem.-Nath. = *Corylus maxima* Mill. = *Corylus pontica* K. Koch = *Corylus tubulosa* Willd. [Betulaceae, Corylaceae].
Common Name(s): Ablano, avellana hembra, avellana macho, avellano, avellano común, avellano de lambert, nochizo [Spanish]. Avelinier, coudrier, noisetier, noisetier franc [French]. Cobnut, common filbert, english filbert, european filbert, european hazel, giant filbert, hazel, hazel-nut, hazel nut tree [English]. Aveleira [Portuguese].
Life form: Tree. **Part(s) Used:** leaf, stem bark / Fresh. **Geographic distribution:** Temperate-Asia. Europe. Cultivated in several places.

Reference(s): Bolte *et al.* 1997; Dorta Soares, n.d.; Gotfredsen, 2009.

Crataegus oxyacantha

Scientific Name(s) / [Botanical Family]: *Crataegus calycina* auct.= *Crataegus curvisepala* Lindm. = *Crataegus oxyacantha* L. = *Crataegus laevigata* (Poiret) DC. = *Crataegus lindmanii* Hrabetova =*Crataegus oxyacantha* auct. = *Crataegus rhipidophylla* Gand. = *Mespilus laevigata* Poir. [Rosaceae].

Common Name(s): Espino albar, espino blanco, espino navarro [Spanish]. Aubépine lisse, aubépine à deux styles, aubépine épineuse, epine blanche [French]. Common hawthorn, english hawthorn, haw, hawthorn, hawthorne, may, mayflower, midland hawthorn, woodland hawthorn [English]. Crataego, espinheiro alvar, pilriteiro [Portuguese].

Life form: Tree. **Part(s) Used:** Fruit mature / Fresh. **Geographic distribution:** Asia-temperate, Europe, North America (United States of America).

Reference(s): Bolte *et al.* 1997; Dorta Soares, n.d.; Tiwari *et al.* 2013.

Crocus

Scientific Name(s) / [Botanical Family]: *Crocus sativus* L. = *Crocus autumnalis* Mill. = *Crocus sativa* L. [Iridaceae].

Common Name(s): Azafrán, azafrí, croco, hupa, rosa del azafrá [Spanish]. Crocus cultivé, safran [French]. Asian saffron, Bulgarian saffron, Greek saffron, Indian saffron, Italian saffron, saffron crocus, true saffron [English]. Açafrão, Flower da Aurora [Portuguese].

Life form: Herb. **Part(s) Used:** Buds / Fresh; flower stigmas / Dried. **Geographic distribution:** Asia, South Europe & cultivated.

Reference(s): Clarke, 2008; Dorta Soares, n.d.; Gotfredsen, 2009; Tiwari *et al.* 2013; American Institute of Homeopathy,

1979.

Cucurbita citrullus

Scientific Name(s) / [Botanical Family]: *Citrullus lanatus* (Thunb.) Matsum. & Nakai = *Citrullus aedulis* Pangalo = *Citrullus colocynthoides* Pangalo = *Citrullus vulgaris* (Schrader) Mansf. var. *citroides* L.H. Bailey = *Colocynthis citrullus* (L.) Kuntze = *Cucurbita citrullus* L. = *Momordica lanata* Thunb. = *Cucurbita citrullus* L. [Cucurbitaceae].
Common Name(s): Melón de agua, sandía [Spanish]. Coloquinte, melon fourrager, pastèque fourragère [French]. Afghan melon, bastard-melon, bitter-melon, egusi-melon, fodder-melon, preserving-melon, watermelon, wild melon [English].
Life form: Herb. **Part(s) Used:** Seeds. **Geographic distribution:** Extensively naturalized & cultivated.
Reference(s): Bharatan *et al.* 2002; Clarke, 2008; Fuentes, 1996; Remedia/at, 2010.

Cucurbita pepo

Scientific Name(s) / [Botanical Family]: *Cucurbita pepo* L. = *Cucurbita ceratoceras* Haberle ex Mart. = *Cucurbita fraterna* L. H. Bailey = *Cucurbita galeottii* Cogn. = *Cucurbita melopepo* L. = *Cucurbita ovifera* L. = *Cucumis pepo* (L.) Dumort. = *Tristemon texanus* Scheele & more scientific synonyms. [Cucurbitaceae].
Common Name(s): Calabacera, calabacilla de ensalada, calabacin común, calabaza, calabaza bellota, calabaza común, purú, semilas de calabaza [Spanish]. Citrouille, courgeron, courgette, pâtisson, pépon [French]. Acorn squash, delicata squash, bitter bottle gourd, dodi marrow, gem squash, marrow, pattypan squash, pumpkin, squash, summer squah, vegetable marrow [English]. Abóbora amarela [Portuguese].
Life form: Herb. **Part(s) Used:** Seed, complete plant / Fresh.

Geographic distribution: North America (United States of America, Mexico). Extensively naturalized & cultivated.
Reference(s): Bharatan *et al.* 2002; Boericke, 1927, 1927b.; Dorta Soares, n.d.; Gotfredsen, 2009; Tiwari *et al.* 2013.

Cundurango

Scientific Name(s) / [Botanical Family]: *Marsdenia cundurango* Rchb. f. = *Marsdenia condurango* Nichols = *Gonobolus cundurango* Triana [Asclepiadaceae].
Common Name(s): Condurango blanco, lechero [Spanish]. Common condorvine, condurango, condor plant, eaglevine [English]. Conduarngo [French]. Condurango [Portuguese].
Life form: Tree. **Part(s) Used:** Bark branch, trunk / Dried.
Geographic distribution: South America (Cordillera of the Andes), Peru, Colombia, Ecuador.
Reference(s): Bharatan *et al.* 2002; Dorta Soares, n.d.; Gotfredsen, 2009.

Cuphea viscosissima

Scientific Name(s) / [Botanical Family]: *Cuphea viscosissima* Jacq. = *Cuphea brownei* Jacq. = *Cuphea petiolata* (L.) Koehne = *Lytrum petiolatum* L. = *Parsonsia petiolata* (L.) Rusby [Lythraceae].
Common Name(s): Blue wax-weed, flux-weed, clammy cuphea, tar-weed [English]. Erva de breu [Portuguese].
Life form: Herb. **Part(s) Used:** Complete plant / Fresh.
Geographic distribution: China, North America (United States of America).
Reference(s): Bharatan *et al.* 2002; Bolte *et al.* 1997; Dorta Soares, n.d.; Gotfredsen, 2009; American Institute of Homeopathy, 1979.

Cupressus australis

Scientific Name(s) / [Botanical Family]: *Cupressus australis* Pers. = *Callitris rhomboidea* R. Br. ex A. Rich. [Cupressaceae].

Common Name(s): Italian cypress, Mediterranean cypress [English]. Cyprčs commun, cyprčs d'Italie [French]. CiprEast [Portuguese]. Ciprés común, ciprés Italian [Spanish].

Life form: Tree. **Part(s) Used:** Fruit, Leaf. **Geographic distribution:** Europe, Oriental Asia. Cultivated.

Reference: Boericke, 1927, 1927b.

Cupressus lawsoniana

Scientific Name(s) / [Botanical Family]: *Chamaecyparis lawsoniana* (A. Murray) Parl. = *Cupressus lawsoniana* A. Murray [Cupressaceae].

Common Name(s): Ginger-pine, Lawson's false cypress, Lawson's-cypress, Oregon-cedar, Port Orford-cedar [English]. Cyprčs de Lawson [French]. CiprEast [Portuguese]. Cedro de Óregon, falso ciprés de Lawson [Spanish].

Life form: Tree. **Part(s) Used:** Fruit, Leaf. **Geographic distribution:** North America (Northwest & Southwest United States of America). Naturalized in Asia, Australia, Europe & New Zealand.

Reference: Allen, 2006-2010.

Cuscuta

Scientific Name(s) / [Botanical Family]: *Cuscuta epithymum* (L.) L. = *Cuscuta europaea* var. *epithymum* L. [Convolvulaceae, Cuscutaceae].

Common Name(s): Clover dodder, dodder, lesser dodder [English]. Cuscute du thym [French]. Cipó-de-chumbo, cuscuta [Portuguese]. Epitimo, zacatlaxcale? [Spanish]. Cipó-de-chumbo, cuscuta [Portuguese].

Life form: Liana, epiphyte. **Part(s) Used:** Complete plant in

bloom / Fresh. **Geographic distribution:** North Africa. Europe Central. Asia. Naturalized in several places.
Reference(s): Bharatan *et al.* 2002; Boericke, 1927, 1927b.; Dorta Soares, n.d.

Cyclamen europaeum

Scientific Name(s) / [Botanical Family]: *Cyclamen hederifolium* Aiton. = *Cyclamen europaeum* Auct. = *Cyclamen neapolitanum* Ten. [Primulaceae].
Common Name(s): Cyclamen, sowbread, spring sowbread [English]. Cyclamen à feuilles de lierre, cyclamen de Naples, Pain de pourceau [French]. Ciclamen napoletano [Italian]. Ciclamen, mitra [Spanish]. Ciclame da Europe, violeta dos alpes; [Portuguese].
Life form: Herb. **Part(s) Used:** Subterraneous parts / Fresh. **Geographic distribution:** South Europe. Naturalized in Great Britain.
Reference(s): Dorta Soares, n.d.; Gotfredsen, 2009; Plants for a future, 2009.

Cydonia vulgaris

Scientific Name(s) / [Botanical Family]: *Cydonia oblonga* Mill. = *Cydonia vulgaris* Pers = *Pyrus cydonia* L. [Rosaceae].
Common Name(s): Quince [English]. Wen po [Chinese]. Cognassier, coing [French]. Marmelo [Portuguese]. Azamboa, cacho, codon, membrillero, membrillo [Spanish].
Life form: Tree. **Part(s) Used:** Fruit, leaf, seeds. **Geographic distribution:** Temperate-Asia. Naturalized & cultivated in several places.
Reference(s): Gotfredsen, 2009; Plants for a future, 2009; Remedia/at, 2010; Tiwari *et al.* 2013; American Institute of Homeopathy, 1979.

Cynara scolymus

Scientific Name(s) / [Botanical Family]: *Cynara scolymus* L. = *Cynara cardunculus* L. [Asteraceae, Compositae].

Common Name(s): Artichoke, artichoke thistle, cardoon, globe artichoke [English]. Artichaut commun, cardon d'Espagne [French]. Alcachofa, cardo, cardo de comer [Spanish]. Alcachofra [Portuguese].

Life form: Herb. **Part(s) Used:** Complete plant / Fresh. **Geographic distribution:** Temperate-Asia. Europe, cultivated.Cosmopolitan.

Reference(s): Dorta Soares, n.d.; Remedia/at, 2010; Tiwari *et al.* 2013.

Cynoglossum officinale

Scientific Name(s) / [Botanical Family]: *Cynoglossum officinale* L. [Boraginaceae].

Common Name(s): Dog's tongue, gypsy Flower, hound's-tongue, rats-and-mice [English]. Cynoglosse officinale, langue de chien [French]. Bizniega, conoglossa, hierba del conejo, lengua de perro, orejas de liebre [Spanish]. Cino glossa, língua de cão [Portuguese].

Life form: Herb. **Part(s) Used:** Leaf, Root / Fresh. **Geographic distribution:** Temperate-Asia. Europe.

Reference(s): De Legarreta, 1961; Dorta Soares, n.d.; American Institute of Homeopathy, 1979.

Cypripedium pubescens

Scientific Name(s) / [Botanical Family]: *Cypripedium pubescens* Willdenow [Orchidaceae].

Common Name(s): American valerian, bleeding heart, Indian shoe, lady's slipper, Moccasin Root, nerve Root, nervine [English]. Sabot [French]. Cipripedium, Sapato de Vênus, valeriana americana [Portuguese].

Life form: Herb. **Part(s) Used:** Subterraneous parts / Fresh. **Geographic distribution:** North America (Canada, United States of America).
Reference(s): Bolte *et al.* 1997; Dorta Soares, n.d.; Gotfredsen, 2009; Tiwari *et al.* 2013.

Cytisus scoparius

Scientific Name(s) / [Botanical Family]: *Cytisus scoparius* (L.) Link = *Spartium scoparium* L. = *Sarothamnus scoparius* (L.) Wimm. ex W. D. J. Koch = *Sarothamnus vulgaris* Wimm. = *Genista scoparia* (L.) Lam. [Fabaceae, Leguminosae].
Common Name(s): Broom tops common, European, Irish, or Scotch broom [English]. Genęt ŕ balais [French]. Giesta, giesta das vassouras [Portuguese]. Cabestro de oro, escoba, escoba negra, hiniesta [Spanish]. Giestam giesta das vassouras [Portuguese].
Life form: Shrub. **Part(s) Used:** Flower & leaf / Fresh; complete plant in bloom / Fresh. **Geographic distribution:** Central, South Russia. Great Britain. West & North de Europe. Japan. Occasionaly in Central & South United States of America. Australia, etc.
Reference(s): Dorta Soares, n.d.; Hering, 2006; Remedia/at, 2010; American Institute of Homeopathy, 1979.

Daphne indica

Scientific Name(s) / [Botanical Family]: *Daphne indica* L. = *Daphne cannabina* Lour. ex Wall. = *Daphne odora* Thunb. = *Wikstroemia indica* C. A. Meyer [Thymelaeaceae].
Common Name(s): Small-leaf salago, sweet-scented spruge laurel, winter daphne [English]. Jinchoge [Japanese].

Life form: Shrub. **Part(s) Used:** Bark, branch.
Geographic distribution: Temperate-Asia. Cultivated. Ornamental.
Reference(s): Remedia/at, 2010; Tiwari *et al.* 2013; American Institute of Homeopathy, 1979.

Datura arborea

Scientific Name(s) / [Botanical Family]: *Datura arborea* L. = *Datura arborea* Ruiz & Pavón = *Datura cornigera* Hook = *Brugmansia arborea* (L.) Lagerth.
Common Name(s): Angel's-trumpet [English]. Açucena-do-brejo, cálice-de-vênus, cartucheira, cartucho-branco, trombetão-branco, trombeta [Portuguese]. Almizclillo, Flor de campanilla, florifundio, floripondio, floripondio blanco del Peru, toloache, trómbita, trompeta [Spanish].
Life form: Herb. **Part(s) Used:** Flower / Fresh. **Geographic distribution:** Central, North & South America (Mexico, United States of America. Peru, Colombia, Bolivia).
Reference(s): Dorta Soares, n.d.; Remedia/at, 2010; Tiwari *et al.* 2013.

Datura candida

Scientific Name(s) / [Botanical Family]: *Datura candida* (Pers.) Saff. = *Brugmansia* x *candida* (Pers.) Saff. [Solanaceae].
Common Name(s): Angel's-trumpet, white angel's-trumpet, tree stramonium [English]. Borrachero, campana, floripondio, toloache [Spanish].
Life form: Shrub. **Part(s) Used:** Flower / Fresh. **Geographic distribution:** Central, North & South America. (Peru. Mexico. United States of America).
Reference: American Institute of Homeopathy, 1979.

Datura ferox

Scientific Name(s) / [Botanical Family]: *Datura ferox* L. [Solanaceae].

Common Name(s): Angel's-trumpet, Chinese datura, fierce thorn-apple, large thorn-apple, long-spine thorn-apple [English]. Grootstinkblaar [African]. Chamico [Portuguese].

Life form: Herb. **Part(s) Used:** Seeds / Dried. **Geographic distribution:** China. This plant are considered as a weed around the world.

Reference(s): Allen, 2006-2010; Bharatan *et al.* 2002; Dorta Soares, n.d.; American Institute of Homeopathy, 1979.

Datura inoxia

Scientific Name(s) / [Botanical Family]: *Datura inoxia* Mill. [Solanaceae].

Common Name(s): Angel's-trumpet, downy thorn-apple, Indian-apple, sacred datura, thorn-apple [English]. Harige stinkblaar [African]. Datura innocente [French]. Datura-européia, trombeta-branca, trombeteira-branca [Portuguese]. Burladora, cacaito, estramonio de fruit redondo, nuez del diablo, toloache [Spanish].

Life form: Shrub. **Part(s) Used:** Seeds. **Geographic distribution:** Extensively naturalized in several places.

Reference(s): Allen, 2006-2010; Bharatan *et al.* 2002; Bolte *et al.* 1997; Clarke, 2008.

Datura metel

Scientific Name(s) / [Botanical Family]: *Datura metel* L. = *Datura alba* Nees = *Datura chlorantha* Hook. = *Datura fastuosa* L. = *Datura metel* var. *fastuosa* (L.) Saff. [Solanaceae].

Common Name(s): Downy thorn-apple, Hindu datura, Hindu thorn-apple, hoary thorn-apple, horn-of-plenty, Indian datura, metel, purple thorn-apple [English]. Babado de viúva, burbiaca

[Portuguese]. Burladora [Spanish].
Life form: Herb. **Part(s) Used:** Seeds/ Dried. **Geographic distribution:** India. Extensively cultivated.
Reference(s): Dorta Soares, n.d.; Remedia/at, 2010.

Datura sanguinea

Scientific Name(s) / [Botanical Family]: *Datura sanguinea* (Ruiz & Pavón) D. Don = *Datura sanguinea* Ruiz & Pavón [Solanaceae].
Common Name(s): Red floripontio, red angel's trumpet [English]. Floripondio rojo, toloache [Spanish].
Life form: Shrub. **Part(s) Used:** Flower. **Geographic distribution:** West South America. Extensively cultivated.
Reference(s): Allen, 2006-2010; Bharatan *et al.* 2002; Bolte *et al.* 1997; Clarke, 2008; Remedia/at, 2010.

Desmodium gangeticum

Scientific Name(s) / [Botanical Family]: *Desmodium gangeticum* (L.) DC. Blanco = *Hedysarum gangeticum* L. = *Meibomia gangetica* (L.) Kuntze [Fabaceae, Leguminosae].
Common Name(s): Sarivan, salpani [English].
Life form: Herb. **Part(s) Used:** Complete plant. **Geographic distribution:** Philippines. South America. South Africa. Temperate Asia.
Reference(s): Allen, 2006-2010; Bharatan *et al.* 2002; Tiwari *et al.* 2013.

Dictamnus albus

Scientific Name(s) / [Botanical Family]: *Dictamnus albus* L. = *Dictamnus caucasicus* (Fisch. & C. A. Mey.) Grossh. = *Dictamnus fraxinellus* Pers. [Rutaceae].
Common Name(s): Bastard dittany, burniningbush, dittany, fraxinella, gasplant, white fraxinella [English]. Dictame blanc [French]. Dittamo [Italian]. Chitán, díctamo blanco, fraxinella,

fresnillo, itamo real [Spanish]. Fraxinella [Portuguese].
Life form: Herb. **Part(s) Used:** Root-bark, leaves fresh, complete plant. **Geographic distribution:** Mexico. Europe (Italy, France) & Russia.
Reference(s): Dorta Soares, n.d.; Zandvoort, 2006.

Digitalis lutea

Scientific Name(s) / [Botanical Family]: *Digitalis lutea* L. [Schrophulariaceae].
Common Name(s): Foxglove, small yellow foxglove, straw foxglove, yellow foxglove [English]. Digitale jaune, digitale à petites fleurs, petite digitale [French]. Digital amarilla [Spanish].
Life form: Herb. **Part(s) Used:** Leaf / Fresh. **Geographic distribution:** Europe. Cultivated in several regions.
Reference(s): Dorta Soares, n.d.

Digitalis purpurea

Scientific Name(s) / [Botanical Family]: *Digitalis purpurea* L. [Schrophulariaceae].
Common Name(s): Annual foxglove, fairy fingers, fairy's gloves, fox glove, purple fox glove, purple glove [English]. Digitale pourprée, gant de Notre-Dame [French]. Calzones de zorra, cartucho, chupamieles, dedal de doncella, dedal de princesa, dedalera, digital, guante de nuestra Señora, gualdaperra, guantelete, San Juán, viluria [Spanish]. Abeleura, dedaleira, dedo de dama, erva dedal [Portuguese].
Life form: Herb. **Part(s) Used:** Leaf / Fresh. **Geographic distribution:** South, Central Europe, England, Norway. Cultivated in several regions.
Reference(s): Dorta Soares, n.d.; Gotfredsen, 2009; Plants for a future, 2009; Tiwari *et al.* 2013; American Institute of Homeopathy, 1979.

Dioscorea villosa

Scientific Name(s) / [Botanical Family]: *Dioscorea villosa* L. = *Dioscorea hirticaulis* Bartlett = *Dioscorea paniculata* auct.= *Dioscorea quaternata* J. F. Gmel. = *Dioscorea villosa* L. var. *hirticaulis* (Bartlett) H. E. Ahles [Dioscoreaceae].

Common Name(s): Colic root, devil's bone, dioscorea, fourleaf yam, huang yao tzu, Mexican wild yam, rheumatism root, wild yam [English]. Espèce d'igname sauvage [French]. Batata, batata silvestre, boniato silvestre, ñame, ñame silvestre, raíz de China. [Spanish]. Cará, inhame selvagem [Portuguese].

Life form: Liana. **Part(s) Used:** Rhizome, leaves before bloom, Complete plant / Fresh. **Geographic distribution:** East North America (United States of America).

Reference(s): Allen, 2006-2010; Dorta Soares, n.d.; Fuentes, 1996; Plants for a future, 2009; Tiwari *et al.* 2013; American Institute of Homeopathy, 1979.

Dipsacus sylveaster

Scientific Name(s) / [Botanical Family]: *Dipsacus sylvestris* Huds. = *Dipsacus silveaster* Huds. = *Dipsacus fullonum* L. = *Dipsacus fullonum sativus* (L.) Thellung [Dipsacaceae].

Common Name(s): Common or wild teasel, venus bath [English]. Cardère sauvage [French]. Baño de Venus, cardencha, cardo de cardadores, peines [Spanish].

Life form: Herb. **Part(s) Used:** Complete plant, flower. **Geographic distribution:** North Africa. Temperate-Asia. North Europe. Naturalized in United States of America, Australia, etc.

Reference(s): Dorta Soares, n.d.; Plants for a future, 2009; American Institute of Homeopathy, 1979.

Dirca palustris

Scientific Name(s) / [Botanical Family]: *Dirca palustris* L. [Thymelaeaceae].

Common Name(s): Leather wood, mouse wood, rope bark, swamp bark, thong bark, wicopy [English]. Bois de plomb [French]. Pau de couro [Portuguese].
Life form: Shrub. **Part(s) Used:** Bark-branches / Fresh.
Geographic distribution: North America (East Canada. North East, North, Central & Southeast United States of America).
Reference(s): Bolte,1997; Dorta Soares, n.d.; Plants for a future, 2009; Seror, 2000; Tiwari *et al.* 2013.

Draconitum foetidum see *Ictodes foetida*

Drosera rotundifolia
Scientific Name(s) / [Botanical Family]: *Drosera rotundifolia* L. [Droseraceae].
Common Name(s): Moor-grass, red-rot, round-leavesundew, round-leaf ed sundew, sun-dew, youth-wort [English]. Drosère [French]. Atrapamoscas, rocío del sol, yerba de la gota, yerba del rocío [Spanish]. Drósera [Portuguese].
Life form: Herb. **Part(s) Used:** Complete plant / Fresh.
Geographic distribution: Temperate-Asia. Europe. North America (Canada-United States of America).
Reference(s): Dorta Soares, n.d.; Tiwari *et al.* 2013; American Institute of Homeopathy, 1979.

Dulcamara
Scientific Name(s) / [Botanical Family]: *Solanum dulcamara* L. [Solanaceae].
Common Name(s): Bitter nightshade, bittersweet, dulcamara, woody nightshade [English]. Douce-amčre, Morelle [French]. Dulcamara europea [Spanish]. Doce amarga, dulcamara [Portuguese].
Life form: Shrub. **Part(s) Used:** Leaf, stem; leaves & branches collected before bloom or / and fructifying. **Geographic distribution:** North Africa. Temperate-Asia. Tropical Asia.

Europe, naturalized in several places.
Reference(s): Comisión Editora de la Farmacopea Homeopática de los Estados Unidos Mexicanos, 1988; Dorta Soares, n.d.; Plants for a future, 2009; Tiwari *et al.* 2013; American Institute of Homeopathy, 1979.

Echinacea angustifolia
Scientific Name(s) / [Botanical Family]: *Echinacea angustifolia* DC. = *Brauneria pallida* (Nutt.) Britton = *Brauneria angustifolia* (DC.) A. Heller = *Rudbeckia pallida* Nutt. [Asteraceae, Compositae].
Common Name(s): Black sampson, black-sampson echinacea, echinacea, Kansas snakeroot, narrow-lefconeflower, narrow-leaf echinacea, narrow-leaf purple-coneflower [English]. Equinácea, rudbeckia [Portuguese].
Life form: Herb. **Part(s) Used:** Complete plant / Fresh.
Geographic distribution: North America (West Canada. North Central, Northwest & South Central, United States of America).
Reference(s): Allen, 2006-2010; Bharatan *et al.* 2002; Dorta Soares, n.d.; Fuentes, 1996; Remedia/at, 2010; Tiwari *et al.* 2013.

Echinacea purpurea
Scientific Name(s) / [Botanical Family]: *Echinacea purpurea* (L.) Moench. = *Rudbeckia purpurea* L. [Asteraceae, Compositae].
Common Name(s): Black sampson, Eastern purple-coneflower, purple-coneflower [English].
Life form: Herb. **Part(s) Used:** Aerial part in bloom, Root / Fresh.
Geographic distribution: East United States of America.
Reference(s): Anshutz, 2008; Bharatan *et al.* 2002; Dorta Soares, n.d.; Tiwari *et al.* 2013.

Elaeagnus

Scientific Name(s) / [Botanical Family]: *Elaeagnus angustifolia* L. = *Elaeagnus iliensis* Musheg. = *Elaeagnus umbellata* Thunb. [Elaeagnaceae].

Common Name(s): Oleander, oleaster, Russian olive, Russian silverberry [English]. Sha zao [Chinese?]. Árbol del paraiso, azofaifo blanco, cinamomo vulgar, oliva silvestre of franceses [Spanish].

Life form: Shrub, Tree. **Part(s) Used:** Mature seeds / Dried.

Geographic distribution: Europe (Mediterranean). Asia (China, Iran, Siria]. Bermudas. North America (Canada, Mexico, United States of America). New Zealand.

Reference(s): Allen, 2006-2010; Bharatan *et al.* 2002; Clarke, 2008; Dorta Soares, n.d.

Elaterium

Scientific Name(s) / [Botanical Family]: *Ecballium elaterium* (L.) A. Rich = *Momordica elaterium* L. [Cucurbitaceae].

Common Name(s): Squirting cucumber [English]. Ecbalie élatère [French]. Cohombrillo [Spanish]. Elatério, pepino do diabo, pepino de São Gregório [Portuguese].

Life form: Liana. **Part(s) Used:** Fruit / Dried; fruit juice sediment.

Geographic distribution: Mediterranean (Europe). Africa. Asia.

Reference(s): Dorta Soares, n.d.; Remedia/at, 2010; Tiwari *et al.* 2013.

Eleutherococcus senticosus

Scientific Name(s) / [Botanical Family]: *Eleutherococcus senticosus* (Rupr. & Maxim.) Maxim. = *Acanthopanax asperatus* Franch. & Sav. = *Acanthopanax asperulatus* Franch. = *Acanthopanax eleutherococcus* (Maxim.) Makino = *Acanthopanax senticosus* (Rupr. & Maxim.) Harms [Araliaceae].

Common Name(s): Eleuthero, Siberian-ginseng [English]. Ci wu jia, zu wu zha [Chinese]. Acanthopanax espinoso, Arbusto del diablo, eleuterococco espinoso, Ginseng espinoso, Ginseng siberiano, matorral del diablo. [Spanish]. Buisson du diable, eleutherococoque [French]. Ezo-ukogi [Japanese]. Čertov kust, dikij perec, svobodnojagodnik koljučij [Russian].
Life form: Herb. **Part(s) Used:** Root / Dried. **Geographic distribution:** Temperate-Asia. Russia. China. Japan.
Reference(s): Bharatan *et al.* 2002; Fuentes, 1996; Remedia/at, 2010.

Ephedra see *Ephedra vulgaris*

Ephedra vulgaris
Scientific Name(s) / [Botanical Family]: *Ephedra vulgaris* Rich. = *Ephedra distachya* L. subsp. *monostachya* = *Ephedra monostachya* L. = *Ephedra helvetica* C. A. Mey. [Ephedraceae].
Common Name(s): Ephedrine, epitonin, sea-grape [English]. Shuang sui ma huang [Chinese]. Agraz marino, ceñudo, efedra, granos de helecho, piorno [Spanish].
Life form: Shrub. **Part(s) Used:** Complete plant / Fresh. Dried leaves collected during bloom. **Geographic distribution:** Europe (Mediterranean). Russian Federation.
Reference(s): Bharatan *et al.* 2002; Dorta Soares, n.d.; Remedia/at, 2010; Tiwari *et al.* 2013.

Equisetum arvense
Scientific Name(s) / [Botanical Family]: *Equisetum arvense* L. [Equisetaceae].
Common Name(s): Bottle-brush, field horsetail. pewterwort, shave-grass [English]. Prêle des champs [French]. Candadillo, cien nudillos, cola de caballo, equiseto menor [Spanish]. Cauda de cavalo, cavalinha, cola de cavalo, lixa vegetal [Portuguese].
Life form: Herb. **Part(s) Used:** Complete plant / Fresh. Plant

whitout root / Dried. **Geographic distribution:** Europe temperate North America & Asia.
Reference(s): Bharatan *et al.* 2002; Dorta Soares, n.d.; Rowe, 2006.

Equisetum hyemale

Scientific Name(s) / [Botanical Family]: *Equisetum hyemale* L. [Equisetaceae].
Common Name(s): Horsetail [English]. Prêle d'hiver [French]. Cola de caballo, equiseto mayor, equiseto mecánico, yerba estañera [Spanish]. Cauda de cavalo [Portuguese].
Life form: Herb. **Part(s) Used:** Complete plant / Fresh. complete plant whitout Root / Dried. **Geographic distribution:** naturalized in several places.
Reference(s): Dorta Soares, n.d.; Plants for a future, 2009; Tiwari *et al.* 2013.

Equisetum limosum

Scientific Name(s) / [Botanical Family]: *Equisetum limosum* L. = *Equisetum fluviatile* L. [Equisetaceae].
Common Name(s): Swamp horsetail, water horsetail [English]. Prêle des eaux courantes [French]. Equiseto fluviatile [Italian].
Life form: Herb. **Part(s) Used:** Complete plant / Fresh. **Geographic distribution:** Europe.
Reference: Dorta Soares, n.d.

Erechites

Scientific Name(s) / [Botanical Family]: *Erechtites hieracifolia* (L.) Raf. ex DC. = *Erechtites hieraciifolius* (L.) Raf. ex DC. = *Senecio hieraciifolius* L. = *Senecio hieracifolia* L. [Asteraceae, Compositae].
Common Name(s): American fireweed, burnweed, fireweed, Malayan groundsel, pilewort [English]. Achicoria de cabra

[Spanish]. Caruru amargo, joio do fogo [Portuguese].
Life form: Herb. **Part(s) Used:** Aerial part in bloom / Fresh.
Geographic distribution: North, Central & South America. Naturalized in several places.
Reference(s): Bharatan *et al.* 2002; Clarke, 2008; Comisión Editora de la Farmacopea Homeopática de los Estados Unidos Mexicanos, 1988; Dorta Soares, n.d.; Guermonprez *et al.* 1989; Müntz, n.d.; Remedia/at, 2010; Tiwari *et al.* 2013.

Erigeron

Scientific Name(s) / [Botanical Family]: *Erigeron paniculatus* Lam. = *Erigeron canadensis* L. = *Conyza canadensis* (L.) Cronquist [Asteraceae, Compositae].
Common Name(s): Butterweed, Canada fleabane, horseweed [English]. Cauda de raposa, erva carniceira, erva pulgueira [Portuguese].
Life form: Herb. **Part(s) Used:** Complete plant / fresh, complete plant in bloom / fresh. **Geographic distribution:** Europe, North America.
Reference(s): Bharatan *et al.* 2002; Dorta Soares, n.d.; Remedia/at, 2010; Tiwari *et al.* 2013.

Eriodictyon californicum

Scientific Name(s) / [Botanical Family]: *Eriodictyon californicum* (Benth.) Hook. = *Eriodictyon californicum* (Hook. & Arn.) Torr. = *Wigandia californica* Hook & Arn. [Hydrophyllaceae].
Common Name(s): California yerba santa, yerba santa [English]. California yerba santa [Spanish].
Life form: Shrub. **Part(s) Used:** Leaf, complete plant / Dried.
Geographic distribution: North America (West United States of America).
Reference(s): Allen, 2006-2010; Dorta Soares, n.d.; Plants for a future, 2009.

Eryngium maritimum

Scientific Name(s) / [Botanical Family]: *Eryngium maritimum* (L.) Hook. = *Eryngium campestre* L. [Umbelliferae].
Common Name(s): Eryngo, sea holly [English]. Cardo corredor de marina, cardo cuerno, eringio marino azul [Spanish].
Life form: Herb. **Part(s) Used:** Complete plant / Fresh.
Geographic distribution: England. Europe. Asia. North Africa.
Reference: Allen, 2006-2010.

Eucalyptus globulus

Scientific Name(s) / [Botanical Family]: *Eucalyptus globulus* Labill. [Myrtaceae].
Common Name(s): Blue gum tree, fever tree [English]. Eucalyptus globuleux, gommier bleu [French]. Eucalipto, eucalipto gigante, eucalipto alcanforero [Spanish]. Eucalipto, gomeiro azul [Portuguese].
Life form: Tree. **Part(s) Used:** Leaf / Dried. **Geographic distribution:** cultivated & naturalized in Europe & America.
Reference(s): Allen, 2006-2010; Dorta Soares, n.d.; Tiwari *et al*. 2013.

Euonymus atropurpurea

Scientific Name(s) / [Botanical Family]: *Euonymus atropurpureus* Jacq. [Celastraceae].
Common Name(s): Bitter-ash, burningbush, eastern wahoo, wahoo [English]. Agracejo, evónimo [Spanish]. Evônimo [Portuguese].
Life form: Shrub. **Part(s) Used:** Root, branch / Fresh. **Geographic distribution:** North America (Canada, United States of America).
Reference(s): Comisión Editora de la Farmacopea Homeopática de los Estados Unidos Mexicanos, 1988; Dorta Soares, n.d.; Rowe, 2006; Tiwari *et al*. 2013.

Euonymus europaea

Scientific Name(s) / [Botanical Family]: *Euonymus europaea* L. = *Euonymus vulgaris* Mill. [Celastraceae].
Common Name(s): Common spindle, European spindletree, spindle [English]. Bonnet de prëtre, fusain d'Europe [French].
Life form: Shrub. **Part(s) Used:** Root, branch / Fresh. **Geographic distribution:** Asia-temperate, Caucasus. Europe. Also cultivated.
Reference: Dorta Soares, n.d.

Eupatorium aromaticum

Scientific Name(s) / [Botanical Family]: *Eupatorium aromaticum* L. = *Eupatorium latidens* Small = *Ageratina aromatica* (L.) Spach. [Asteraceae, Compositae].
Common Name(s): Hemp agrimony, lesser snakeroot [English].
Life form: Herb. **Part(s) Used:** Leaf, complete plant in bloom / Fresh. **Geographic distribution:** North America (East United States of America).
Reference(s): Bharatan *et al.* 2002; Dorta Soares, n.d.; Tiwari *et al.* 2013.

Eupatorium cannabinum

Scientific Name(s) / [Botanical Family]: *Eupatorium cannabinum* L. [Asteraceae, Compositae].
Common Name(s): Hemp agrimony [English]. Eupatoire chanvrine [French]. Alfabaca, alfavaca, altabaca, altarraga, atabaca, canabina de agua, cañamazo, cáñamo silvestre, eupatorio de Avicena [Spanish]. Eupatório [Portuguese].
Life form: Herb. **Part(s) Used:** Leaf, complete plant in bloom / Fresh. **Geographic distribution:** Asia, Europe. Cultivated & naturalized in China & North America (Canada).
Reference(s): Comisión Editora de la Farmacopea Homeopática de los Estados Unidos Mexicanos, 1988; Dorta Soares, n.d.

Eupatorium perfoliatum

Scientific Name(s) / [Botanical Family]: *Eupatorium perfoliatum* L. = *Eupatorium chapmanii* Small = *Eupatorium perfoliatum* var. *colpophilum* Fernald & Griscom = *Eupatorium perfoliatum* var. *cuneatum* Fernald & Griscom [Asteraceae].

Common Name(s): Boneset, common boneset, thorough-wort [English]. Eupatoire perfoliée, herbé à la fièvre [French]. Arregla huesos, hierba de la fiebre [Spanish]. Cura ossos [Portuguese].

Life form: Herb. **Part(s) Used:** Leaf, bud / Fresh. **Geographic distribution:** North America (Canada, United States of America).

Reference(s): Bharatan *et al*. 2002; Bolte *et al*. 1997; Dorta Soares, n.d.; Plants for a future, 2009; Tiwari *et al*. 2013.

Eupatorium purpureum

Scientific Name(s) / [Botanical Family]: *Eupatorium purpureum* L. = *Eupatoriadelphus purpureus* (L.) R. Middle King & H.Rob. = *Cunigunda purpurea* Lunell = *Cunigunda purpurea* (L.) Lundell [Asteraceae, Compositae].

Common Name(s): Gravel root, green-stem joe-pye-weed, Joe pye weed, trumpet weed (queen of the meadow) [English]. Racine à la gravelle [French]. Joio trompeto, rainha dos prados [Portuguese]. Eupatoria purpúrea, eupatorio, reina de los prados [Spanish].

Life form: Herb. **Part(s) Used:** Root / Fresh. **Geographic distribution:** North America (North East, North, Central & Southeast United States of America).

Reference(s): Allen, 2006-2010; Bharatan *et al*. 2002; Comisión Editora de la Farmacopea Homeopática de los Estados Unidos Mexicanos, 1988; Dorta Soares, n.d.; Tiwari *et al*. 2013.

Euphorbia corollata

Scientific Name(s) / [Botanical Family]: *Euphorbia corollata* L.

[Euphorbiaceae].
Common Name(s): Blooming spurge, emetic root, Floring spurge, posion-milkweed [English]. Tithymale fleuri [French].
Life form: Herb. **Part(s) Used:** Root / Fresh. **Geographic distribution:** North America (East Canada, United States of America).
Reference(s): Allen, 2006-2010; Bharatan *et al.* 2002; Comisión Editora de la Farmacopea Homeopática de los Estados Unidos Mexicanos, 1988; Dorta Soares, n.d.; Tiwari *et al.* 2013.

Euphorbia cyparissias

Scientific Name(s) / [Botanical Family]: *Euphorbia cyparissias* L. = *Euphorbia cyparissias* (L.) Haw. [Euphorbiaceae].
Common Name(s): Cypress spurge [English]. Esula Minor, lechetrezna, mirabel lechero [Spanish].
Life form: Shrub. **Part(s) Used:** Complete plant in bloom / Fresh.
Geographic distribution: Temperate-Asia. Europe. Cultivated & naturalized in several places.
Reference(s): Allen, 2006-2010; Bharatan *et al.* 2002; Comisión Editora de la Farmacopea Homeopática de los Estados Unidos Mexicanos, 1988; Dorta Soares, n.d.; Remedia/at, 2010; Tiwari *et al.* 2013.

Euphorbia esula

Scientific Name(s) / [Botanical Family]: *Euphorbia esula* L. = *Euphorbia cyparissias* L. = *Euphorbia discolor* Ledeb. = *Euphorbia distincta* Stschegl. = *Euphorbia glomerulans* (Prokh.) Prokh. = *Euphorbia gmelinii* Steud. = *Euphorbia jaxartica* Prokh. = *Euphorbia kaleniczenkii* Czern. Ex Trautv. = *Euphorbia leoncroizatii* Oudejans = *Euphorbia lunulata* Bunge = *Euphorbia maackii* Meinsh. = *Euphorbia tommasiniana* Bertol. etc. [Euphorbiaceae].
Common Name(s): Faitours-grass, leaf and spurge, wolf's milk

[English]. Ru jiang da ji [Chinese]. Leiteira-folhosa [Portuguese].
Life form: Shrub. **Part(s) Used:** Complete plant in bloom / Fresh.
Geographic distribution: Temperate-Asia. Europe. Cultivated & naturalized in several places.
Reference: Dorta Soares, n.d.

Euphorbia helioscopia

Scientific Name(s) / [Botanical Family]: *Euphorbia helioscopia* L. [Euphorbiaceae].
Common Name(s): Coapatli, golondrina, hierba de la golondrina [Spanish]. Sun spurge, wolf's milk [English]. Euphorbe réveil-matin [French]. Leteira-do-sol, maleteira [Portuguese]. Lecherina, lechetrezna común, lechocino [Spanish].
Life form: Herb. **Part(s) Used:** Complete plant in bloom / Fresh.
Geographic distribution: Africa, Temperate-Asia, Europe. Naturalized in several places.
Reference: Dorta Soares, n.d.

Euphorbia pilosa

Scientific Name(s) / [Botanical Family]: *Euphorbia pilosa* L. = *Euphorbia procera* M. Bieb. [Euphorbiaceae].

Common Name(s): Mao da ji [Chinese]. Spurge [English].
Life form: Herb. **Part(s) Used:** Root / Fresh. **Geographic distribution:** Temperate-Asia, Russian Federation, Europe.
Reference: Dorta Soares, n.d.

Euphorbia prostrata

Scientific Name(s) / [Botanical Family]: *Chamaesyce prostrata* (Aiton) Small = *Euphorbia prostrata* Aiton [Euphorbiaceae].
Common Name(s): Coapatli, golondrina, hierba de la golondrina [Spanish]. Prostrate sandmat, swallow wort [English].
Life form: Herb. **Part(s) Used:** Root / Fresh. **Geographic distribution:** North America (United States of America, Mexico).

Central America. South America. Tropics. Naturalized in Temperate-Asia, Europe & several places.
Reference(s): Bharatan *et al.* 2002; Rowe, 2006.

Euphorbia pulcherrima

Scientific Name(s) / [Botanical Family]: *Euphorbia pulcherrima* Willd. ex Klotzch = *Euphorbia eritrophylla* Bertol. = *Euphorbia erytrophylla* Bertol. = *Euphorbia fastuosa* Sessé & Mociño = *Euphorbia coccinea* Raf. = *Poinsettia pulcherrima* (Willd. ex Klotzsch) Graham [Euphorbiaceae].
Common Name(s): Christmas star, poinsettia. [English]. Fleur de feu, fleur de Pâques [French]. Catalina, flor de pascua, flor de fuego, flor de nochebuena, nochebuena, paño de Holanda [Spanish]. Asa de papagaio, cardeal, flor de papagaio [Portuguese].
Life form: Herb. **Part(s) Used:** Flower, stem / Fresh; flowers / Dried. **Geographic distribution:** Mexico. Cultivated in several countries as ornamental.
Reference(s): Bharatan *et al.* 2002; Dorta Soares, n.d.

Euphrasia officinalis

Scientific Name(s) / [Botanical Family]: *Euphrasia officinalis* L. = *Euphrasia rostkoviana* Hayne [Orobanchae, Scrophulariaceae].
Common Name(s): Eyebright, large-flowered eybright, red eyebright, meadow eyebright [English]. Euphraise officinale [French]. Eufrasia oficinal, eufrasia vulgar, furasia, mujares [Spanish]. Eufrásia [Portuguese].
Life form: Herb. **Part(s) Used:** Complete plant, flower / Fresh.
Geographic distribution: China, North America. Europe.
Reference(s): Bharatan *et al.* 2002; Dorta Soares, n.d.; Gotfredsen, 2009; Remedia/at, 2010; Tiwari *et al.* 2013.

Eysenhardtia polystachya

Scientific Name(s) / [Botanical Family]: *Eysenhardtia polystachya* (Ortega) Sarg. = *Dalea fruticosa* G. Don = *Eysenhardtia amorphoides* Kunth = *Psoralea fruticosa* Kellog = *Psoralea fruticosa* Sessé & Mociño = *Psoralea stipularis* Sessé & Mociño = *Varennea polystachya* Ortega = *Viborquia polystachya* Ortega = *Wiborgia amorphodes* (Kunth) Kuntze = *Wiborgia polystachya* (Ortega) Kuntze [Fabaceae, Leguminosae].

Common Name(s): Kidneywood [English]. Palo azul, palo dulce, palo santo, vara dulce [Spanish].

Life form: Tree. **Part(s) Used:** Wood / Fresh. **Geographic distribution:** North America (Southeast United States of America, North Mexico). Cultivated.

Reference(s): Comisión Editora de la Farmacopea Homeopática de los Estados Unidos Mexicanos, 1988; Plants for a future, 2009.

Fabiana imbricata see *Pichi pichi*

Fagopyrum

Scientific Name(s) / [Botanical Family]: *Fagopyrum esculentum* Moench. = *Fagopyrum sagittatum* Gilib. = *Polygonum fagopyrum* L. [Polygonaceae].

Common Name(s): Buckwheat, japanese buckwheat, notch-seeded buckwheat [English]. Qiao mai {Chinese]. Blé noir sarrasin, bouquette, sarrasin commun [French]. Alforfón, grano sarraceno, grano turco, trigo sarraceno [Spanish]. Trigo mourisco, trigo negro, trigo sarraceno[Portuguese].

Life form: Herb. **Part(s) Used:** Aerial parts in bloom / Fresh.

Geographic distribution: North America. Temperate-Asia. Europe. Cultivated in several places.
Reference(s): Bharatan *et al.* 2002; Dorta Soares, n.d.; Gotfredsen, 2009; Tiwari *et al.* 2013.

Fagus

Scientific Name(s) / [Botanical Family]: *Fagus sylvatica* L. = *Fagus moesiaca* (K. Malý) Czeczott = *Fagus orientalis* Lipsky = *Fagus sylvatica* var. *moesiaca* K. Malý [Fagaceae].
Common Name(s): Beech, common beech, European beech [English]. Le hétre (le fayard) [French]. Fabeta, fabuco, fago, faya, haya [Spanish].
Life form: Tree. **Part(s) Used:** Fruit. **Geographic distribution:** Temperate-Asia. Europe.
Reference: Bharatan *et al.* 2002.

Ferula

Scientific Name(s) / [Botanical Family]: *Ferula communis* L. = *Ferula communis* L. subsp. *glauca* (L.) Rouy & E. G. Camus = *Ferula glauca* L. = *Ferula neapolitana* Ten. [Apiaceae, Umbelliferae].
Common Name(s): Giant anise fennel, giant fennel [English]. Ferula communis [Italian].
Life form: Herb. **Part(s) Used:** Root / Dried. **Geographic distribution:** Temperate-Asia. Europe.
Reference(s): Bharatan *et al.* 2002; Dorta Soares, n.d.

Filix

Scientific Name(s) / [Botanical Family]: *Dryopteris filix-mas* (L.) Schott = *Aspidium filix-mas* (L.) Sw. = *Polypodium filix-mas* L. [Dryopteridaceae, Polypodiaceae].
Common Name(s): Aspidium, basket fern, male fern, marginal shield-fern [English]. Fougère mâle. Fougère mâle du chêne

[French]. Samambaia [Portuguese]. Helecho macho [Spanish]. Feto macho [Portuguese].
Life form: Herb. **Part(s) Used:** Rhizome / Fresh; complete plant / collected between july and september months. **Geographic distribution:** cultivated in several places, ornamental.
Reference(s): Allen, 2006-2010; Bharatan *et al.* 2002; Bolte *et al.* 1997; Dorta Soares, n.d.; Tiwari *et al.* 2013.

Foeniculum anethum

Scientific Name(s) / [Botanical Family]: *Foeniculum vulgare* Mill. = *Foeniculum dulce* Mill. = *Foeniculum capillaceum* Gilb. = *Foeniculum officinale* All.= *Anethum foeniculum* L. = *Anethum piperitum* Ucria. [Apiaceae, Umbelliferae].
Common Name(s): Bitter fennel, common fennel, fennel, French fennerl, sweet cumin, sweet fennel, wild fennel [English]. Anet, aneth, fenouil amer, fenouil [French]. Fenojo, hinojo, hinojo común [Spanish]. Erva douce, fiôlho, funcho-amargo [Portuguese].
Life form: Herb. **Part(s) Used:** Complete plant / Fresh. Mature fruits / Dried; seeds. **Geographic distribution:** cultivated & naturalized in several places.
Reference(s): Bharatan *et al.* 2002; Dorta Soares, n.d.; Gotfredsen, 2009.

Foenum-graecum

Scientific Name(s) / [Botanical Family]: *Trigonella foenum-graecum* L. = *Trigonella tibetana* (Alef.) Vassilcz. [Fabaceae, Leguminosae].
Common Name(s): Fenugreek, Greek hay, Greek-clover [English]. Fenugrec [French]. Alhova, alholva, alforva, fenogreco [Spanish]. Alforvas, feno greco [Portuguese].
Life form: Herb. **Part(s) Used:** Seeds / Dried. **Geographic distribution:** Temperate-Asia. East Europe. Cultivated &

naturalized in several places.
Reference(s): Bolte *et al.* 1997; Dorta Soares, n.d.; Fuentes, 1996; Plants for a future, 2009.

Fragaria

Scientific Name(s) / [Botanical Family]: *Fragaria vesca* L. [Rosaceae].

Common Name(s): Alpine strawberry, english strawberry, european strawberry, perpetual strawberry, steawberie, strawberry, wild european strawberry, wild strawberry, wild strawberry, wood strawberry, woods strawberry [English]. Frasier des bois, fraises des bois [French]. Frutilla silvestre, fraguera, fresa, fresa silvestre, fresal común, madroncillo, maibeta [Spanish]. Morango, morangeiro [Portuguese].

Life form: Herb. **Part(s) Used:** Mature fruits / Fresh. **Geographic distribution:** Africa. Temperate-Asia. East Europe. North America. Cultivated & naturalized in several places.

Reference(s): Bharatan *et al.* 2002; Dorta Soares, n.d.

Fraxinus

Scientific Name(s) / [Botanical Family]: *Fraxinus americana* L. = *Fraxinus alba* Marsh. [Oleaceae].

Common Name(s): American ash, American white ash, ash, cane ash, white ash [English]. Frêne blanc, frêne blanc d'amérique [French]. Fresno, fresno americano [Spanish]. Freixo blanco [Portuguese].

Life form: Tree. **Part(s) Used:** New bark / Fresh; leaves / Dried collected in bloom. **Geographic distribution:** North America (Canada, United States of America). Cultivated in several places.

Reference(s): Bharatan *et al.* 2002; Dorta Soares, n.d.; Tiwari *et al.* 2013.

Fraxinus excelsior

Scientific Name(s) / [Botanical Family]: *Fraxinus excelsior* L.

[Oleaceae].
Nombre(s) comun(es):Ash, black ash, European ash [English]. Frêne commun [French]. Fresno, fresno americano [Spanish]. Freixo blanco [Portuguese].
Life form: Tree. **Part(s) Used:** New bark / Fresh; equal parts of bark & leaves / Fresh. **Geographic distribution:** Temperate-Asia. Europe. Cultivated in several places.
Reference(s): Bharatan *et al.* 2002; Dorta Soares, n.d.

Fumaria officinalis

Scientific Name(s) / [Botanical Family]: *Fumaria officinalis* L. [Fumariaceae, Papaveraceae].
Common Name(s): Common fumitory, drug fumitory, earth smoke, fumatory, wax-dolls [English]. Fumeterre officinal [French]. Camisitas del niño Jesús, conejitos, cuello de paloma, fumaria, fumoterra, gitanillas, palomilla, perejilera, zapaticos del Señor [Spanish]. Erva molarinha, fel da terra, fumaria [Portuguese].
Life form: Herb. **Part(s) Used:** Flower / Dried. **Geographic distribution:** Temperate-Asia, North Africa, Europe, naturalized in China, Nueva Zelandia, North America, South America.
Reference(s): Bharatan *et al.* 2002; Bolte *et al.* 1997; Dorta Soares, n.d.; Fuentes, 1996; Plants for a future, 2009.

Galega

Scientific Name(s) / [Botanical Family]: *Galega officinalis* L. = *Galega bicolor* Boiss. & Hausskn. ex Regel = *Galega patula* Steven. = *Galega vulgaris* Bauh. [Fabaceae, Leguminosae].
Common Name(s): French lilac / galega, galega officinalis, goat's rue, goats rue, goat's-rue, Italian fitch, professor-weed [English]. Galega officinal, rue de chèvre [French]. Galega officinalis, ruda

cabruna [Spanish]. Falso anil, galega [Portuguese].
Life form: Herb. **Part(s) Used:** Flowers; complete plant / Dried.
Geographic distribution: Africa, Asia-temperate, Europe. Cultivated & naturalized in several places.
Reference(s): Bharatan *et al.* 2002; Dorta Soares, n.d.; Tiwari *et al.* 2013.

Galium aparine

Scientific Name(s) / [Botanical Family]: *Galium aparine* L. = *Galium vaillanti* DC. = *Galium spurium* var. *vaillanti* (DC.) G. Beck [Rubiaceae].
Common Name(s): Bedstraw, catchweed bedstraw, cleavers, goose grass, goosebill, everlasting friendship, scarthgrass [English]. Gaillet gratteron [French]. Amigo de caminantes, amor de hortelano, cadillo, galio de flor blanca, pasto del ganso [Spanish]. Amor de hortelão, erva de pato, pega pega [Portuguese].
Life form: Herb. **Part(s) Used:** Complete plant in bloom / Fresh.
Geographic distribution: North America. England. This specie are considered wickedness around the world.
Reference(s): Bharatan *et al.* 2002; Bolte *et al.* 1997; Dorta Soares, n.d.; Gotfredsen, 2009.

Galium odoratum

Scientific Name(s) / [Botanical Family]: *Galium odoratum* (L.) Scopoli. = *Asperula odorata* L. [Rubiaceae].
Common Name(s): Hay plant, sweet woodruff, sweetscented bedstraw, wild baby's breath, woodruff-asperule [English]. Asperule odorant, gaillet odorant, petit muguet des bois [French]. Asperilla olorosa, aspérula olorosa, bregandia, hepática estrellada, rubilla, yerba estrellada [Spanish]. Aspérula, farinha dos bosques [Portuguese].
Life form: Herb. **Part(s) Used:** Complete plant. **Geographic**

distribution: Temperate-Asia. Siberia. North & Central Europe. North Africa. North America introduced. Cultivated & naturalized in several regions.
Reference(s): Bharatan *et al.* 2002; Boericke, 1927, 1927b.; Bolte *et al.* 1997; Clarke, 2008; Plants for a future, 2009.

Galium verum

Scientific Name(s) / [Botanical Family]: *Galium verum* L. = *Galium glabratum* Klok [Rubiaceae].
Common Name(s): Cheese-rennet, cheese-running, lady's bedstraw, yellow spring bedstraw [English]. Gaillet jaune, gaillet vrai [French]. Cuajaleche, galio, hierba sanjuanera, presera, Sanjuanera [Spanish]. Gálio-amareli, gálio-verdadeiro [Portuguese].
Life form: Herb. **Part(s) Used:** Complete plant / Fresh; leaves collected before bloom / Dried. **Geographic distribution:** North Africa. Europe. Temperate-Asia. North America. Naturalized in several places.
Reference(s): Bolte *et al.* 1997; Bharatan *et al.* 2002; Dorta Soares, n.d.; Gotfredsen, 2009; Plants for a future, 2009.

Ganoderma lucidum

Scientific Name(s) / [Botanical Family]: *Polyporus lucidus* (Curtis = Fr.) Fr. = *Ganoderma lucidum* (Curtis = Fr.) P. Karst. = *Fomes lucidus* (Curtis) Fr. [Coriolaceae, Polyporaceae].
Common Name(s): Varnished conk [English]. Ling shi [Chinese].
Life form: Fungi. **Part(s) Used:** Complete mushroom / Dried.
Geographic distribution: Cosmopolitan.
Reference: Gotfredsen, 2009.

Gaultheria

Scientific Name(s) / [Botanical Family]: *Gaultheria procumbens* L. = *Gaultheria humilis* Salisb. = *Gaultheria repens* Raf. nom. illeg.

[Ericaceae].

Common Name(s): Chá da montanha [Portuguese]. Gaulteria, té del Canadá [Spanish]. Aromatic wintergreen, Canada tea, checkerberry, creeping wintergreen, mountain-tea, teaberry, wintergreen [English]. Gaultherie, petit thé des bois [French].

Life form: Shrub. **Part(s) Used:** Leaves / Dried. **Geographic distribution:** North America (Canada. North East, Central North, South, United States of America).

Reference(s): Bharatan *et al.* 2002; Dorta Soares, n.d.; Tiwari *et al.* 2013.

Gelsemium

Scientific Name(s) / [Botanical Family]: *Gelsemium sempervirens* (L.) Ait. f. = *Gelsemium sempervirens* (L.) J. St.-Hill = *Bignonia sempervirens* L. [Loganiaceae, Gelsemiaceae].

Common Name(s): Gelsemio, jazmín amarillo, jazmín de Carolina, jazmín silvestre, raíz de Gelsemio [Spanish]. Carolina-jasmine, false jessamine, false jasmine, gelsemium, woodbine, wild yellow jasmine [English]. Gelsémine [French]. Jasmim amarelo, jasmim da Carolina, jasmim do campo [Portuguese].

Life form: Shrub. **Part(s) Used:** Root / Fresh; leaves / Dried collected in bloom.

Geographic distribution: North America (Southeast & South Central United States of America), Mexico. Central America.

Reference(s): Bharatan *et al.* 2002; Dorta Soares, n.d.; Remedia/at, 2010; Tiwari *et al.* 2013.

Genista tinctoria

Scientific Name(s) / [Botanical Family]: *Genista tinctoria* L. = *Genista anxantica* Griseb. = *Genista multibracteata* Tausch = *Genista ovata* Waldst. & Kit. = *Genista patula* M. Bieb. [Fabaceae, Leguminosae].

Common Name(s): Dyer's broom, dyer's greenweed,

greenwood, woad, wood-waxen, whin [English]. Genêt des teinturiers [French]. Flor de teñir, genestra, hiniesta, retama de tinte [Spanish].
Life form: Shrub. **Part(s) Used:** Complete plant / Fresh.
Geographic distribution: Europe. West Asia. Cultivated in United States of America.
Reference(s): Bharatan *et al.* 2002; Bolte *et al.* 1997; Dorta Soares, n.d.; Plants for a future, 2009; Tiwari *et al.* 2013; American Institute of Homeopathy, 1979.

Gentiana cruciata

Scientific Name(s) / [Botanical Family]: *Gentiana cruciata* L. [Gentianaceae].
Common Name(s): Cross-leaved gentian, cross gentian, crosswort [English]. Gentiane croisette [French]. Crujía, genciana de hojas en forma de cruz, genciana de verano, genciana menor [Spanish].
Life form: Herb. **Part(s) Used:** Root / Fresh. **Geographic distribution:** Temperate-Asia. Europe.
Reference(s): Bharatan *et al.* 2002; Comisión Editora de la Farmacopea Homeopática de los Estados Unidos Mexicanos, 1988; Dorta Soares, n.d.; Plants for a future, 2009; Tiwari *et al.* 2013.

Gentiana lutea

Scientific Name(s) / [Botanical Family]: *Gentiana lutea* L. = *Swertia lutea* Vest [Gentianaceae].
Common Name(s): Bitter root, bitterwort, gentian, Gentian, yellow gentian [English]. Gentiane, gentiane jaune. grande gentiane, grande gentiane [French]. Genciana, gengiba, genciana amarilla, junciana, quina de Europe, raíz de genciana, xaranzana [Spanish]. Genciana, Genciana amarela [Portuguese].
Life form: Herb. **Part(s) Used:** Root / Fresh. **Geographic**

distribution: Temperate-Asia. Europe (Alpes). Also cultivated.
Reference(s): Allen, 2006-2010; Bharatan *et al.* 2002; Bolte *et al.* 1997; Dorta Soares, n.d.; Tiwari *et al.* 2013; American Institute of Homeopathy, 1979.

Gentiana quinquefolia

Scientific Name(s) / [Botanical Family]: *Gentianella quinquefolia* (L.) Small. = *Gentiana quinquefolia* (L.) Small. = *Gentiana quinqueflora* (L.) emend Sm. [Gentianaceae].
Common Name(s): Ague weed, five flowered gentian, gall of the earth, stiff gentian [English].
Life form: Herb. **Part(s) Used:** Root. **Geographic distribution:** East North America (Canada [Ôntario], United States of America [Maine, Tennessee & Florida]).
Reference(s): Allen, 2006-2010; Bharatan *et al.* 2002; Bolte *et al.* 1997; Comisión Editora de la Farmacopea Homeopática de los Estados Unidos Mexicanos, 1988; Dorta Soares, n.d.; Gotfredsen, 2009; American Institute of Homeopathy, 1979.

Geranium

Scientific Name(s) / [Botanical Family]: *Geranium maculatum* L. [Geraniaceae].
Common Name(s): Alum bloom, spotted cranesbill, wild geranium [English]. Geranio, geranio silvestre, geranio manchado [Spanish]. Gerânio, pedra ume caá [Portuguese].
Life form: Herb. **Part(s) Used:** Rhizome / Fresh; Bulb, subterraneous parts / Fresh. **Geographic distribution:** North America (East Canada. North East, North, Central & Southeast United States of America).
Reference(s): Bolte *et al.* 1997; Bharatan *et al.* 2002; Dorta Soares, n.d.; Gotfredsen, 2009; Plants for a future, 2009; Tiwari *et al.* 2013.

Geranium robertianum

Scientific Name(s) / [Botanical Family]: *Geranium robertianum* L. [Geraniaceae].

Common Name(s): Herb Robert [English]. Géranium herbe à Robert [French]. Geranio, hierba de San Roberto [Spanish]. Bico de cegonha, bico de pombo, cicuta vermelha, erva Roberto [Portuguese].

Life form: Herb. **Part(s) Used:** Aerial part in recently bloom / Fresh. **Geographic distribution:** Europe (United Kingdom). Japan & Himalaya.

Reference(s): Bharatan *et al.* 2002; Comisión Editora de la Farmacopea Homeopática de los Estados Unidos Mexicanos, 1988; Dorta Soares, n.d.; Remedia/at, 2010.

Ginseng

Scientific Name(s) / [Botanical Family]: *Panax pseudoginseng* Wall. var. *elegantior* (Burkill) G. Hoo & C. J. Tseng = *Panax quinquefolius* L. = *Panax americanus* Raf. = *Aralia quinquefolia* (L.) Decne. & Planch.

Common Name(s): American-ginseng, ginseng, Chinese physic, elegant pseudoginseng, western ginseng, five–fingers garantogen, gensang, ninsin, red berry, shang [English]. Xi yang shen, xiu li jia ren shen [Chinese]. Ginseng d'America ique, racine de ginseng [French].

Life form: Herb. **Part(s) Used:** Root / Dried. **Geographic distribution:** North, Central & West United States of America. Cultivated in China.

Reference(s): Bharatan *et al.* 2002; Gotfredsen, 2009; Remedia/at, 2010; Plants for a future, 2009; Tiwari *et al.* 2013.

Gnaphalium

Scientific Name(s) / [Botanical Family]: *Gnaphalium polycephalum* Wall. ex DC. = *Gnaphalium polycephalum* Spreng.

ex DC. = *Gnaphalium polycephalum* Willd. ex Spreng. = *Gnaphalium polycephalum* Michx. [Asteraceae] = *Gnaphalium domingense* Lam. = *Pterocaulon cylindrostachyum* C. B. Clarke = *Helichrysum nudifolium* (L.) Less? [Asteraceae, Compositae].
Common Name(s): Cud weed-old balsa, everlasting, fragant everlasting, life everlasting, old field balsam [English]. Immortelle le cotonničre [French]. Gordolobo, siempreviva [Spanish]. Erva branca [Portuguese].
Life form: Herb. **Part(s) Used:** Complete plant / Fresh.
Geographic distribution: North America (Canada, United States of America).
Reference(s): Bharatan *et al.* 2002; Clarke, 2008; Dorta Soares, n.d.; Müntz, n.d.; Tiwari *et al.* 2013; American Institute of Homeopathy, 1979.

Gnaphalium arenarium

Scientific Name(s) / [Botanical Family]: *Helichrysum arenarium* (L.) Moench. = *Gnaphalium arenarium* L. [Asteraceae, Compositae].
Common Name(s): Everlasting flower, sandy everlasting, yellow chasteweed, yellow everlasting daisy [English].
Life form: Herb. **Part(s) Used:** Complete plant. **Geographic distribution:** Temperate-Asia. Europe.
Reference(s): Allen, 2006-2010; Bharatan *et al.* 2002; Boericke, 1927, 1927b.; Comisión Editora de la Farmacopea Homeopática de los Estados Unidos Mexicanos, 1988.

Gnaphalium polycephalum

Scientific Name(s) / [Botanical Family]: *Gnaphalium polycephalum* Michx. [Asteraceae, Compositae].
Common Name(s): Common everlasting, Indian posey, Indian tobacco [English]. Gnaphalie à plusieurs têtes [French].
Life form: Herb. **Part(s) Used:** Complete plant / Fresh.

Geographic distribution: North America (Canada, United States of America).
Reference(s): Bolte *et al.* 1997; Dorta Soares, n.d.; Plants for a future, 2009; Tiwari *et al.* 2013.

Granatum

Scientific Name(s) / [Botanical Family]: *Punica granatum* L. [Punicaceae, Lythraceae].
Common Name(s): Pomegranate [English]. Le Grenadier [French]. Granado dulce, granado, mangrano [Spanish]. Milgreira, româ, româzeiro [Portuguese].
Life form: Tree. **Part(s) Used:** Stem-bark, root-bark / Dried; bark with inmature fruits / Fresh. **Geographic distribution:** Temperate-Asia. Europe. Cultivated & naturalized in several places.
Reference(s): Bharatan *et al.* 2002; Dorta Soares, n.d.; Tiwari *et al.* 2013; American Institute of Homeopathy, 1979.

Gratiola officinalis

Scientific Name(s) / [Botanical Family]: *Gratiola officinalis* L. [Scrophulariaceae].
Common Name(s): Hedge hyssop [English]. Gratiolw officinale [French]. Hierba del pobre, graciola [Spanish]. Graça de Deus, graciola, graciosa [Portuguese].
Life form: Herb. **Part(s) Used:** Complete plant / Fresh. **Geographic distribution:** Europe. North America. Australia subtropical.
Reference(s): Allen, 2006-2010; Bharatan *et al.* 2002; Dorta Soares, n.d.; Fuentes, 1996; Tiwari *et al.* 2013.

Grindelia robusta

Scientific Name(s) / [Botanical Family]: *Grindelia robusta* Nutt. = *Grindelia bracteosa* J. T. Howell = *Grindelia camporum* Greene = *Grindelia camporum* var. *bracteosa* [Asteraceae, Compositae].
Common Name(s): Great valley gumweed, grindelia, gumweed,

wild sunflower [English]. Grindélia [French]. Grindelia [Spanish].
Life form: Herb, Shrub. **Part(s) Used:** Flower / Dried; Complete plant in bloom / Fresh. **Geographic distribution:** North America (East & Southwest United States of America, Mexico).
Reference(s): Bharatan *et al.* 2002; Comisión Editora de la Farmacopea Homeopática de los Estados Unidos Mexicanos, 1988; Dorta Soares, n.d.; Plants for a future, 2009; Tiwari *et al.* 2013.

Grindelia squarrosa

Scientific Name(s) / [Botanical Family]: *Grindelia squarrosa* (Pursh.) Dunal. [Asteraceae, Compositae].
Common Name(s): Grindelia [Spanish]. Gum plant, rosin weed, snake-headed grindelia [English]. Grindélia [French]. Malmequer do campo [Portuguese].
Life form: Herb. **Part(s) Used:** Flower / Dried. **Geographic distribution:** North America (United States of America).
Reference(s): Bharatan *et al.* 2002; Comisión Editora de la Farmacopea Homeopática de los Estados Unidos Mexicanos, 1988; Dorta Soares, n.d.; Plants for a future, 2009.

Gymnocladus canadensis

Scientific Name(s) / [Botanical Family]: *Gymnocladus dioica* (L.) K. Koch. = *Gymnocladus canadensis* Lam. = *Guilandina dioica* L. [Fabaceae, Leguminosae].
Common Name(s): American, coffe tree, chicot, Kentucky coffee tree, Kentucky mahogany [English]. Cafeeiro americano [Portuguese].
Life form: Tree. **Part(s) Used:** Fruit (pulp that surrounds the seeds) / Fresh; seeds / Fresh-Dried. **Geographic distribution:** North America (East & Central United States of America).
Reference(s): Bharatan *et al.* 2002; Dorta Soares, n.d.; Plants for a future, 2009; American Institute of Homeopathy, 1979.

Hamamelis

Scientific Name(s) / [Botanical Family]: *Hamamelis virginiana* L. = *Hamamelis androgyna* Walt = *Hamamelis caroliniana* Walt [Hamamelidaceae].

Common Name(s): Ameiro mosqueado, aveleira de bruxa, aveleira de feiticeira [Portuguese]. Witch-hazel [English]. Café du diable, hamémelis [French].

Life form: Tree. **Part(s) Used:** Flower / Fresh. **Geographic distribution:** North America (Canada, United States of America, Mexico). Extensively cultivated.

Reference(s): Dorta Soares, n.d.; Tiwari *et al.* 2013.

Helianthus

Scientific Name(s) / [Botanical Family]: *Helianthus annuus* L = *Helianthus aridus* Rydb. = *Helianthus lenticularis* Douglas ex Lindl. [Asteraceae, Compositae].

Common Name(s): Annual sunflower, common garden sunflower, common sunflower, girasol, sunflower, turnsole [English]. Grand soleil, helianthe, tournesol [French]. Girassol [Portuguese]. Acahual, andani, chimálatl, chimalitl, copa de Júpiter, Flor del sol, giganta, gigantón, lampote, girasol, maíz de Tejas, maíz de Texas, mirasol, rosa de Jericó, sol de las Indias [Spanish].

Life form: Herb. **Part(s) Used:** Flower / Fresh; mature seeds / Dried. **Geographic distribution:** North America. Extensively cultivated & naturalized.

Reference(s): Bharatan *et al.* 2002; Comisión Editora de la Farmacopea Homeopática de los Estados Unidos Mexicanos, 1988; Dorta Soares, n.d.; Tiwari *et al.* 2013.

Heliotropium

Scientific Name(s) / [Botanical Family]: *Heliotropium arborescens* L. = *Heliotropium peruvianum* L. [Boraginaceae].
Common Name(s): Cherry pie, heliotrope [English]. Heliotropo [Spanish].
Life form: Herb. **Part(s) Used:** Complete plant / Fresh.
Geographic distribution: America, cultivated.
Reference(s): Allen, 2006-2010; Bharatan *et al.* 2002; Comisión Editora de la Farmacopea Homeopática de los Estados Unidos Mexicanos, 1988.

Helleborus

Scientific Name(s) / [Botanical Family]: *Helleborus niger* L. = *Helleborus grandiflorus* Salisb. [Ranunculaceae].
Common Name(s): Black hellebore, christmas rose, snowrose [English]. Hellébore noir, la rose d'hiver [French]. Flower do Natal, rosa de Janeiro [Portuguese]. Eléboro negro, heléboro negro [Spanish].
Life form: Herb. **Part(s) Used:** Root / Fresh / Dried; leaf in bloom / Dried. **Geographic distribution:** Europe, North East United States of America, naturalized in several places.
Reference(s): Allen, 2006-2010; Bharatan *et al.* 2002; Bolte *et al.* 1997; Dorta Soares, n.d.; Plants for a future, 2009; Tiwari *et al.* 2013; American Institute of Homeopathy, 1979.

Helleborus foetidus

Scientific Name(s) / [Botanical Family]: *Helleborus foetidus* L. [Ranunculaceae].
Common Name(s): Bear's foot, setterwort, stinking hellebore [English]. Hellébore fétide [French]. Eléboro [Spanish]. Erva besteira, fava de lobo, heléboro fétido [Portuguese].
Life form: Herb. **Part(s) Used:** Root / Fresh / Dried; leaf collected in bloom / Dried.

Geographic distribution: Europe (North, Central, Southeast & Southwest). Introduced in United States of America.
Reference(s): Allen, 2006-2010; Bharatan *et al.* 2002; Comisión Editora de la Farmacopea Homeopática de los Estados Unidos Mexicanos, 1988; Dorta Soares, n.d.; Gotfredsen, 2009; Plants for a future, 2009; Remedia/at, 2010; American Institute of Homeopathy, 1979.

Helleborus orientalis

Scientific Name(s) / [Botanical Family]: *Helleborus orientalis* Lam. [Ranunculaceae].
Common Name(s): Hellebore, lenten-rose [English]. Heléboro [Spanish].
Life form: Herb. **Part(s) Used:** Root / Dried.
Geographic distribution: Temperate-Asia. Southeast Europe & Greece. Minor Asia. Naturalized in several countries and introduced in United States of America.
Reference(s): Bharatan *et al.* 2002; Bolte *et al.* 1997; Dorta Soares, n.d.; American Institute of Homeopathy, 1979.

Helleborus viridis

Scientific Name(s) / [Botanical Family]: *Helleborus viridis* L. [Ranunculaceae].
Common Name(s): Green hellebore, grione, niesswurz [English]. Ellébore vert, hellébore verte [French]. Eléboro, eléboro verde [Spanish]. Heléboro verde [Portuguese].
Life form: Herb. **Part(s) Used:** Root, rhizome / Dried; Buds youngs. **Geographic distribution:** Europe, and introduced in United States of America.
Reference(s): Allen, 2006-2010; Bharatan *et al.* 2002; Bolte *et al.* 1997; Clarke, 2008; Dorta Soares, n.d.

Helonias dioica

Scientific Name(s) / [Botanical Family]: *Helonias dioica* (Walter) Pursh = *Chamaelirium luteum* (L.) A. Gray = *Melanthium dioicum* Walter [Melanthiaceae, Chionographidaceae, Liliaceae].

Common Name(s): Blazing-star, devil's-bit, fairy-wand, false unicorn, false unicorn-root, helonias [English]. Etoile de feu [French].

Life form: Herb. **Part(s) Used:** Root / Fresh. **Geographic distribution:** North America (East Canada. North East, North, Central & Southeast United States of America).

Reference(s): Allen, 2006-2010; Bharatan *et al.* 2002; Bolte *et al.* 1997; Dorta Soares, n.d.; Remedia/at, 2010; Tiwari *et al.* 2013.

Hepatica

Scientific Name(s) / [Botanical Family]: *Hepatica triloba* Gilib. = *Hepatica triloba* var. *acuta* Pursh = *Hepatica triloba* var. *acutiloba* (DC.) R. Warner = *Hepatica nobilis* Schreber = *Anemone hepatica* L. [Ranunculaceae].

Common Name(s): American liver-wort, hepatica, kidneywort, liver leaf [English]. Hépatique à trois lobes, hépatique [French]. Hepática [Spanish].

Life form: Herb. **Part(s) Used:** Leaf / Fresh. **Geographic distribution:** North America (East United States of America).

Reference(s): Comisión Editora de la Farmacopea Homeopática de los Estados Unidos Mexicanos, 1988; Tiwari *et al.* 2013.

Heracleum see *Branca ursina*

Hoitzia coccinea

Scientific Name(s) / [Botanical Family]: *Loeselia coccinea* (Cav.) G. Don. = *Loeselia mexicana* (Lam.) Brand. = *Hoitzia coccinea* Cav. = *Hoitzia mexicana* Lam. [Polemoniaceae].

Common Name(s): Cuachile, chuparosa, espinosilla, Flor del

chupamirto [Spanish]. Mexican false-calico [English].
Life form: Herb. **Part(s) Used:** Complete plant / Fresh.
Geographic distribution: North America (Mexico).
Reference(s): Farias, 2001; Tiwari *et al.* 2013.

Hoya carnosa

Scientific Name(s) / [Botanical Family]: *Hoya carnosa* (L. f.) R. Br. = *Asclepias carnosa* L. f. [Asclepiadaceae].
Common Name(s): Honeyplant, porcelain flower, waxplant [English]. Flor de cera, Flor de nácar, cerilla [Spanish].
Life form: Liana. **Part(s) Used:** Flower?. **Geographic distribution:** Temperate & tropical Asia. Cultivated.
Reference(s): Bharatan *et al.* 2002; Comisión Editora de la Farmacopea Homeopática de los Estados Unidos Mexicanos, 1988; De Legarreta, 1961; Müntz, n.d.; American Institute of Homeopathy, 1979.

Humulus lupulus

Scientific Name(s) / [Botanical Family]: *Humulus lupulus* L. [Cannabaceae, Urticaceae].
Common Name(s): Bine, European hop, hop [English]. Pi-jiu-hua [Chinese]. Houblon [French]. Lúparo, vinho-do-North [Portuguese]. Lúpulino, lúpulo [Spanish].
Life form: Shrub. **Part(s) Used:** Complete plant / Fresh.
Geographic distribution: Extensively cultivated & naturalized.
Reference(s): Bharatan *et al.* 2002; Bolte *et al.* 1997; Dorta Soares, n.d.; Müntz, n.d.; Seror, 2000.

Hydrangea

Scientific Name(s) / [Botanical Family]: *Hydrangea arborescens* L. = *Hydrangea cinerea* Small. = *Hydrangea radiata* Walter = *Viburnum alnifolium* Marshall = *Viburnum americanum* Mill. [Hydrangeaceae, Saxifragaceae].

Common Name(s): Annabelle, seven bark, smooth hydrangea, tree hydrangea, wild hydrangea [English]. Hortensia de Virginie [French]. Hortensia [Spanish]. Sete casas [Portuguese].
Life form: Shrub. **Part(s) Used:** Subterraneous parts / Fresh; leaf & branches before bloom / Fresh / Dried. **Geographic distribution:** North America (United States of America).
Reference(s): Bharatan *et al.* 2002; Comisión Editora de la Farmacopea Homeopática de los Estados Unidos Mexicanos, 1988; Dorta Soares, n.d.; Tiwari *et al.* 2013.

Hydrastis

Scientific Name(s) / [Botanical Family]: *Hydrastis canadensis* L. [Ranunculaceae].
Common Name(s): Golden seal, orange-root, yellow pucoon [English]. Fard inolien, hydrastis du Canada [French]. Hidrastis, raíz de oro, raíz amarilla, sello de oro [Spanish]. Cânhamo do Canada, Hisdraste do Canada, raiz amarela, selo de ouro [Portuguese].
Life form: Herb. **Part(s) Used:** Root / Fresh / Dried. Root collected in summer/ Fresh. **Geographic distribution:** North America (East Canada. North East, North, Central & Southeast United States of America).
Reference(s): Remedia/at, 2010; Bharatan *et al.* 2002; Dorta Soares, n.d.; Tiwari *et al.* 2013; American Institute of Homeopathy, 1979.

Hydrophyllum virginicum

Scientific Name(s) / [Botanical Family]: *Hydrophyllum virginianum* L. [Hydrophyllaceae].
Common Name(s): Burr flowers, waterleaf [English].
Life form: Herb. **Part(s) Used:** Complete plant / Fresh. Complete plant collected during bloom. **Geographic distribution:** North America (Canada, United States of America).

Reference(s): Allen, 2006-2010; Bharatan *et al.* 2002; Bolte *et al.* 1997; Comisión Editora de la Farmacopea Homeopática de los Estados Unidos Mexicanos, 1988; Dorta Soares, n.d.; American Institute of Homeopathy, 1979.

Hydropiper see *Polygonum hydropiperoides*

Hyoscyamus

Scientific Name(s) / [Botanical Family]: *Hyoscyamus niger* L = *Hyoscyamus vulgaris* Bubani = *Hyoscyamus vulgaris* Neck. = *Hyoscyamus lethalis* Salisb. [Solanaceae].
Common Name(s): Stinking roger, henbane, hog-bean, belene, hen-bell, poison tobaco [English]. Jusquiame noire [French]. Beleño, beleño negro [Spanish]. Erva louca, meimendro, meimendro negro [Portuguese].
Life form: Herb. **Part(s) Used:** Complete plant / Fresh. Complete plant in bloom / Fresh. **Geographic distribution:** Western Asia & Himalaya. America. Europe.
Reference(s): Bharatan *et al.* 2002; Dorta Soares, n.d.; Tiwari *et al.* 2013; American Institute of Homeopathy, 1979.

Hypericum

Scientific Name(s) / [Botanical Family]: *Hypericum perforatum* L. = *Hypericum nachitschevanicum* Grossh = *Hypericum vulgare* Lam. [Hypericaceae, Clusiaceae].
Common Name(s): Goatweed, klamathweed, perforate St. John's-wort, racecourseweed, St. John's-wort, tiptonweed [English]. Mille-pertuis [French]. Hipericón [Spanish]. Guan ye lian qiao [Chinese].
Life form: Herb. **Part(s) Used:** Complete plant, flower / Fresh. **Geographic distribution:** Europe. North Africa. West Asia. Cultivated & naturalized in several world parts.
Reference(s): Allen, 2006-2010; Bharatan *et al.* 2002; Bolte *et al.* 1997; Dorta Soares, n.d.; Tiwari *et al.* 2013.

Hyssopus officinalis

Scientific Name(s) / [Botanical Family]: *Hyssopus officinalis* L. [Lamiaceae, Labiatae].
Common Name(s): Hyssop [English]. Hysope officinale [French]. Hissopo [Portuguese]. Hisopo [Spanish].
Life form: Herb. **Part(s) Used:** Aerial part in bloom / Fresh.
Geographic distribution: North Africa, Temperate-Asia. Europe.
Reference(s): Allen, 2006-2010; Bharatan *et al.* 2002; Comisión Editora de la Farmacopea Homeopática de los Estados Unidos Mexicanos, 1988; Dorta Soares, n.d.; Plants for a future, 2009; American Institute of Homeopathy, 1979.

Iberis amara

Scientific Name(s) / [Botanical Family]: *Iberis amara* L. [Brassicaceae, Cruciferae].
Common Name(s): Bitter candytuft, rocket candytuft, wild candytuft [English]. Iberis amer, thlaspi blanc [French]. Carraspique blanco, ibéride [Spanish].
Life form: Herb. **Part(s) Used:** seeds / Dried. **Geographic distribution:** South Europe-Siberia, England.
Reference(s): Bharatan *et al.* 2002; Müntz, n.d.; Tiwari *et al.* 2013.

Ictodes foetida

Scientific Name(s) / [Botanical Family]: *Symplocarpus foetidus* (L.) W. Salisb. Ex Nutt. = *Draconitum foetidum* L. = *Pothos foetidus* (L.) Michx. = *Ictodes foetidus* Bigelow [Araceae].
Common Name(s): Skunk cabbage [English]. Pothos fétide [French]. Dragoncillo fétido [Spanish].
Life form: Herb. **Part(s) Used:** Root, Complete plant / Fresh.
Geographic distribution: North America (East United States of

America).
Reference(s): Bharatan *et al.* 2002; Comisión Editora de la Farmacopea Homeopática de los Estados Unidos Mexicanos, 1988; Müntz, n.d.; Gofredsen, 2009; Plants for a future, 2009; Tiwari *et al.* 2013; American Institute of Homeopathy, 1979.

Ignatia

Scientific Name(s) / [Botanical Family]: *Ignatia amara* L. = *Strychnos ignatii* P. J. Bergius [Loganiaceae].
Common Name(s): Ignatius bean, St. Ignatius bean [English]. Fęves de Saint-Ignace [French]. Haba de San Ignacio [Spanish].
Life form: Shrub. **Part(s) Used:** seeds / Dried. **Geographic distribution:** Temperate-Asia (China).
Reference(s): Bharatan *et al.* 2002; Comisión Editora de la Farmacopea Homeopática de los Estados Unidos Mexicanos, 1988; Remedia/at, 2010; Tiwari *et al.* 2013.

Ilex aquifolium

Scientific Name(s) / [Botanical Family]: *Ilex aquifolium* L. [Aquifoliaceae].
Common Name(s): English holly, European holly, Oregon holly [English]. Azevim, azevinho, pica-folha [Portuguese].
Life form: Herb. **Part(s) Used:** Leaf / Fresh / Dried. Leaves & fruits / Fresh. **Geographic distribution:** North Africa. Asia-temperate. Europe. Naturalized Australasia & United States of America.
Reference(s): Bolte *et al.* 1997; Bharatan *et al.* 2002; Dorta Soares, n.d.; Tiwari *et al.* 2013; American Institute of Homeopathy, 1979.

Illicium anisatum

Scientific Name(s) / [Botanical Family]: *Illicium anisatum* L. [Illiciaceae, Magnoliaceae].

Common Name(s): Sacred anise tree, star anise, star anise [English]. Anise étoilé [French]. Anís estrella, badiana [Spanish].
Life form: Shrub, Tree. **Part(s) Used:** seeds / Dried. **Geographic distribution:** China, Japan.
Reference(s): Bharatan *et al.* 2002; Comisión Editora de la Farmacopea Homeopática de los Estados Unidos Mexicanos, 1988; Fuentes, 1996; Plants for a future, 2009; Remedia/at, 2010; Tiwari *et al.* 2013; American Institute of Homeopathy, 1979.

Illicium verum see *Illicium anisatum*

Imperatoria
Scientific Name(s) / [Botanical Family]: *Peucedanum ostruthium* (L.) W. D. J. Koch = *Peucedanum officinale* L. = *Imperatoria ostruthium* L. = *Imperatoria major* Gray [Apiaceae, Umbelliferae].
Common Name(s): Hog's fennel, masterwort [English]. Impératoire, peucédan officinal, benzoin Francais, Impératoire Peucédan ostruthium [French]. Imperatoria romana, servato [Spanish]. Imperatoria [Portuguese].
Life form: Herb. **Part(s) Used:** Root / Fresh / Dried. **Geographic distribution:** Central & South Europe.
Reference(s): Bharatan *et al.* 2002; Dorta Soares, n.d.

Inula helenium
Scientific Name(s) / [Botanical Family]: *Inula helenium* L. = *Aster helenium* (L.) Scop. = *Helenium grandiflorum* Giln. = *Corvisartia helenium* (L.) Mérat [Asteraceae, Compositae].
Common Name(s): Elecampane, scab wort. velvet-dock, yellow starwort [English]. Aunée commune, grande aunée, inule [French]. Énula campana, ínula campana, ínula [Portuguese]. Raíz del moro [Spanish].
Life form: Herb. **Part(s) Used:** Flower / Dried; Root / Fresh

collected in the autumn of the second year of growth of the plant. **Geographic distribution:** Asia. Europe. United States of America. Naturalized in several places.
Reference(s): Allen, 2006-2010; Bharatan *et al.* 2002; Clarke, 2008; Dorta Soares, n.d.; Gotfredsen, 2009; Plants for a future, 2009; Tiwari *et al.* 2013.

Ipomoea

Scientific Name(s) / [Botanical Family]: *Ipomoea purpurea* (L.) Roth = *Ipomoea diversifolia* Lindl. = *Ipomoea hirsuta* J. Jacq. = *Ipomoea mexicana* A. Gray = *Pharbitis purpurea* (L.) Voigt = *Convolvulus purpureus* L. [Convolvulaceae].
Common Name(s): Common morning-glory, purperwinde, tall morning-glory [English]. Aurora, campanilla, manto de la vírgen, mecapatli, metlancasis, quiebra plato, chail, yerba morada [Spanish].
Life form: Herb. **Part(s) Used:** Root / Fresh. **Geographic distribution:** America. China. Africa. Pantropical (the species spreads over an area around the tropical zone of the planet).
Reference(s): Bharatan *et al.* 2002; Boericke, 1927, 1927b.; American Institute of Homeopathy, 1979.

Ipomoea stans

Scientific Name(s) / [Botanical Family]: *Ipomoea stans* Cav. = *Calystegia spithamaea* (L.) Pursh. subsp. *stans* (Michx.) Brummitt = *Convolulus firmus* Spreng. = *Convolulus stans* H.B.K. [Convolvulaceae].
Common Name(s): Cacastlapa, espanta lobos, espanta vaqueros, limpia tunas, pegajosa, tanibata, tlaxcapan, tumba vaqueros [Spanish].
Life form: Herb. **Part(s) Used:** Root / Fresh; bark / Dried.
Geographic distribution: North & Central Mexico.
Reference(s): Bharatan *et al.* 2002; Dorta Soares, n.d.; Müntz,

n.d.

Iris

Scientific Name(s) / [Botanical Family]: *Iris versicolor* L. = *Iris caurina* Herb. ex Hook. = *Iris flaccida* Spach = *Iris picta* Mill. = *Iris sativa* Mill. [Iridaceae].
Common Name(s): Blue flag, flag lily, liver lily [English]. Glad'eu bleu [French]. Lirio azul [Spanish-Portugués].
Life form: Herb. **Part(s) Used:** Root / Fresh; root fresh collected before bloom or at the summer, or spring initiation. **Geographic distribution:** Europe. North Africa. North India. United States of America.
Reference(s): Bharatan *et al.* 2002; Dorta Soares, n.d.; American Institute of Homeopathy, 1979.

Iris florentina

Scientific Name(s) / [Botanical Family]: *Iris florentina* L. = *Iris* x *germanica* L. nothovar. *florentina* Dykes = *Iris germanica* var. *florentina* Dykes [Iridaceae].
Common Name(s): Florentine iris, orris, orris-root [English]. Fleur de Lys, iris de Florence. [French]. Iris-florentino [Portuguese]. Lirio blanco, lirio de Florencia, omixóchitl [Spanish]. Lírio branco, lírio florentino [Portuguese].
Life form: Herb. **Part(s) Used:** Root / Fresh. **Geographic distribution:** Europe. Extensively cultivated.
Reference(s): Bharatan *et al.* 2002; Dorta Soares, n.d.; American Institute of Homeopathy, 1979.

Iris germanica

Scientific Name(s) / [Botanical Family]: *Iris germanica* L. [Iridaceae].
Common Name(s): Flag iris, flag lily. German iris [English]. Fleur de Lys [French].

Life form: Herb. **Part(s) Used:** Root / Fresh?. **Geographic distribution:** Europe, Russia. Extensively cultivated.
Reference(s): Allen, 2006-2010; Bharatan *et al.* 2002; Dorta Soares, n.d.; Tiwari *et al.* 2013.

Iris versicolor

Scientific Name(s) / [Botanical Family]: *Iris versicolor* L. [Iridaceae].
Common Name(s): Blue flag varied-color iris, liver lilym water flag [English]. Glad'eu bleu, Iris versicolore [French]. Lirio, lirio azul [Spanish] Lírio azul [Portuguese].
Life form: Herb. **Part(s) Used:** Root / Fresh or Dried collected before bloom or at the end summer, or spring initiation.
Geographic distribution: Europe. North Africa. North India. North America (United States of America).
Reference(s): Allen, 2006-2010; Bharatan *et al.* 2002; Dorta Soares, n.d.; Tiwari *et al.* 2013.

Jacaranda mimosifolia

Scientific Name(s) / [Botanical Family]: *Jacaranda mimosifolia* D. Don = *Jacaranda chelonia* Griseb. = *Jacaranda filicifolia* (D. Don sec.) ex Seem. = *Jacaranda ovalifolia* R. Br. [Bignoniaceae].
Common Name(s): Jacaranda [English]. Jacaranda [French, Spanish]. Carona-guassú, jacaranda-mimoso, jacaranda roxo [Portuguese].
Life form: Tree. **Part(s) Used:** Flower. **Geographic distribution:** Cosmopolitan cultivated.
Reference(s): Bharatan *et al.* 2002; Müntz, n.d.

Jalapa

Scientific Name(s) / [Botanical Family]: *Ipomoea purga* (Wender) Hayne = *Ipomoea jalapa* Schiede & Deppe ex G. Don = *Convolvulus purga* Wender = *Convolvulus jalapa* L. = *Convolvulus officinalis* Pelletan ex Steud. = *Exogonium purga* (Wender) Benth. [Convolvulaceae].

Common Name(s): Jalap, Jalap root [English]. Jalap [French]. Jalapa [Portuguese]. Jalapa, Jalapa de Veracruz, jalapa hembra, jalapa limoncillo, limoncillo, mechoacán, purga, tolonpatl [Spanish]. Batata de pura, Jalapa, Jalapa verdadeira [Portuguese].

Life form: Herb. **Part(s) Used:** Tuber, root / Dried. **Geographic distribution:** North America (Mexico). Naturalized in various places of the neotropical region.

Reference(s): Bharatan *et al.* 2002; Dorta Soares, n.d.; Tiwari *et al.* 2013.

Jequirity see *Abrus precatorius*

Juglans cinerea

Scientific Name(s) / [Botanical Family]: *Juglans cinerea* L. = *Juglans cathartica* F. Michxaux = *Juglans oblonga* Miller [Juglandaceae].

Common Name(s): Butternut, lemon walnut, oil nut, oil nut bark, white walnut [English]. Noyer cerdré [French]. Nogal blanco americano, nogal ceniciento [Spanish].

Life form: Tree. **Part(s) Used:** Root-bark, inner bark branches / Fresh; bark & fruit mature / Dried. **Geographic distribution:** North America (Canada. East, North East, North, Central & Southeast United States of America).

Reference(s): Bharatan *et al.* 2002; Dorta Soares, n.d.; Tiwari *et al.* 2013; American Institute of Homeopathy, 1979.

Juglans nigra

Scientific Name(s) / [Botanical Family]: *Juglans nigra* L. [Juglandaceae].

Common Name(s): American black walnut, black walnut [English]. Noyer noir [French]. Nogueira-preta [Portuguese]. Nogal, nogal americano, nogal negro [Spanish].

Life form: Tree. **Part(s) Used:** Leaf, fruit / Fresh. **Geographic distribution:** North America (Canada, East, North East, North, Central & Southeast United States of America). Cultivated in Caucasus, Central Asia, Russia.

Reference(s): Allen, 2006-2010; Bolte *et al.* 1997; Müntz, n.d.; American Institute of Homeopathy, 1979.

Juglans regia

Scientific Name(s) / [Botanical Family]: *Juglans regia* L. = *Juglans duclouxiana* Dode = *Juglans fallax* Dode = *Juglans orientis* Dode = *Juglans kamaonia* (C. DC.) Dode = *Juglans sinensis* (C. DC.) Dode = *Juglans regians* var. *sinensis* (C. DC.) Dode = *Nux juglans* Tourn. [Juglandaceae].

Common Name(s): Common walnut, english walnut, Greek nut, European walnut, nut tree, walnut [English]. Noix royale, noix commune, noyer [French]. Hojas de nogal, nogal, nogal común, nogal europeo, nogal inglés, nuez de Castilla, quaucacaotl [Spanish]. Nogueira [Portuguese].

Life form: Tree. **Part(s) Used:** Leaf, Fruit / Fresh; equal parts of fruit-bark and leaves / Fresh; leaves & green fruits. **Geographic distribution:** Temperate-Asia. Europe, Iran. Mexico. Cultivated.

Reference(s): Bharatan *et al.* 2002; Dorta Soares, n.d.; Hutchens, 1991; Tiwari *et al.* 2013.

Juncus effusus

Scientific Name(s) / [Botanical Family]: *Juncus effusus* L. [Juncaceae].

Common Name(s): Bulrush, common rush, soft rush [English]. Jonc commune [French]. Junco [Portuguese]. Junquera [Spanish]. Junco, junco de asvieira, junco manso [Portuguese].
Life form: Herb. **Part(s) Used:** Root, rhizome / Fresh; rhizome collected in spring / Fresh. **Geographic distribution:** Arctic & temperate zones of the world. Cosmopolitan.
Reference(s): Allen, 2006-2010; Bharatan *et al.* 2002; Bolte *et al.* 1997; Dorta Soares, n.d.; Tiwari *et al.* 2013; American Institute of Homeopathy, 1979.

Juniperus communis

Scientific Name(s) / [Botanical Family]: *Juniperus communis* L. = *Juniperus depressa* (Pursh) Raf. [= *Juniperus communis* var. *depressa*] = *Juniperus hemisphaerica* C. Presl [= *Juniperus communis* var. *communis*] = *Juniperus nipponica* Maxim. [= *Juniperus communis* var. *nipponica*] = *Juniperus oblonga* M. Bieb. [= *Juniperus communis* var. *saxatilis*] = *Juniperus sibirica* Burgsd. [= *Juniperus communis* var. *saxatilis*] = *Juniperus suecica* Mill. [=*Juniperus communis* var. *communis*] [Cupressaceae].
Common Name(s): Common juniper, dwarf juniper, juniper, malchangel, mountain juniper, prostrate juniper [English]. Genévrier, geničvre commun [French]. Ginepro [Italian]. Zimbreiro [Portuguese]. Enebro [Spanish]. Zimbreiro [Portuguese]. Xien bei ci bai [Chinese].
Life form: Shrub, Tree. **Part(s) Used:** Fruit / Fresh. **Geographic distribution:** North Africa (Morocco). Temperate-Asia. Europe. North America (Canada, United States of America). Cultivated.
Reference(s): Bharatan *et al.* 2002; Dorta Soares, n.d.; Tiwari *et al.* 2013; American Institute of Homeopathy, 1979.

Juniperus oxycedrus

Scientific Name(s) / [Botanical Family]: *Juniperus oxycedrus* L. [Cupressaceae].

Common Name(s): Cade juniper, prickly cedar, prickly juniper, red-berry juniper [English]. Genévrier cade, genévrier epineux, oxycèdre [French]. Enebro de bayas rojas [Spanish].
Life form: Shrub, tree. **Part(s) Used:** wood oil / Fresh.
Geographic distribution: North Africa. Temperate-Asia. South Europe.
Reference(s): Bharatan *et al.* 2002; Boericke, 1927, 1927b.; Clarke, 2008; Müntz, n.d.

Juniperus sabina

Scientific Name(s) / [Botanical Family]: *Juniperus sabina* (L.) Endl. = *Juniperus chinensis* var. *arenaria* E. H. Wilson = *Juniperus lycia* L. = *Juniperus prostrata* Pers. = *Sabina officinalis* Garcke. [Cupressaceae].
Common Name(s): Sabina, sabino [Spanish]. Juniper, sabina, savin, savin juniper [English]. Cha zi yuan bai [Chinese]. Sabine [French]. Sabina, zimbro [Portuguese].
Life form: Shrub, tree. **Part(s) Used:** Leaf, branch / Fresh; Leaves & inflorescences / Fresh; Leaves & fruits. **Geographic distribution:** North America. North Africa. Temperate-Asia. Europe. Russia.
Reference(s): Bharatan *et al.* 2002; Dorta Soares, n.d.; Müntz, n.d.; Remedia/at, 2010.

Juniperus virginiana

Scientific Name(s) / [Botanical Family]: *Juniperus virginiana* (L.) Endl. = *Juniperus foetida* var. *virginiana* (L.) Spach [Cupressaceae].
Common Name(s): Eastern red cedar, juniper, pencil-cedar, redjuniper, savin [English]. Cčdre de Virginie, genévrier de Virginie [French]. Enebro [Spanish]. Cedro da Virginia, cedro vermelho [Portuguese].
Life form: Tree. **Part(s) Used:** Leaf, stem / Fresh; Fruits / Fresh;

Buds / Fresh; Oil. **Geographic distribution:** North America (East Canada. North Central, Southeast & South Central United States of America).

Reference(s): Bharatan *et al.* 2002; Dorta Soares, n.d.; Guermonprez *et al.* 1989; Müntz, n.d.

Justicia adhatoda

Scientific Name(s) / [Botanical Family]: *Justicia adhatoda* L. = *Adhatoda adhatoda* (L.) Huth = *Adhatoda pubescens* Moench. = *Adhatoda vasica* Nees = *Adhatoda zeylanica* Medik.= *Dianthera latifolia* Salisb.= *Gendarussa adhatoda* Steud. [Acanthaceae].

Common Name(s): Malabar-nut, Malabar-nut-tree, pavettia, vasaka, Adotodai [English]. Noiz de Malabar, noyer des Indes [French]. Nuez de Malabar [Spanish]. Nogueira da Índia [Portuguese]. Adulsa [Others].

Life form: Herb. **Part(s) Used:** Leaf / Fresh; bark fruit mature / Fresh. **Geographic distribution:** Temperate & tropical-Asia. Extensively cultivated in tropics.

Reference(s): Allen, 2006-2010; Bharatan *et al.* 2002; Comisión Editora de la Farmacopea Homeopática de los Estados Unidos Mexicanos, 1988; Dorta Soares, n.d.; Tiwari *et al.* 2013; American Institute of Homeopathy, 1979.

Kalmia latifolia

Scientific Name(s) / [Botanical Family]: *Kalmia latifolia* L. [Ericaceae].

Common Name(s): Calico-bush, mountain-laurel, spoonwood [English]. Kalmie [French]. Loureiro das montanhas [Portuguese].

Life form: Shrub, Tree. **Part(s) Used:** Leaf / Fresh; leaves collected during the bloom / Fresh. **Geographic distribution:**

North America (North & Southeast United States of America).
Reference(s): Bharatan *et al.* 2002; Dorta Soares, n.d.; Müntz, n.d.; Tiwari *et al.* 2013.

Karwinskia humboldtiana
Scientific Name(s) / [Botanical Family]: *Karwinskia humboldtiana* (Roem. & Schult.) Zucc. = *Rhamnus humboldtiana* Roem. & Schult. [Rhamnaceae].
Common Name(s): Crippler [English]. Cachila, cacachila, cacachila china, capulín, capulín cimarrón, capulín de zorra, capulincillo, carbullo, cholchonote, coyotillo, diente de molino, frutillo, itzil, himoli, jimoli, margarita, negrito, palo negrito, piojillo, tullidor, tullidora, yagalán [Spanish].
Life form: Shrub. **Part(s) Used:** Pounded seeds / Dried.
Geographic distribution: North America (South Central United States of America & Mexico).
Reference(s): Bharatan *et al.* 2002; Dorta Soares, n.d.; Müntz, n.d.; American Institute of Homeopathy, 1979.

Laburnum anagyroides
Scientific Name(s) / [Botanical Family]: *Cytisus laburnum* L. = *Laburnum anagyroides* Medik. = *Laburnum laburnum* (L.) Dorfler [Fabaceae, Leguminosae].
Common Name(s): Golden-chain, golden-chaintree, peatree [English]. Fa ux-ébénier [French]. Chuva de ouro, codeço bastardo [Portuguese].
Life form: Shrub, tree. **Part(s) Used:** Flowers & leaves in equal parts / Fresh. **Geographic distribution:** Europe (Central, Southeast & Southwest). Cultivated in United States of America & Central Europe.

Reference(s): Bharatan *et al.* 2002; Dorta Soares, n.d.; American Institute of Homeopathy, 1979.

Lachnanthes tinctoria

Scientific Name(s) / [Botanical Family]: *Lachnanthes caroliniana* (Lam.) Dandy = *Lachnanthes carolina* (Lam.) Dandy = *Lachnanthes tinctoria* (Walter ex J. F. Gmel.) Elliott [Haemodoraceae].
Common Name(s): Carolina red root [English]. Racine rouge [French]. Lachnante [Spanish]. Erva espiritual [Portuguese].
Life form: Herb. **Part(s) Used:** Complete plant / Fresh.
Geographic distribution: North America (East Canada. North East & Southeast United States of America).
Reference(s): Bharatan *et al.* 2002; Dorta Soares, n.d.; Müntz, n.d.; Tiwari *et al.* 2013; American Institute of Homeopathy, 1979.

Lactuca

Scientific Name(s) / [Botanical Family]: *Lactuca sativa* L. = *Lactuca scariola* var. *sativa* Moris [Asteraceae, Compositae].
Common Name(s): Garden lettuce, head lettuce, lettuce [English]. Laitue cultivée, salade [French]. Lechuga [Spanish]. Alface [Portuguese].
Life form: Herb. **Part(s) Used:** Complete plant / Fresh.
Geographic distribution: Extensively cultivated.
Reference(s): Bharatan *et al.* 2002; Dorta Soares, n.d.; Gotfredsen, 2009; Müntz, n.d.; Plants for a future, 2009; Tiwari *et al.* 2013; American Institute of Homeopathy, 1979.

Lactuca virosa

Scientific Name(s) / [Botanical Family]: *Lactuca virosa* L. = *Lactuca serriola* L = *Lactuca sinuata* Forssk. [Asteraceae, Compositae].

Common Name(s): Poisonous lettuce, prickly letucce, wild lettuce [English]. Laitue vireuse [French]. Alface brava, lactucário alemâo [Portuguese].
Life form: Herb. **Part(s) Used:** Complete plant / Fresh. complete plant at begining of bloom. **Geographic distribution:** Asia, West & South Europe, Siberia. Naturalized in New England. North Africa (Morocco).
Reference(s): Allen, 2006-2010; Bharatan *et al.* 2002; Dorta Soares, n.d.

Lamium

Scientific Name(s) / [Botanical Family]: *Lamium album* L. = *Lamium archangelica* Garsault = *Lamium barbatum* Siebold & Zucc. = *Lamium brachyodon* (Bordz.) Kuprian. = *Lamium capitatum* Sm. in Rees = *Lamium dumeticola* Klok. = *Lamium niveum* Hort. ex Rchb. = *Lamium parietariaefolium* Benth. [Lamiaceae, Labiatae].
Common Name(s): Blind nettle, snowflake, white dead-nettle, white-nettle [English]. Ortie morte, lamier maculé, l'ortie blanche [French]. Ortiga maculata [Spanish]. Lamio branco, pé de gallina, urtiga branca [Portuguese].
Life form: Herb. **Part(s) Used:** Flower, leaf / Fresh. **Geographic distribution:** Temperate-Asia. Europe. Naturalized in several places from temperate regions.
Reference(s): Allen, 2006-2010; Bharatan *et al.* 2002; Dorta Soares, n.d.; Plants for a future, 2009; Tiwari *et al.* 2013; American Institute of Homeopathy, 1979.

Lamium laevigarum see *Lamium*

Lamium maculatum see *Lamium*

Lapathum acutum

Scientific Name(s) / [Botanical Family]: *Rumex obtusifolius* L. =

Rumex sylvestris Wallr. [Polygonaceae].

Common Name(s): Bitter dock, broad-leaf dock, broad-leaved dock [English]. Dun ye suan mo [Chinese]. Patience sauvage [French]. Labaca, língua-de-vaca-amarga, labaça-de-vaca-amarga [Portuguese)]. Acedera obtusifolia, consólida brava, romaza de leaves grandes, vinagrillo [Spanish].

Life form: Herb. **Part(s) Used:** Root / Fresh. **Geographic distribution:** North Africa. Temperate-Asia. Europe. Extensively naturalized in several places.

Reference: Bharatan *et al.* 2002.

Lappa major

Scientific Name(s) / [Botanical Family]: *Arctium lappa* L. = *Arctium majus* (Gaertn.) Bernh. = *Lappa major* Gaertn. = *Lappa arctium* Hill. [Asteraceae, Compositae].

Common Name(s): Burdock, edible burdock, great burdock, lappa [English]. Niu bang zi [Chinese]. Bardane comestible, glouteron, grande bardane [French]. Bardana-maior [Portuguese]. Bardana lampazo mayor, lapa [Spanish].

Life form: Herb. **Part(s) Used:** Root, seeds / Fresh. **Geographic distribution:** Europe. North Asia. Naturalized in United States of America.

Reference(s): Allen, 2006-2010; Bharatan *et al.* 2002; Müntz, n.d.; Remedia/at, 2010.

Lariciformes officinalis

Scientific Name(s) / [Botanical Family]: *Lariciformes officinalis* (Vill. = Fr.) Kotl. & Pouz. = *Fomitopsis officinalis* (Villars. = Fr.) Bondartsev & Singer = *Fomes laricis* Jacq. Fomes *officinalis* (Villars. = Fr.) Kotlaba = *Boletus laricis* Jacquin = *Polyporus officinalis* Vill. = *Boletus purgans* Pers. [Formitopsidaceae, Polyporaceae].

Common Name(s): Chinese agaricus, female agaric, larch agaric,

purging agaric, white agaric [English]. Polypore officinal [French]. Agárico blanco, agárico de alerce, agárico largo, hongo blanco [Spanish].
Life form: Fungi. **Part(s) Used:** Complete mushroom / Dried?.
Geographic distribution: North America (Canada-United States of America). Europe.
Reference(s): Bharatan *et al.* 2002; Fuentes, 1996; Tiwari *et al.* 2013; American Institute of Homeopathy, 1979.

Lathyrus

Scientific Name(s) / [Botanical Family]: *Lathyrus sativus* L. [Fabaceae, Leguminosae].
Common Name(s): Chickling-pea, chickling-vetch, dogtooth-pea, grass peavine, grass-pea, Indian-pea, khesari. Riga-pea, wedge-peavine [English]. Gesse commune, gesse cultivée, lentille d'Espagne, pois carré [French]. Almorta, alverja, chícharo, frijolillo, guija [Spanish]. Chícharo [Portuguese].
Life form: Herb. **Part(s) Used:** seeds / Dried. **Geographic distribution:** Extensively cultivated & naturalized in Europe, Temperate-Asia & North Africa.
Reference(s): Bharatan *et al.* 2002; Comisión Editora de la Farmacopea Homeopática de los Estados Unidos Mexicanos, 1988; Dorta Soares, n.d.; Müntz, n.d.; Tiwari *et al.* 2013.

Laurocerasus officinalis

Scientific Name(s) / [Botanical Family]: *Prunus laurocerasus* L. = *Padus laurocerasus* Mill. = *Laurocerasus officinalis* Middle Roem. [Rosaceae].
Common Name(s): Cherry laurel, English laurel [English]. Laurier-amande, Laurier-cerise [French]. Loureiro-cerejeira [Portuguese]. Laurel cerezo, lauroceraso [Spanish].
Life form: Shrub. **Part(s) Used:** Leaf / Fruit? **Geographic distribution:** Temperate-Asia South Europe. naturalized in

several regions in Tropical Asia, Australia, United States of America.

Reference(s): Bharatan *et al.* 2002; Dorta Soares, n.d.; Müntz, n.d.; Tiwari *et al.* 2013; American Institute of Homeopathy, 1979.

Laurus nobilis

Scientific Name(s) / [Botanical Family]: *Laurus nobilis* L. [Lauraceae].
Common Name(s): Laurel, laurel de poeta [Spanish]. Bay laurel, bay leaf, laurel [English]. Laurier, laurier sauce [French]. Loureiro, louro, sempre verde [Portuguese].
Life form: Tree. **Part(s) Used:** Leaf / Fresh. **Geographic distribution:** North Africa. Asia-temperate, Southwest Europe.
Reference(s): Bharatan *et al.* 2002; Dorta Soares, n.d.; American Institute of Homeopathy, 1979; Zandvoort, 2006.

Lavandula angustifolia

Scientific Name(s) / [Botanical Family]: *Lavandula angustifolia* Mill. = *Lavandula officinalis* Chaix ex Vill. = *Lavandula spica* L. = *Lavandula vera* DC. [Lamiaceae, Labiatae].
Common Name(s): Lavender, lavandula [English]. Lavande spic [French]. Lavanda [Spanish].
Life form: Herb. **Part(s) Used:** Flower / Fresh. **Geographic distribution:** Southeast & Southwest Europe. Naturalized in several regions in Europe & Africa.
Reference(s): Müntz, n.d.; Tiwari *et al.* 2013.

Leccinum testaceoscabrum

Scientific Name(s) / [Botanical Family]: *Leccinum testaceoscabrum* (Sécretan) Singer = *Leccinum versipelle* (Fr.& Hök) Snell [Boletaceae].
Common Name(s): Orange birch bolete, fries snell [English].

Life form: Fungi. **Part(s) Used:** Complete plant. **Geographic distribution:** North America. Europe.
Reference: Müntz, n.d.

Ledum palustre

Scientific Name(s) / [Botanical Family]: *Ledum palustre* L. = *Rhododendron tomentosum* Harmaja [Ericaceae].
Common Name(s): Crystal-tea, marsh-tea, wild rosemary [English]. Romarin sauvage [French]. Romero silvestre [Spanish]. Ledum [Portuguese].
Life form: Shrub. **Part(s) Used:** Complete plant / Fresh; Leaf during the bloom / Dried. **Geographic distribution:** North, Central & East Europe, Asia, Labrador peninsula to Alaska, Aleutianan Islands.
Reference: Bharatan *et al.* 2002; Dorta Soares, n.d.; Müntz, n.d.; Tiwari *et al.* 2013.

Lemna

Scientific Name(s) / [Botanical Family]: *Lemna minor* L. [Lemnaceae].
Common Name(s): Common duckweed, duckmeat, duckweed [English]. Petite lentille d'eau, lentille d'eau [French]. Lenticchia d'acqua comune [Italian]. Chichicastle, lentejas de agua, lentejilla de agua [Spanish].
Life form: Herb. **Part(s) Used:** Complete plant / Fresh. **Geographic distribution:** naturalized in several places.
Reference(s): Bharatan *et al.* 2002; Dorta Soares, n.d.; Müntz, n.d.; Plants for a future, 2009; Remedia/at; Tiwari *et al.* 2013; American Institute of Homeopathy, 1979.

Lentinula edodes

Scientific Name(s) / [Botanical Family]: *Lentinula edodes* (Berk.) Pegler & Hiratake = *Agaricus edodes* Berk. & 10 scientific

synonyms more [Marasmiaceae].
Common Name(s): Golden oaks, Japanese forest mushroom, oak mushroom, shiitake [English]. Dong gu, dong xun [Chinese].
Life form: Fungi. **Part(s) Used:** Complete. **Geographic distribution:** East Asia (China, Japan) - Oceania.
Reference(s): Bharatan *et al.* 2002; Müntz, n.d.; Plants for a future, 2009.

Lentinus edodes see *Lentinula edodes*

Leontopodium alpinum
Scientific Name(s) / [Botanical Family]: *Gnaphalium leontopodium* L. = *Leontopodium alpinum* Cass. [Asteraceae, Compositae].
Common Name(s): Austrian flower, common edelweiss, edelweiss, flower of Salzburg and Tyrol, stella alpina [English]. Edelweiss des Alpes, étoile des Alpes [French]. Flor de nieve, leontopodio [Spanish].
Life form: Herb. **Part(s) Used:** Complete plant? / Fresh?.
Geographic distribution: Europe (Alpes).
Reference: Müntz, n.d.

Leonurus
Scientific Name(s) / [Botanical Family]: *Leonurus cardiaca* L [Lamiaceae, Labiatae].
Common Name(s): Motherwort [English]. Agripaume cardiaque, léonure [French]. Agripalma, marihuanilla [Spanish]. Agripalma, cauda de Leâom corado de frade [Portuguese].
Life form: Herb. **Part(s) Used:** Aerial part during the bloom / Fresh. **Geographic distribution:** Europe. Temperate-Asia. North America.
Reference(s): Gotfredsen, 2009; Dorta Soares, n.d.; Müntz, n.d.; Tiwari *et al.* 2013.

Leptandra virginica

Scientific Name(s) / [Botanical Family]: *Veronicastrum virginicum* (L.) Farw. = *Leptandra virginica* (L.) Nutt. [Complete plant ginaceae]. [Scrophulariaceae].

Common Name(s): Blackroot, bowman's-root, Culver's-root, tall speedwell. Racine de leptandra [French]. Raíz de Bowman, raíz de Culver, raíz negra [Spanish].

Life form: Herb. **Part(s) Used:** Root / Fresh. **Geographic distribution:** North America (East & West Canada. United States of America).

Reference(s): Bharatan *et al.* 2002; Müntz, n.d.; Plants for a future, 2009; Tiwari *et al.* 2013.

Lespedeza capitata

Scientific Name(s) / [Botanical Family]: *Lespedeza capitata* Michx. [Fabaceae, Leguminosae].

Common Name(s): Bushclover, round-head bush-clover [English].

Life form: Herb. **Part(s) Used:** Aerial part in bloom / Fresh; seeds / Dried. **Geographic distribution:** North America (Canada, United States of America).

Reference(s): Bharatan *et al.* 2002; Dorta Soares, n.d.; Tiwari *et al.* 2013; American Institute of Homeopathy, 1979.

Liatris

Scientific Name(s) / [Botanical Family]: *Liatris spicata* (L.) Willd. = *Serratula spicata* L. [Asteraceae, Compositae].

Common Name(s): Blazing-star, button snakewort, gayfeather, marsh blazing-star, prairie-pine [English]. Serrátula [Portuguese].

Life form: Herb. **Part(s) Used:** Subterraneous parts / Fresh.
Geographic distribution: North America (East Canada, United States of America).

Reference(s): Bharatan *et al.* 2002; Dorta Soares, n.d.; Müntz, n.d.

Lilium tigrinum

Scientific Name(s) / [Botanical Family]: *Lilium tigrinum* Ker Gawl. = *Lilium lancifolium* Thunb.
Common Name(s): Devil lily, easter lily, kentan, martagon, tiger lily [English]. Juan dan [Chinese]. Lis élégant [French]. Lirio del Japón, lirio de tigre [Spanish]. Lírio de tigre, lírio tigrino laços de ouro [Portuguese].
Life form: Herb. **Part(s) Used:** Complete plant / Fresh.
Geographic distribution: China & Japan. Cultivated & naturalized in temperate areas.
Reference(s): Bharatan *et al.* 2002; Dorta Soares, n.d.; Remedia/at, 2010; Tiwari *et al.* 2013.

Linaria vulgaris

Scientific Name(s) / [Botanical Family]: *Linaria vulgaris* Mill. = *Antirrhinum linaria* L. [Plantaginaceae]. [Scrophulariaceae, Veronicaceae].
Common Name(s): Butter-and-eggs, common toadflax, toadfax, wild snapdragon, yellow toadflax [English]. Linaire vulgaire [French]. Linho de sapo [Portuguese].
Life form: Herb. **Part(s) Used:** Complete plant / Fresh.
Geographic distribution: West Asia. Europe. Naturalized in America.
Reference(s): Bharatan *et al.* 2002; Dorta Soares, n.d.; Tiwari *et al.* 2013; American Institute of Homeopathy, 1979.

Linum catharticum

Scientific Name(s) / [Botanical Family]: *Linum catharticum* L. = *Cathartolinum catharticum* Small = *Nezera cathartica* Nieuwl [Linaceae].

Common Name(s): Fairy flax, mountain flax, purging flax, white flax [English]. Lin purgatif [French]. Lino catártico [Spanish]. Linho purgativo [Portuguese].
Life form: Herb. **Part(s) Used:** Complete plant / Fresh.
Geographic distribution: North Africa. Temperate-Asia. North East United States of America. Europe. Naturalized in several places of temperate regions.
Reference(s): Bharatan *et al.* 2002; Dorta Soares, n.d.; Müntz, n.d.; Plants for a future, 2009; American Institute of Homeopathy, 1979.

Linum usitatissimum

Scientific Name(s) / [Botanical Family]: *Linum usitatissimum* L. = *Linum angustifolium* Huds. = *Linum humile* Mill. [Linaceae].
Common Name(s): Flax, linseeds [English]. Lin [French]. Linhaça, linho [Portuguese]. Gueeche becueza xtilla, queeche-pecueza, queeche-pe-cueze-castilla, linaza, lino [Spanish].
Life form: Herb. **Part(s) Used:** Aerial part in bloom / Fresh.
Geographic distribution: Europe. Cultivated in other regions.
Reference(s): Allen, 2006-2010; Bharatan *et al.* 2002; Dorta Soares, n.d.; Gotfredsen, 2009; Plants for a future, 2009; Tiwari *et al.* 2013.

Lippia mexicana

Scientific Name(s) / [Botanical Family]: *Lippia dulcis* Trevir. = *Phyla dulcis* (Trevir.) Moldenke = *Phyla scaberrima* (A. Juss. ex Pers.) Moldenke. = *Zapania scaberrima* A. Juss. ex Pers [Verbenaceae].
Common Name(s): Aztec sweetherb, honeynerb, Mexican lippia, sweet herb [English]. Hierba dulce, neuclixihuítl, orégano, orozuz, orozuz del país, yerba dulce. [Spanish]. Verbena mexicana [Portuguese].
Life form: Herb. **Part(s) Used:** Complete plant / Fresh.

Geographic distribution: North America (Mexico, United States of America). Central & South America.
Reference(s): Bharatan *et al.* 2002; Dorta Soares, n.d.; Müntz, n.d.

Lithospermum officinale

Scientific Name(s) / [Botanical Family]: *Lithospermum officinale* L. [Boraginaceae].
Common Name(s): Common gromwell, gromwell, pearl gromwell [English]. Steinhirse. Ti hsueh, tzu tan, tzu ts'ao, ya hsien ts'ao [Chinese]. Grémil officinal, herbe aux perles, millet d'amour, perločre [French]. Mijo de sol [Spanish].
Life form: Herb. **Part(s) Used:** Leaf. **Geographic distribution:** Temperate-Asia. Europe. Naturalized in several places.
Reference(s): Bharatan *et al.* 2002; Comisión Editora de la Farmacopea Homeopática de los Estados Unidos Mexicanos, 1988; De Legarreta, 1961; American Institute of Homeopathy, 1979.

Lobelia

Scientific Name(s) / [Botanical Family]: *Lobelia inflata* L. [Campanulaceae, Lobeliaceae].
Common Name(s): Asthma root, bladder-podded lobelia, bugle weed, Indian tobacco [English]. Herbe de lobélie enflée, lobélie gonflée [French]. Lobélia, tabaco indiano [Portuguese]. Hierba del asma, tabaco indio [Spanish].
Life form: Herb. **Part(s) Used:** Complete plant / Fresh. seeds / Dried; complete plant in bloom. **Geographic distribution:** North America (East Canada. North East, North, Central & Southeast United States of America).
Reference(s): Bharatan *et al.* 2002; Bolte *et al.* 1997; Dorta Soares, n.d.; Seror, 2000; Tiwari *et al.* 2013.

Lobelia cardinalis

Scientific Name(s) / [Botanical Family]: *Lobelia cardinalis* L. [Campanulaceae, Lobeliaceae].

Common Name(s): Cardinal Flower, red cardinal plant, red lobelia [English]. Lobélie écarlate [French]. Lóbelia [Portuguese]. Cardenal de maceta, lobelia [Spanish].

Life form: Herb. **Part(s) Used:** Complete plant / Fresh.

Geographic distribution: North America (East Canada, Mexico. United States of America). Central America.

Reference(s): Bharatan *et al.* 2002; Dorta Soares, n.d.; Müntz, n.d.; Tiwari *et al.* 2013; American Institute of Homeopathy, 1979.

Lobelia dortmanna

Scientific Name(s) / [Botanical Family]: *Lobelia dortmanna* L. [Campanulaceae, Lobeliaceae].

Common Name(s): Wasser-lobelie. Water lobelia [English]. Lobélie de Dortmann [French].

Life form: Herb. **Part(s) Used:** Complete plant / Fresh.

Geographic distribution: North America (North East United States of America). Cultivated.

Reference(s): Bharatan *et al.* 2002; Gotfredsen, 2009; Müntz, n.d.; Plants for a future, 2009; American Institute of Homeopathy, 1979.

Lobelia erinus

Scientific Name(s) / [Botanical Family]: *Lobelia erinus* L. [Campanulaceae, Lobeliaceae].

Common Name(s): Wild lobelia, edging lobelia [English]. Lobélie à fleurs blanches ou bleues [French].

Life form: Herb. **Part(s) Used:** Complete plant / Fresh.

Geographic distribution: South Africa. Naturalized in several places.

Reference: Bharatan *et al.* 2002.

Lobelia purpurascens

Scientific Name(s) / [Botanical Family]: *Lobelia corolata* Wall. = *Lobelia purpurascens* Wall. = *Lobelia zeylanica* L. [Campanulaceae, Lobeliaceae].
Common Name(s): Purple lobelia, white root [English].
Life form: Herb. **Part(s) Used:** Complete plant / Fresh.
Geographic distribution: Temperate-Asia. Naturalized in several places. Cultivated (Australia). Pacific islands (Fiji).
Reference: Bharatan *et al.* 2002.

Lobelia siphilitica

Scientific Name(s) / [Botanical Family]: *Lobelia siphilitica* L. [Campanulaceae, Lobeliaceae].
Common Name(s): Bladder-podded cardinal flower, blue cardinal flower, blue lobelia, great blue lobelia, great lobelia [English]. Lobélia antisyphilitique, lobélie géante [French]. Lobélia sifilítica [Portuguese].
Life form: Herb. **Part(s) Used:** Complete plant / Fresh.
Geographic distribution: East North America (Canada. United States of America).
Reference(s): Bharatan *et al.* 2002; Boericke, 1927, 1927b.; Clarke, 2008; Dorta Soares, n.d.; Müntz, n.d.; Tiwari *et al.* 2013.

Lobelia syphilitica see *Lobelia siphilitica*

Lolium

Scientific Name(s) / [Botanical Family]: *Lolium temulentum* L. = *Lolium robustum* Rchb. [Poaceae = Gramineae].
Common Name(s): Bearded darnel, bearded ryegrass, darnel, poison darnel [English]. Ivraie énivrante [French]. Joio, sizânia [Portuguese]. Bayico, raygrás [Spanish].

Life form: Herb. **Part(s) Used:** Mature fruit, seeds / Dried; Complete plant collected in bloom. **Geographic distribution:** Europe. West Asia. North Africa & India. United States of America. Extensively naturalized.
Reference(s): Bharatan *et al.* 2002; Dorta Soares, n.d.; Müntz, n.d.; Plants for a future, 2009; Tiwari *et al.* 2013; American Institute of Homeopathy, 1979.

Lonicera

Scientific Name(s) / [Botanical Family]: *Lonicera xylosteum* L. = *Lonicera xylosteum* Georgi = *Lonicera xylosteum* Sibth. & Sm. = *Lonicera xylosteum* Lour. [Caprifoliaceae].
Common Name(s): Dwarf honeysuckle, fly woodbine [English]. La chčvre-feuille des haies, chévrefeuille des buissons [French].
Life form: Shrub. **Part(s) Used:** Fruit mature / Dried. **Geographic distribution:** East Europe-North Asia. Introduced in United States of America.
Reference(s): Bharatan *et al.* 2002; Dorta Soares, n.d.; Müntz, n.d.; Remedia/at, 2010; American Institute of Homeopathy, 1979.

Lonicera caprifolium

Scientific Name(s) / [Botanical Family]: *Lonicera caprifolium* L. [Caprifoliaceae].
Common Name(s): Honeysuckle, italian woodbine, italian honeysuckle [English]. Chévrefeuille commun, lonicéra [French]. Lonicera, madreselva [Spanish]. Madressilva, maravilha [Portuguese].
Life form: Herb. **Part(s) Used:** Complete plant / Fresh; fruit. **Geographic distribution:** Europe. Extensively cultivated & naturalized in several places.
Reference(s): Allen, 2006-2010; Bharatan *et al.* 2002; Dorta Soares, n.d.; Seror, 2000.

Lupulina see Lupulus humulus

Lupulinum see Lupulus humulus

Lupulus humulus

Scientific Name(s) / [Botanical Family]: *Humulus lupulus* L. [Cannabaceae, Urticaceae].

Common Name(s): Bine, common hop, European hop, hop, hops [English]. Pi jiu hua [Chinese]. Houblon [French]. Lúpulo [Spanish].

Life form: Herb. **Part(s) Used:** Flower / Fresh. **Geographic distribution:** North America. Europe. Extensively cultivated & naturalized in several places.

Reference(s): Bharatan *et al.* 2002; Müntz, n.d.; Tiwari *et al.* 2013.

Lycium berberis

Scientific Name(s) / [Botanical Family]: *Berberis lycium* Royle [Berberidaceae].

Common Name(s): Barberry, Indian Bareberry [English]. Ishkeen, kashmal [Indian].

Life form: Shrub. **Part(s) Used:** Aerial part in bloom / Fresh.

Geographic distribution: East Asia (North India, Pakistan, Himalayas).

Reference(s): Bharatan *et al.* 2002; American Institute of Homeopathy, 1979.

Lycopersicum

Scientific Name(s) / [Botanical Family]: *Solanum lycopersicum* (L.) H. Karst. = *Lycopersicon lycopersicum* (L.) H. Karst. = *Lycopersicon esculentum* Mill. [Solanaceae].

Common Name(s): Tomato [English]. Tomate [French]. Tomatateiro [Portuguese]. Aadi maxi, bachuga, be-thoxi, bi-

tuixi, pe-toxhi, jitomate, jitomate guajillo, tomate [Spanish].
Life form: Herb. **Part(s) Used:** Aerial part in early bloom; fruit / Fresh. **Geographic distribution:** naturalized & cultivated in several places.
Reference(s): Bharatan *et al.* 2002; Müntz, n.d.; Plants for a future, 2009; Tiwari *et al.* 2013.

Lycopodium

Scientific Name(s) / [Botanical Family]: *Lycopodium selago* L. [Lycopodiaceae].
Common Name(s): Fir clubmoss [English].
Life form: Herb. **Part(s) Used:** Complete plant / Dried.
Geographic distribution: Arctic & North temperate region. Spain & Himalayas.
Reference(s): Plants for a future, 2009; Remedia/at, 2010.

Lycopodium clavatum

Scientific Name(s) / [Botanical Family]: *Lycopodium clavatum* L. [Lycopodiaceae].
Common Name(s): Antler herb, clubmoss, common club moss, elk-moss, running-pine, stag's-horn clubmoss [English]. Lycopode in massue [French]. Licopodio [Spanish]. Musgo terrestre, pé de lobo [Portuguese].
Life form: Herb. **Part(s) Used:** Spores ("seeds"), sporangium / Dried; "pollen" / Dried. **Geographic distribution:** Temperate-Asia. Europe, England. North America (Canada, Mexico. United States of America). South America.
Reference(s): Bharatan *et al.* 2002; Dorta Soares, n.d.; Plants for a future, 2009; Tiwari *et al.* 2013.

Lycopus

Scientific Name(s) / [Botanical Family]: *Lycopus europaea* L. [Lamiaceae, Labiatae].

Common Name(s): Bugleweed, European bugleweed, gypsywort [English]. Ou di sun [Chinese]. Lycope de Virginie, lycope d'Europe [French]. Menta de lobo, pie de lobo americano [Spanish].
Life form: Herb. **Part(s) Used:** Complete plant / Fresh.
Geographic distribution: Temperate-Asia. Europe. East United States of America. Naturalized in several places.
Reference(s): Allen, 2006-2010; Bharatan *et al.* 2002; Dorta Soares, n.d.; Fuentes, 1996; Plants for a future, 2009; American Institute of Homeopathy, 1979.

Lycopus

Scientific Name(s) / [Botanical Family]: *Lycopus virginicus* L. [Lamiaceae, Labiatae].
Common Name(s): Bugleweed, Virginia water horehound, water bugle, water horehound [English]. Lycope de Virginie [French]. Erva consolida [Portuguese].
Life form: Herb. **Part(s) Used:** Complete plant / Fresh.
Geographic distribution: North America (North East, North Central, Southeast & South Central United States of America).
Reference(s): Bharatan *et al.* 2002; Gotfredsen, 2009; Dorta Soares, n.d.; Müntz, n.d.; Tiwari *et al.* 2013.

Lysimachia

Scientific Name(s) / [Botanical Family]: *Lysimachia nummularia* L. [Myrsinaceae]. [Primulaceae].
Common Name(s): Creeping-Jenny, moneywort [English]. Lysimaque nummularire [French].
Life form: Herb. **Part(s) Used:** Aerial part in early bloom; leaf / Fresh. **Geographic distribution:** Temperate-Asia. Europe. United States of America.
Reference(s): Bharatan *et al.* 2002; Dorta Soares, n.d.; Müntz, n.d.; American Institute of Homeopathy, 1979.

Macrozamia spiralis

Scientific Name(s) / [Botanical Family]: *Macrozamia spiralis* (Salisb. ex C. W. Konig & Sims) Miq. = *Zamia spiralis* ex C. W. Konig & Sims [Zamiaceae].
Common Name(s): Burrawang [English].
Life form: Shrub. **Part(s) Used:** seeds?. **Geographic distribution:** Australia.
Reference(s): Bharatan *et al.* 2002; Müntz, n.d.; Seror, 2000.

Magnolia glauca

Scientific Name(s) / [Botanical Family]: *Magnolia glauca* L. = *Magnolia virginiana* L. [Magnoliaceae].
Common Name(s): Laurel magnolia, sweet magnolia, sweet bay. Magnolia [French]. Flor del corazón [Spanish].
Life form: Shrub, Tree. **Part(s) Used:** Flower / Fresh. **Geographic distribution:** East North America (United States of America). Taiwan, China.
Reference(s): Bharatan *et al.* 2002; Boericke, 1927, 1927b.; Bolte *et al.* 1997; Clarke, 2008; Dorta Soares, n.d.; Müntz, n.d.

Magnolia grandiflora

Scientific Name(s) / [Botanical Family]: *Talauma mexicana* (DC.) G. Don. = *Magnolia mexicana* DC. [Magnoliaceae].
Common Name(s): Magnolia [English]. Magnolie [French]. Anonilla, Flor del corazón, magnolia, semíramis, yoloxóchitl, yolotxóchitl [Spanish].
Life form: Tree. **Part(s) Used:** Flower / Fresh. **Geographic distribution:** Mexico. Cultivated.

Reference(s): Bharatan *et al.* 2002; Bolte *et al.* 1997; Clarke, 2008; Dorta Soares, n.d.; Plants for a future, 2009; American Institute of Homeopathy, 1979.

Magnolia virginiana see *Magnolia glauca*

Mahonia aquifolium see *Berberis aquifolium*

Malva silvestris

Scientific Name(s) / [Botanical Family]: *Malva sylvestris* L. [Malvaceae].
Common Name(s): Cheeses, high mallow, malve wilde, tall malow [English]. Mauve des bois, mauve sauvage [French]. Malva [Spanish].
Life form: Herb. **Part(s) Used:** Aerial part in recently bloom / Fresh. **Geographic distribution:** cultivated & naturalized in several places.
Reference(s): Dorta Soares, n.d.; Schumacher, 2007; Tiwari *et al.* 2013.

Mandragora

Scientific Name(s) / [Botanical Family]: *Mandragora officinarum* L. = *Mandragora autumnalis* = *Atropa mandragora* Sibth. & Sm [Solanaceae].
Common Name(s): Devil's Apple, mandrake, spring mandrake [English]. Mandragore [French]. Mandrágora [Spanish, Italian].
Life form: Shrub. **Part(s) Used:** Complete plant (without root) / Dried. **Geographic distribution:** North Africa. Temperate-Asia. Europe. Naturalized in several places.
Reference(s): Bharatan *et al.* 2002; Dorta Soares, n.d.; Müntz, n.d.; Tiwari *et al.* 2013.

Manzanita

Scientific Name(s) / [Botanical Family]: *Arctostaphylos pungens*

Kunth = *Arctostaphylos manzanita* Parry [Ericaceae].

Common Name(s): Manzanita, pointleaf manzanita, Mexican manzanita [English]. Manzanitas, pendicua, pingüica, tepezquite [Spanish].

Life form: Shrub. **Part(s) Used:** Fruit, Leaf. **Geographic distribution:** United States of America (New Mexico, Texas, California), Mexico.

Reference(s): Bharatan *et al.* 2002; Clarke, 2008; Müntz, n.d.

Marrubium vulgare

Scientific Name(s) / [Botanical Family]: *Marrubium vulgare* L. [Lamiaceae, Labiatae].

Common Name(s): Horehound, white horehound [English]. Marrube blanc, marrube vulgaire [French]. Marroio [Portuguese]. Marrubio, marrubio blanco, marrubio común, vitsiqua [Spanish].

Life form: Herb. **Part(s) Used:** Leaf, aerial part in recently bloom / Fresh. **Geographic distribution:** Cultivated & naturalized in several places.

Reference(s): Bharatan *et al.* 2002; Dorta Soares, n.d.; Plants for a future, 2009; Provings, 2008-2009.

Mate

Scientific Name(s) / [Botanical Family]: *Ilex paraguariensis* A. St.-Hil. [Aquifoliaceae].

Common Name(s): Brazilian-tea, mate, Paraguayan-tea, yerba-mate [English]. Thé du Paraguay [French]. Erva-mate [Portuguese]. Hierba mate, mate, yerba mate [Spanish].

Life form: Herb. **Part(s) Used:** Leaf / Dried. **Geographic distribution:** South America (Brazil, Argentine, Paraguay, Uruguay).

Reference(s): Bharatan *et al.* 2002; Dorta Soares, n.d.; Müntz, n.d.; Tiwari *et al.* 2013.

Mathiola

Scientific Name(s) / [Botanical Family]: *Matthiola graeca* Sweet = *Matthiola incana* (L.) R. Br. = *Cheiranthus incanus* L. [Brassicaceae, Cruciferae].

Common Name(s): Brompton stock, gillyflower, hoary stock, Stock gilliflower [English]. Alelí, alelí blanco, alhelí blanco, alhelí encarnado [Spanish].

Life form: Herb. **Part(s) Used:** Complete plant / Fresh.

Geographic distribution: Temperate-Asia. South Europe. South America. Extensively cultivated.

Reference: Müntz, n.d.

Matricaria maritima

Scientific Name(s) / [Botanical Family]: *Matricaria maritima* L. = *Tripleurospermum maritimum* (L.) W. D. J. Koch subsp. *maritimum* [Asteraceae, Compositae].

Common Name(s): Coastal scentless mayweed, sea mayweed [English].

Life form: Herb. **Part(s) Used:** Aerial part in early bloom?.

Geographic distribution: Europe.

Reference(s): Bharatan *et al.* 2002; Clarke, 2008.

Matricaria parthenium see *Pyrethrum parthenium*

Melaleuca alternifolia

Scientific Name(s) / [Botanical Family]: *Melaleuca alternifolia* (Maiden & Betche) Cheel [Myrtaceae].

Common Name(s): Narrow leaf paperbark, tea tree, teebaum [English]. Árbol del té [Spanish].

Life form: Shrub, tree. **Part(s) Used:** Leaf / Fresh. **Geographic distribution:** Australia.

Reference: Müntz, n.d.

Melilotus

Scientific Name(s) / [Botanical Family]: *Melilotus officinalis* Willd. = *Trifolium officinalis* L. [Fabaceae, Leguminosae].

Common Name(s): Melilot, ribbed melilot, sweet clover, tall melilot, tall yellow sweetclover [English]. Mélilot jaune, mélilot officinal [French]. Coroa do rei, trevo-cheiroso [Portuguese]. Meliloto amarillo, trébol de olor, trébol oloroso [Spanish].

Life form: Herb. **Part(s) Used:** Complete plant / Fresh.

Geographic distribution: Europe. North Temperate-Asia. Naturalized in British Islands. New Zealand. United States of America, Canada & South America.

Reference(s): Bharatan *et al.* 2002; Dorta Soares, n.d.; Müntz, n.d.; Tiwari *et al.* 2013.

Melilotus alba

Scientific Name(s) / [Botanical Family]: *Melilotus alba* Lam. = *Melilotus alba* Medik. = *Middle albus* Desr. = *Melilotus albus* Medik. = *Trifolium officinalis* L. = *Sertula alba* (Medik.) Kuntze [Fabaceae, Leguminosae].

Common Name(s): Bokharaclover, honeyclover, white melilot, white sweet clover [English]. Mélilot blanc, méliot blanc [French]. Coronilla blanca, trébol dulce, trébol de Santa María, [Spanish]. Meliloto branco, trevo doce [Portuguese].

Life form: Herb. **Part(s) Used:** Complete plant / Fresh.

Geographic distribution: Europe, Russia.

Reference(s): Bharatan *et al.* 2002; Clarke, 2008; Dorta Soares, n.d.; Tiwari *et al.* 2013; American Institute of Homeopathy, 1979.

Melissa

Scientific Name(s) / [Botanical Family]: *Melissa officinalis* L. [Lamiaceae, Labiatae].

Common Name(s): Balm, bee balm, lemon balm, melissa [English]. Citronelle, mélisse officinale [French]. Erva-cidreira verdadeira, melissa [Portuguese]. Citraria, melisa, toronjil, totonjil extranjero [Spanish].
Life form: Herb. **Part(s) Used:** bud, leaf. **Geographic distribution:** Minor Asia, Europe (Mediterranean). Extensively cultivated in temperate regions.
Reference(s): Bharatan *et al.* 2002; Clarke, 2008; Dorta Soares, n.d.; American Institute of Homeopathy, 1979.

Menispermum

Scientific Name(s) / [Botanical Family]: *Menispermum canadense* L. = *Menispermum angulatum* Moench. [Menispermaceae].
Common Name(s): Canada moon seeds, moon seeds, yellow parilla [English]. Menisperme du Canada [French]. Parilla [Spanish]. Salsaparilha do Texas, semente lua [Portuguese].
Life form: Shrub. **Part(s) Used:** Root, complete plant / Fresh.
Geographic distribution: North America (East & West Canada. North East, North, Central & Southeast United States of America).
Reference(s): Bharatan *et al.* 2002; Bolte *et al.* 1997; Dorta Soares, n.d.; Fuentes, 1996; Plants for a future, 2009.

Mentha

Scientific Name(s) / [Botanical Family]: *Mentha x piperita* L. = *Mentha aquatica* × *Middle spicata*]. = *Mentha lavanduliodora* ined. = *Mentha officinalis* Hull [Lamiaceae, Labiatae].
Common Name(s): Brandy mint, mint, peppermint [English]. Menthe poivrée, menthe poivrée [French]. Bete, bi-ti, nocuana-biti, nocuana-pete, nocuana-piti, menta, menta negra, menta piperita, pete [Spanish]. Hortelâ, menta inglesa [Portuguese].
Life form: Herb. **Part(s) Used:** Complete plant / Fresh.

Geographic distribution: Europe. Cosmopolitan cultivated.
Reference(s): Bharatan *et al.* 2002; Bolte *et al.* 1997; Clarke, 2008; Dorta Soares, n.d.; Müntz, n.d.; Tiwari *et al.* 2013; American Institute of Homeopathy, 1979.

Mentha piperita see *Mentha*

Mentha pulegium
Scientific Name(s) / [Botanical Family]: *Mentha pulegium* L. [Lamiaceae, Labiatae].
Common Name(s): European Pennyroyal, pennyroyal [English]. Menthe pouliot, pouliot [French]. Poejo, hortelâ-miúda [Portuguese]. Poleo [Spanish]. Erva de Sâo Lourenço, poejo [Portuguese].
Life form: Herb. **Part(s) Used:** Aerial part / Fresh; leaves collected in bloom / Dried. **Geographic distribution:** Africa. Temperate-Asia. Europe. Cultivated in several places. Cosmopolitan.
Reference(s): Bharatan *et al.* 2002; Clarke, 2008; Dorta Soares, n.d.; Müntz, n.d.

Mentha viridis
Scientific Name(s) / [Botanical Family]: *Mentha spicata* L. = *Mentha viridis* (L.) L. [Labiatae].
Common Name(s): Brandy mint, mint, peppermint [English]. Menthe poivre, menthe poivrée [French]. Hortelâ-comum [Portuguese]. Alfabieso, caxtalalhka'jna, hierba buena, hierbabuena de comer, menta romana, té de olor, yerbabuena [Spanish].
Life form: Herb. **Part(s) Used:** Complete plant / Fresh.
Geographic distribution: Africa, Temperate-Asia. Europe. Cultivated. Cosmopolitan. Naturalized in temperate regions.
Reference(s): Bharatan *et al.* 2002; Clarke, 2008; Müntz, n.d.; Tiwari *et al.* 2013.

Menyanthes

Scientific Name(s) / [Botanical Family]: *Menyanthes trifoliata* L. [Menyanthaceae].

Common Name(s): Bitterklee, bog-bean, buck bean, common bog-bean, marsh-trefoil, water trefoil [English]. Ményanthe trifolié, trefle des marais, trèfle-d'eau [French]. Trébol de agua [Spanish]. Soldanela d'agua [Portuguese].

Life form: Herb. **Part(s) Used:** Complete plant / Fresh.

Geographic distribution: North Africa, Temperate-Asia Europe, North America (Canada-United States of America).

Reference(s): Bharatan *et al.* 2002; Dorta Soares, n.d.; Remedia/at, 2010.

Mercurialis

Scientific Name(s) / [Botanical Family]: *Mercurialis annua* L. [Euphorbiaceae].

Common Name(s): Annual mercury, herb mercury [English].

Life form: Herb. **Part(s) Used:** Complete plant / Fresh.

Geographic distribution: North Africa. Europe. Naturalized in several places.

Reference(s): Bharatan *et al.* 2002; Bolte *et al.* 1997; Clarke, 2008; Dorta Soares, n.d.; Gotfredsen, 2009; Müntz, n.d.

Mercurialis perennis

Scientific Name(s) / [Botanical Family]: *Mercurialis perennis* L. [Euphorbiaceae].

Common Name(s): Dogs's mercury [English]. Mercuriale vivace [French]. Mercurial perenne [Spanish].

Life form: Herb. **Part(s) Used:** Complete plant / Fresh.

Geographic distribution: Africa. Temperate-Asia. Europe.

Reference(s): Bharatan *et al.* 2002; Dorta Soares, n.d.; Müntz, n.d.; Plants for a future, 2009; Tiwari *et al.* 2013.

Mezereum

Scientific Name(s) / [Botanical Family]: *Daphne mezereum* L. [Thymelaceae].

Common Name(s): February daphne, mezereon, paradise-plant [English]. Lauréole gentile [French]. Laureola hembra, olivareta, leño gentil, torvisco, mecerón, matacabras, mezereo [Spanish].

Life form: Shrub. **Part(s) Used:** Bark / Fresh. **Geographic distribution:** Temperate-Asia. Europe. Naturalized in several places.

Reference(s): Bharatan *et al.* 2002; Comisión Editora de la Farmacopea Homeopática de los Estados Unidos Mexicanos, 1988; Müntz, n.d.; Tiwari *et al.* 2013; American Institute of Homeopathy, 1979.

Millefolium

Scientific Name(s) / [Botanical Family]: *Achillea millefolium* L. = *Achillea borealis* Bong. Krause = *Achillea lanulosa* Nutt = *Achillea laxiflora* Pollard & Cockerell = *Chamaemelum millefolium* E. H.L. [Asteraceae, Compositae].

Common Name(s): Bloodwort, carpenter's weed, common yarrow, milfoil, nosebleed, soldier's woundwort, staunchweed, thousand leaf, thousand seal, thousand weed, thousandleaf, woundwort, yarrow, yarrow bloodwort, yarrow milfoil [English]. Achillée, herbe à Dinde, herbe aux militaires [French]. Miel en rama, mil en rama [Spanish]. Aquiléia, erva carpinteiro, milefólio [Portuguese].

Life form: Herb. **Part(s) Used:** Aerial part in recently bloom / Fresh. **Geographic distribution:** America. Asia. Europe. cultivated, Cosmopolitan.

Reference(s): Bharatan *et al.* 2002; Dorta Soares, n.d.; Müntz, n.d.; Plants for a future, 2009; Tiwari *et al.* 2013; American Institute of Homeopathy, 1979.

Mimosa humilis

Scientific Name(s) / [Botanical Family]: *Mimosa dormiens* Humb. et Bonpl. ex Willd. = *Mimosa humilis* Humb. et Bonpl. [Fabaceae, Leguminosae].
Common Name(s): Sensitive plant [English]. Malicia das mulheres, mimosa, sensitiva [Portuguese].
Life form: Herb. **Part(s) Used:** Leaf / Fresh. **Geographic distribution:** North, Central & South America.
Reference(s): Bharatan *et al.* 2002; Clarke, 2008; Dorta Soares, n.d.; Fuentes, 1996; Gotfredsen, 2009; Müntz, n.d.; Remedia/at, 2010.

Mimosa pudica

Scientific Name(s) / [Botanical Family]: *Mimosa pudica* L. [Fabaceae, Leguminosae].
Common Name(s): Sensitive plant, shameplant, touch-me-not [English]. Sensitive [French]. Dormidera, dormilón, dormilona, pinahuihuixtle, quececupatli, sensitiva, ten vergûenza, vergonzosa, xmutz [Spanish].
Life form: Herb. **Part(s) Used:** Leaf / Fresh. **Geographic distribution:** Temperate & pantropical (the species spreads over an area around the tropical zone of the planet).
Reference(s): Bharatan *et al.* 2002; Remedia/at, 2010; Tiwari *et al.* 2013.

Mitchella

Scientific Name(s) / [Botanical Family]: *Mitchella repens* L. [Rubiaceae].
Common Name(s): Checker berry, deer berry, one berry, partridge-beans, partridge-berry, squaw vine, winter clover [English]. Vino squaw [Spanish].
Life form: Herb, Shrub. **Part(s) Used:** Complete plant / Fresh.

Geographic distribution: North & Central America. (North & East United States of America), Japan.
Reference(s): Bharatan *et al.* 2002; Clarke, 2008; Dorta Soares, n.d.; Müntz, n.d.; Tiwari *et al.* 2013.

Momordica charantia

Scientific Name(s) / [Botanical Family]: *Momordica charantia* L. [Cucurbitaceae].
Common Name(s): Balsam-apple, balsam-pear, bitter gourd, bitter melon, bitter-cucumber, carilla gourd [English]. Concombre africain, margose, momordique [French]. Bálsamo, balsamito, cundeamor, cundeamor de Yucatán, yakunah-ax [Spanish].
Life form: Herb. **Part(s) Used:** Fruit / Fresh. **Geographic distribution:** Temperate-Asia. Cultivated.
Reference(s): Bharatan *et al.* 2002; Clarke, 2008; Dorta Soares, n.d.; Müntz, n.d.; Tiwari *et al.* 2013; American Institute of Homeopathy, 1979.

Monotropa uniflora

Scientific Name(s) / [Botanical Family]: *Monotropa uniflora* L. [Pyrolaceae].
Common Name(s): Bird's nest, corpse plant, ghost plant, Indian pipe [English]. Pipa de indio, plantita albina [Spanish]. Akino-ginryoso, ginryoso-modoki [Japanese].
Life form: Herb. **Part(s) Used:** Complete plant / Fresh. **Geographic distribution:** Temperate-Asia. North America (Alaska. Canada. Mexico. United States of America).
Reference(s): Dorta Soares, n.d.; Müntz, n.d.

Morus nigra

Scientific Name(s) / [Botanical Family]: *Morus nigra* L. [Moraceae].

Common Name(s): Black mulberry, common mulberry [English]. Mûrier noir [French]. Amoreira negra, amoreira prieta [Portuguese]. Moral, moral negro, morera negra [Spanish].
Life form: Tree. **Part(s) Used:** Leaf, fruit. **Geographic distribution:** Southwest Asia. Extensively cultivated.
Reference: American Institute of Homeopathy, 1979.

Myosotis arvensis

Scientific Name(s) / [Botanical Family]: *Myosotis arvensis* (L.) Hill. = *Myosotis scorpiodes* L. var. *arvensis* L. [Boraginaceae].
Common Name(s): Field forgot-me-not, field scorpion-grass [English]. Myosotis des champs [French]. No me olvides [Spanish]. Nâo-me-esqueças [Portuguese].
Life form: Herb. **Part(s) Used:** Complete plant / Fresh.
Geographic distribution: North Africa. Temperate-Asia. Europe. North America (Northwest & North East of United States of America).
Reference(s): Bharatan *et al.* 2002; Bolte *et al.* 1997; Dorta Soares, n.d.; Gotfredsen, 2009; Müntz, n.d.; Plants for a future, 2009.

Myosotis symphytifolia

Scientific Name(s) / [Botanical Family]: *Myosotis symphytifolia?* = *Myosotis palustris* (L.) Nath. = *Myosotis scorpioides* L. [Boraginaceae].
Common Name(s): Black root, forget-me-not, water forget-me-not [English]. Myosotis faux scorpion [French]. No me olvides [Spanish].
Life form: Herb. **Part(s) Used:** Complete plant / Fresh.
Geographic distribution: Temperate-Asia. Europe. United States of America (California, Indiana). Europe. Naturalized in several places.
Reference(s): Bharatan *et al.* 2002; Bolte *et al.* 1997; Clarke,

2008; Zandvoort, 2006.

Myrica cerifera

Scientific Name(s) / [Botanical Family]: *Myrica cerifera* L. = *Morella cerifera* (L.) Small [Myricaceae].
Common Name(s): Bayberry, candle-berry, southern bayberry, stemw shrub, wax, wax myrtle [English]. Arbre à suif [French]. Árbol de la cera, arrayán, huancanala, otocamay [Spanish]. Fruit das baiaas, louro bravo [Portuguese].
Life form: Shrub. **Part(s) Used:** Bark-Root / Fresh. **Geographic distribution:** North East United States of America. Cultivated in Central & South America.
Reference(s): Bharatan *et al.* 2002; Boericke, 1927, 1927b.; Bolte *et al.* 1997; Clarke, 2008; Dorta Soares, n.d.; Müntz, n.d.; Tiwari *et al.* 2013; Zandvoort, 2006.

Myrtus communis

Scientific Name(s) / [Botanical Family]: *Myrtus communis* L. [Myrtaceae].
Common Name(s): Common myrtle, myrtle, true myrtle [English]. Myrte commun [French]. Mirto [Spanish]. Mirta, murta, murta cheirosa [Portuguese].
Life form: Tree. **Part(s) Used:** Leaf, stem / Fresh. **Geographic distribution:** West Asia. Naturalized in Europe. Cultivated in other regions.
Reference(s): Bharatan *et al.* 2002; Bolte *et al.* 1997; Clarke, 2008; Dorta Soares, n.d.; Müntz, n.d.; Tiwari *et al.* 2013; American Institute of Homeopathy, 1979.

Nabalus see *Nabalus serpentaria*

Nabalus albus

Scientific Name(s) / [Botanical Family]: *Prenanthes alba* L. = *Nabalus albus* (L.) Hook. [Asteraceae, Compositae].
Common Name(s): Rattlesnake-root, white rattlesnake- root, lions's foot, white-lettuce [English]. Lechuga blanca [Spanish].
Life form: Herb. **Part(s) Used:** Complete plant / Fresh.
Geographic distribution: North America (Canada, United States of America).
Reference(s): Clarke, 2008; Müntz, n.d.; American Institute of Homeopathy, 1979.

Nabalus serpentaria

Scientific Name(s) / [Botanical Family]: *Prenanthes serpentaria* Pursh = *Prenanthes integrifolia* (Cass.) Small = *Nabalus integrifolius* Cass. = *Nabalus serpentarius* (Pursh) Hook. [Asteraceae, Compositae].
Common Name(s): Cankerweed, lions's foot, rattlesnake root, white lettuce [English]. Pied d'Leon, laitue blanche [French].
Life form: Herb. **Part(s) Used:** Complete plant / Fresh.
Geographic distribution: North America (Canada. East United States of America).
Reference(s): Bharatan *et al.* 2002; Müntz, n.d.; Remedia/at, 2010; Tiwari *et al.* 2013.

Narcissus poeticus

Scientific Name(s) / [Botanical Family]: *Narcissus poeticus* L. = *Narcissus angustifolius* Curtis = *Narcissus poeticus* subsp. *radiiflorus* = *Narcissus hellenicus* Pugsley = *Narcissus poeticus* subsp. *poeticus* = *Narcissus poeticus* var. *recurvus* (Haw.) Baker = *Narcissus poeticus* subsp. *poeticus* = *Narcissus* poeticus var.

verbanensis Herb. = *Narcissus poeticus* subsp. *poeticus* = *Narcissus radiiflorus* Salisb. = *Narcissus poeticus* subsp. *radiiflorus* = *Narcissus recurvus* Haw. = *Narcissus poeticus* subsp. *poeticus.* [Amaryllidaceae, Liliaceae].

Common Name(s): Narcissus, pheasant's-eye, poet's narcissus [English]. Claudinette, narcisse, narcisse poetes, oeil de faisan [French]. Narciso [Spanish, Italian]. Narciso blanco, trompón [Spanish].

Life form: Herb. **Part(s) Used:** Bulb / Fresh. **Geographic distribution:** Europe. Cultivated & naturalized in several places. **Reference(s):** Bharatan *et al.* 2002; Müntz, n.d.; American Institute of Homeopathy, 1979; Zandvoort, 2006.

Narcissus pseudonarcissus

Scientific Name(s) / [Botanical Family]: *Narcissus pseudonarcissus* L. = All the names listed below should be considered -to date- as a subspecies (subsp.) of *Narcissus pseudonarcissus* L. = *Narcissus albescens* Pugsley = *Narcissus alpestris* Pugsley = *Narcissus confusus* Pugsley = *Narcissus eugeniae* Fern. Casas = *Narcissus gayi* (Hénon) Pugsley = *Narcissus hispanicus* Gouan = *Narcissus leonensis* Pugsley = *Narcissus macrolobus* (Jord.) Pugsley = *Narcissus major* Curtis = *Narcissus moleroi* Fern. Casas = *Narcissus moschatus* L. = *Narcissus nevadensis* Pugsley = *Narcissus nobilis* (Haw.) Schult. f. = *Narcissus pallidiflorus* Pugsley = *Narcissus portensis* Pugsley = *Narcissus pseudonarcissus* subsp. *tortuosus* (Haw.) A. Fern. = *Narcissus radinganorum* Fern. Casas = *Narcissus tortuosus* Haw. = *Ajax gayi* Hénon = *Ajax macrolobus* Jord. = *Ajax nobilis* Haw. [Amaryllidaceae, Liliaceae].

Common Name(s): Buttercup, common daffodil, daffodil, lent-lily, Tenby daffodil, trumpet narcissus, wild daffodil [English]. Faux narcisse narcisse faux narcisse, narcisse jaune [French]. Narciso [Spanish]. Narciso, narciso dos prados [Portuguese].

Life form: Herb. **Part(s) Used:** Bulb or also complete plant in

bloom / Fresh. **Geographic distribution:** Temperate-Asia. Europe. Naturalized in several places.
Reference(s): Allen, 2006-2010; Bharatan *et al.* 2002; Dorta Soares, n.d.; Müntz, n.d.; Plants for a future, 2009; Tiwari *et al.* 2013.

Nasturtium

Scientific Name(s) / [Botanical Family]: *Rorippa nasturtium-aquaticum* (L.) Hayek = *Nasturtium officinale* R. Br. = *Nasturtium aquaticum* Garsault = *Sisymbrium nasturtium-aquaticum* L. [Brassicaceae, Cruciferae].
Common Name(s): Berro, cresson, watercress [English]. Cresson de fontaine, cresson d'eau [French]. Berro [Spanish]. Agrião, agrião das hortas [Portuguese].
Life form: Herb. **Part(s) Used:** Aerial part in recently bloom / Fresh. **Geographic distribution:** Several parts of the temperate region of the North hemisphere, cultivated & naturalized in several places.
Reference(s): Allen, 2006-2010; Bharatan *et al.* 2002; Clarke, 2008; Dorta Soares, n.d.; Müntz, n.d.; Tiwari *et al.* 2013.

Nelumbo nucifera

Scientific Name(s) / [Botanical Family]: *Nelumbo nucifera* Gaertn. [Nelumbaceae].
Common Name(s): Lotus flower, pink lotus lily, sacred lotus [English]. Fčve d'Egypte, lotus indien [French]. Flor de loto, habas de Egipto, loto sagrado, nelumbio, rosa del Nilo [Spanish].
Life form: Herb. **Part(s) Used:** Fruit, leaf?. **Geographic distribution:** Temperate-Asia & tropical. Australia. East Europe. India. Naturalized in several places.
Reference(s): Bharatan *et al.* 2002; Müntz, n.d.

Nepeta

Scientific Name(s) / [Botanical Family]: *Nepeta cataria* L. = *Cataria vulgaris* Moench [Lamiaceae, Labiatae].

Common Name(s): Cataria, cat-mint, catnip [English]. Cataire, menthe des chats [French]. Erba-de-gatta [Italian]. Erva-gateira [Portuguese]. Hierba gatera, menta de gato [Spanish].

Life form: Herb. **Part(s) Used:** Flower. **Geographic distribution:** Temperate-Asia. Europe. Extensively cultivated & naturalized.

Reference(s): Bharatan *et al.* 2002; Bolte *et al.* 1997; Müntz, n.d.

Nigella sativa

Scientific Name(s) / [Botanical Family]: *Nigella sativa* L. [Ranunculaceae].

Common Name(s): Black caraway, black cumin, fennel flower, blessed seeds, culture devil-in-the-bush [English]. Nigelle de Vrčte, toute épice [French]. Agenuz, ajenuz, arañuel, arañuela, neguilla, toda especia [Spanish]. Alvipre, cuminho preto, nigela [Portuguese].

Life form: Herb. **Part(s) Used:** Mature seeds / Dried. **Geographic distribution:** Temperate-Asia. Extensively cultivated & naturalized from Mediterranean to Central Asia & East United States of America.

Reference(s): Bharatan *et al.* 2002; Dorta Soares, n.d.

Nolana paradoxa

Scientific Name(s) / [Botanical Family]: *Nolana paradoxa* Lindl. = *Nolana acuminata* (Miers) Miers ex Dunal = *Nolana atriplicifolia* D. Don = *Nolana rupicola* Gaudich. = *Sorema acuminata* Miers [Solanaceae, Nolanaceae].

Common Name(s): Blue bird, snowbird [English]. Suspiro de mar [Spanish].

Life form: Herb. **Part(s) Used:** Aerial part in early bloom.

Geographic distribution: North America (Mexico). South America (Chile, Peru).
Reference: Müntz, n.d.

Nuphar

Scientific Name(s) / [Botanical Family]: *Nuphar lutea* (L.) Sm. = *Nuphar luteum* (L.) Sibth. & Sm. = *Nymphaea umbilicalis* Salisb. = *Nymphozanthus luteus* (L.) Fernald [Nymphaeaceae].
Common Name(s): Brandy-bottle, European pond lily, frog lily, yellow pond-lily [English]. Nénufar jaune, nénuphar commun [French]. Nenúfar, nenúfar amarillo [Spanish]. Aguapé de Flower amarela, gigola amarela [Portuguese].
Life form: Herb. **Part(s) Used:** Rhizome/ Fresh; flowers / Dried.
Geographic distribution: Europe. Cultivated in other regions.
Reference(s): Bharatan *et al.* 2002; Dorta Soares, n.d.; Müntz, n.d.; Tiwari *et al.* 2013.

Nuphar luteum

Scientific Name(s) / [Botanical Family]: *Nuphar lutea* (L.) Sibth. & Sm. = *Nuphar minor* Dumort = *Nuphar sericea* Lang. = *Nymphaea lutea* L. [Nymphaeaceae].
Common Name(s): Nixen-blume, yellow piond-lily. Nenuphar jaune [French].
Life form: Herb. **Part(s) Used:** Root / Fresh. **Geographic distribution:** North Africa, Temperate-Asia. Europe, cultivated in several places from temperate regions.
Reference(s): Bharatan *et al.* 2002; Bolte *et al.* 1997; Dorta Soares, n.d.; American Institute of Homeopathy, 1979.

Nymphaea

Scientific Name(s) / [Botanical Family]: *Nymphaea odorata* Aiton = *Castalia lekophylla* Small = *Castalia minor* (Sims) Nyar = *Castalia odorata* (Aiton) Woodv. & Wood = *Castalia pudica*

Salisb. = *Leuconymphaea odorata* (Aiton) Kuntze &. [Nymphaeaceae].

Common Name(s): Beaverroot, cow cabbage, asweet water lilly, tuberous water lilly, white water-lily, etc. [English]. Nymphéa tubéreux [French]. Ninfea blanca [Spanish]. Aguapé, bandeja d'água, lírio d'água, nenúfar [Portuguese].

Life form: Herb. **Part(s) Used:** Rhizome or Leaves collected before bloom / Fresh. **Geographic distribution:** North America (Canada. United States of America. Mexico). Naturalized in several places.

Reference(s): Allen, 2006-2010; Bharatan *et al.* 2002; Dorta Soares, n.d.; Müntz, n.d.; Tiwari *et al.* 2013.

Nymphaea alba

Scientific Name(s) / [Botanical Family]: *Nymphaea alba* L. = *Castalia alba* (L.) Woodv. & Wood = *Castalia minoriflora* Simonk. = *Castalia speciosa* Salisb. = *Leuconymphaea alba* (L.) Kuntze & 21 scientific synonyms & varieties or also forms more. [Nymphaeaceae].

Common Name(s): White water-lily [English]. Nymphéa blanc [French]. Ninfea blanca [Spanish]. Aguapé granco, lírio d'água, ninféia [Portuguese].

Life form: Herb. **Part(s) Used:** Dried leaves collected before bloom / Fresh. **Geographic distribution:** Europe & cultivated in several places from temperate regions.

Reference(s): Allen, 2006-2010; Bharatan *et al.* 2002; Bolte *et al.* 1997; Dorta Soares, n.d.; Müntz, n.d.; American Institute of Homeopathy, 1979.

Ocimum

Scientific Name(s) / [Botanical Family]: *Ocimum basilicum* L. [Lamiaceae, Labiatae].
Common Name(s): Basil, sweet basil [English]. Basilic [French]. Alfavaca, manjericão [Portuguese]. Albaca, albacarón, albahaca, albacar [Spanish]. Alfavaca, basilicum grande, erva real [Portuguese].
Life form: Herb. **Part(s) Used:** Aerial parts collected before bloom / Fresh. **Geographic distribution:** Asia. Extensively cultivated in temperate places.
Reference(s): Dorta Soares, n.d.; Müntz, n.d.; Tiwari *et al.* 2013.

Oenanthe aquatica

Scientific Name(s) / [Botanical Family]: *Oenanthe aquatica* (L.) Poir. = *Oenanthe phellandrium* Lam. = *Phellandrium aquaticum* L. [Apiaceae, Umbelliferae].
Common Name(s): Fine-leaf water-dropwort, water dropwort, water-fennel, water-hemlock. Ciguë aquatique, oenanthe aquatique, phellandre [French]. Hinojo de agua [Spanish]. Cicuta aquática, erva pombinha [Portuguese].
Life form: Herb. **Part(s) Used:** Fruit, seeds / Dried. **Geographic distribution:** Temperate-Asia. Europe.
Reference(s): Bharatan *et al.* 2002; Dorta Soares, n.d.; Fuentes, 1996; Müntz, n.d.; Plants for a future, 2009.

Oenanthe crocata

Oenanthe crocata L. = *Oenanthe apiifolia* Brot. = *Oenanthe gallaecica* Pau & Merino = *Oenanthe macrosciadia* Willk. = *Phellandrium plinii* Bubani [Apiaceae, Umbelliferae].
Common Name(s): Dead tongue, drop water, hemlock water drop [English]. Oenanthe safranée [French]. Acibuta, acibutas, aciguta, apio bravo, nabo del diablo [Spanish]. Salsa leitosa

[Portuguese].
Life form: Herb. **Part(s) Used:** Root or rhizome; rhizome with the complete plant collected at initiation of bloom / Fresh.
Geographic distribution: Europe (Great Britain, France, Italy & Spain). India.
Reference(s): Bharatan *et al.* 2002; Dorta Soares, n.d.; Müntz, n.d.; Tiwari *et al.* 2013.

Oenothera

Scientific Name(s) / [Botanical Family]: *Oenothera biennis* L. = *Oenothera gauroides* Hornem. [Onagraceae].
Common Name(s): Common evening-primrose, German-rampion, scabish [English]. Onagra [French]. Capa de San José, onagra, enotera, hierba del asno, zécora [Spanish]. Boa tarde, círio do North, erva dos burros [Portuguese].
Life form: Herb. **Part(s) Used:** Complete plant / Fresh; flowers / Dried. **Geographic distribution:** North America (Canada, United States of America, Mexico). South America (Peru). Extensively naturalized in temperate & subtropical places.
Reference(s): Bharatan *et al.* 2002; Dorta Soares, n.d.; Müntz, n.d.; American Institute of Homeopathy, 1979.

Oleander

Scientific Name(s) / [Botanical Family]: *Nerium oleander* L. [Apocynaceae].
Common Name(s): Oleander, rose bay, rose-laurel [English]. Laurier rose, le laurier rose, oleandre [French]. Adelfa, laurel rosa, rosa laurel [Spanish]. Adelfa rosada, epirradeira, loendro [Portuguese].
Life form: Shrub. **Part(s) Used:** Leaf / Fresh; leaves / Dried collected during the bloom. **Geographic distribution:** North & West Africa. Temperate-Asia. South Europe. Cultivated & naturalized in several places.

Reference(s): Bharatan *et al.* 2002; Dorta Soares, n.d.; Müntz, n.d.; Tiwari *et al.* 2013; American Institute of Homeopathy, 1979.

Oleum cajeputum see *Cajuputi*

Oleum cajuputi see *Cajuputum*

Oleum europaeum

Scientific Name(s) / [Botanical Family]: *Olea europaea* L. = *Olea europaea* Thunb. [Oleaceae].
Common Name(s): Olive, olive leaf [English]. Olivier d'Europe [French]. Aceituno, olivo [Spanish]. Oliveira [Portuguese].
Life form: Tree. **Part(s) Used:** Leaf, fruit, branch with leaves / Fresh; Fresh leaves collected during fructifying. **Geographic distribution:** Mediterranean & nearest Orient. Cultivated & naturalized in several places.
Reference(s): Allen, 2006-2010; Bharatan *et al.* 2002; Bolte *et al.* 1997; Dorta Soares, n.d.; Fuentes, 1996; Müntz, n.d.; Remedia/at, 2010.

Ononis

Scientific Name(s) / [Botanical Family]: *Ononis spinosa* L. = *Ononis antiquorum* L. = *Ononis campestris* W. D. J. Koch & Ziz. = *Ononis repens* subsp. *antiquorum* (L.) Greuter [Fabaceae, Leguminosae].
Common Name(s): Restharrow, spiny rest-harrow [English]. Bugrane, ononis épineux [French]. Abreojos, aznallo, detienebuey, gatuña, peine de asno [Spanish]. Unha-de-gato [Portuguese].
Life form: Shrub. **Part(s) Used:** Fresh complete plant collected before bloom; flower or subterraneous parts / Dried. **Geographic distribution:** Temperate-Asia. Europe. East United States of America.

Reference(s): Bharatan *et al.* 2002; Dorta Soares, n.d.; Müntz, n.d.; Rowe, 2006; Seror, 2000; Tiwari *et al.* 2013.

Onosmodium

Scientific Name(s) / [Botanical Family]: *Onosmodium virginianum* (L.) A. DC. = *Onosmodium hispidum* Michx. = *Lithospermum virginianum* L. [Boraginaceae].
Common Name(s): Eastern false gromwell, false gromwell wild, Job's tears [English]. Grémil de Virginie [French]. Lágrimas de Jó [Portuguese]. Lágrimas de Job [Spanish].
Life form: Herb. **Part(s) Used:** Complete plant / Fresh.
Geographic distribution: North America (North East & Southeast United States of America).
Reference(s): Bharatan *et al.* 2002; Clarke, 2008; Dorta Soares, n.d.; Müntz, n.d.; Tiwari *et al.* 2013.

Opium

Scientific Name(s) / [Botanical Family]: *Papaver somniferum* L. [Papaveraceae].
Common Name(s): Breadseeds poppy, edibleseeds ed poppy, garden poppy, medicinal poppy, opium poppy, poppyseeds poppy, white poppy [English]. Opium [French]. Adormidera, amapola, amapola de opio, guia-guiña, nocuana-bizuono-huceochoga-becala, quie-guiña [Spanish]. Dormideira, ópio, papaoula, papaoula amarela [Portuguese].
Life form: Herb. **Part(s) Used:** Flower, leaf / Dried. **Geographic distribution:** Asia Minor. Europe cultivated. Cosmopolitan.
Reference(s): Bharatan *et al.* 2002; Boericke, 1927, 1927b.; Bolte *et al.* 1997; Dorta Soares, n.d.; Müntz, n.d.; Tiwari *et al.* 2013; American Institute of Homeopathy, 1979.

Opuntia alba spina

Scientific Name(s) / [Botanical Family]: *Opuntia microdasys*

(Lehm.) Pfeiff. = *Cactus microdasys* Lehm. [Cactaceae].
Common Name(s): Angel's-wings, bunny-ear prickly-pear, bunny-ears prickly-pear, golden-bristle [English]. Cegador, ciega borrego, nopal cegador, nopal real, nopalillo cegador, tlatocanochtli, tlatoc-nochtli [Spanish].
Life form: Shrub. **Part(s) Used:** Complete plant / Fresh.
Geographic distribution: North America. Cultivated & naturalized in several places.
Reference(s): Boericke, 1927, 1927b.; Bolte *et al.* 1997; Fuentes, 1996; Müntz, n.d.; Tiwari *et al.* 2013.

Opuntia ficus-indica

Scientific Name(s) / [Botanical Family]: *Opuntia ficus-indica* (L.) Mill. = *Cactus ficus-indica* L. = *Cactus opuntia* L. [Cactaceae].
Common Name(s): Barbary-fig, Indian-fig, Indian-fig prickly-pear, mission cactus, mission prickly-pear, prickly pear [English]. Figuier d'Inde, figuier de Barbarie [French]. Orelha-de-onca [Portuguese]. Chumba, chumbera, nopal, nopal de Castilla, nopal pelón, nopal sin espinas, tuna, tuna de Castilla [Spanish].
Life form: Shrub. **Part(s) Used:** Complete plant / Fresh.
Geographic distribution: America. Naturalized in Europe.
Reference(s): Bharatan *et al.* 2002; Remedia/at, 2010.

Opuntia microdasys see *Opuntia alba-spina*

Opuntia vulgaris see *Opuntia ficus-indica*

Orchis mascula

Scientific Name(s) / [Botanical Family]: *Orchis mascula* (L.) L. [Orchidaceae].
Common Name(s): Early purple orchid, salep [English]. Satirión manchado, compañon, orquídea macho [Spanish].
Life form: Epiphyte. **Part(s) Used:** Tuber. **Geographic distribution:** Temperate-Asia. Europe.

Reference(s): Allen, 2006-2010; Bharatan *et al.* 2002; Rowe, 2006; American Institute of Homeopathy, 1979.

Oreodaphne california see *Oreodaphne californica*

Oreodaphne californica

Scientific Name(s) / [Botanical Family]: *Oreodaphne californica* (Hook. & Arn.) Nees = *Laurus regia* Douglas = *Laurus regalis* Hort. = *Tetranthera californica* Hook. & Arn. [Lauraceae].
Common Name(s): Balsam of heaven, California laurel, mountain laurel, spice-bush [English]. Benjuí, bálsamo del cielo, laurel de California [Spanish]. Loureiro da California [Portuguese].
Life form: Tree. **Part(s) Used:** Leaf collected before bloom / Fresh-Dried. **Geographic distribution:** Southwest North America (United States of America).
Reference(s): Dorta Soares, n.d.; Müntz, n.d.

Origanum

Scientific Name(s) / [Botanical Family]: *Origanum majorana* L. = *Majorana hortensis* Moench = *Majorana majorana* (L.) H. Karst [Lamiaceae, Labiatae].
Common Name(s): Sweet marjoram [English]. Marjolaine des jardins [French]. Majerona, manjerona [Portuguese]. Mejorana, orégano [Spanish].
Life form: Herb. **Part(s) Used:** Leaf, aerial part in recently bloom / Fresh. **Geographic distribution:** Temperate-Asia. Europe. Extensively cultivated & sometimes naturalized in mediterranean's region.
Reference(s): Bharatan *et al.* 2002; Bolte *et al.* 1997; Clarke, 2008; Dorta Soares, n.d.; Müntz, n.d.

Origanum vulgare

Scientific Name(s) / [Botanical Family]: *Origanum vulgare* L. = *Origanum glandulosum* Desf. & 6 synonyms más. [Lamiaceae, Labiatae].

Common Name(s): Wild marjoram [English]. Origan vulgaire [French]. Orégano [Spanish]. Manjerona selvagem, orégano [Portuguese].

Life form: Herb. **Part(s) Used:** Complete plant with flowers / Fresh. **Geographic distribution:** Asia, North Africa. Europe, cultivated in several places.

Reference(s): Bharatan *et al.* 2002; Dorta Soares, n.d.; Fuentes, 1996; Guermonprez *et al.* 1989; Müntz, n.d.; Plants for a future, 2009; Tiwari *et al.* 2013.

Ornithogalum umbellatum

Scientific Name(s) / [Botanical Family]: *Ornithogalum umbellatum* L. = *Ornithogalum angustifolium* Boreau, = *Scilla campestris* Savi [Hyacinthaceae, Liliaceae].

Common Name(s): Nap-at-noon, sleepy-dick, star-of-Bethlehem [English]. Dame de onze heures, ornithogale in ombelle [French]. Bella di undici ore [Italian]. Estrela-de-Belém, leite de galinha [Portuguese]. Dama de las once, estrella de Belén, leche de gallina, leche de pájaro, ornitógalo [Spanish].

Life form: Herb. **Part(s) Used:** Complete plant / fresh; bulb & leaves / Fresh. **Geographic distribution:** Temperate-Asia. Europe (Mediterranean).

Reference(s): Bharatan *et al.* 2002; Dorta Soares, n.d.; Müntz, n.d.; Tiwari *et al.* 2013.

Orthosiphon stamineus

Scientific Name(s) / [Botanical Family]: *Orthosiphon aristatus* (Blume) Miq. = *Orthosiphon spiralis* auct. = *Orthosiphon stamineus* Benth = *Clerodendranthus spicatus* (Thunb.) C. Y. Wu

ex H. W. Li = *Clerodendrum spicatum* Thunb. [Lamiaceae, Labiatae].
Common Name(s): Cat's-whiskers, Java-tea [English]. Thé de Java [French]. Té de riñón [Spanish]. Bariflora, chá de Java [Portuguese].
Life form: Herb. **Part(s) Used:** Leaf collected before bloom / Dried. **Geographic distribution:** Temperate-Asia (China). Tropical-Asia (Indo-China, Malasia). Australia.
Reference(s): Bharatan *et al.* 2002; Dorta Soares, n.d.; Müntz, n.d.

Ostrya

Scientific Name(s) / [Botanical Family]: *Ostrya virginiana* (Mill.) K. Koch = *Carpinus virginiana* Mill. [Betulaceae].
Common Name(s): Hop-hornbeam, ironwood, lever-wood [English]. Guapaque [Spanish].
Life form: Tree. **Part(s) Used:** Branches and woood / Dried; marrow's wood. **Geographic distribution:** North America (East Canada & United States of America).
Reference(s): Bharatan *et al.* 2002; Dorta Soares, n.d.; Fuentes, 1996; Müntz, n.d.

Ostrya virginica see *Ostrya*

Oxalis acetosa

Scientific Name(s) / [Botanical Family]: *Oxalis acetosella* L. = *Oxalis montana* Raf. [Oxalidaceae].
Common Name(s): Cuckoo-bread, European wood-sorrel, Irish shamrock, wood-sorrel [English]. Alleluia [French]. Acetosella [Italian]. Azedinha [Portuguese]. Acederilla, agritos [Spanish]. Azeda, azeda de trës folhaas, azeda dos bosques [Portuguese].
Life form: Herb. **Part(s) Used:** Complete plant in bloom / Fresh; flower / Dried. **Geographic distribution:** Temperate-Asia. Europe. North America.

Reference(s): Bharatan *et al.* 2002; Bolte *et al.* 1997; Clarke, 2008; Dorta Soares, n.d.; Müntz, n.d.; Tiwari *et al.* 2013.

Oxydendrum arboreum

Scientific Name(s) / [Botanical Family]: *Oxydendrum arboreum* (L.) DC. = *Andromeda arborea* L. [Ericaceae].
Common Name(s): Elk tree, sorrel tree, sour wood [English]. Oxidendro [Spanish]. Árvore azeda [Portuguese].
Life form: Tree. **Part(s) Used:** Leaf / Fresh. **Geographic distribution:** North America (East Canada & United States of America).
Reference(s): Bharatan *et al.* 2002; Dorta Soares, n.d.; Müntz, n.d.

Oxytropis see also *Astragalus lambertii*

Oxytropis

Scientific Name(s) / [Botanical Family]: *Oxytropis lambertii* Pursh = *Aragallus lambertii* (Pursh) Green = *Astragalus lambertii* (Pursh) Spreng. [Fabaceae, Leguminosae]. This remedy includes *Oxytropis campestris* Hook.
Common Name(s): Hierba loca [Spanish]. Lambert's crazyweed, lambert's locoweed, "loco" weed, purple locoweed, rattle-weed [English].
Life form: Herb. **Part(s) Used:** Complete plant (without root) / Fresh. **Geographic distribution:** North America (West Canada. North Central, Northwest, South Central & Southwest United States of America. North Mexico).
Reference(s): Bharatan *et al.* 2002; Müntz, n.d.; Tiwari *et al.* 2013; American Institute of Homeopathy, 1979.

Oxytropis campestris see *Astragallus lamberti*

Oxytropis lambertii see *Astragalus lambertii*

Ozothamnus diosmifolius

Scientific Name(s) / [Botanical Family]: *Ozothamnus diosmifolius* (Vent.) DC. [Asteraceae, Compositae].
Common Name(s): Riceflower, white-dogwood [English].
Life form: Shrub. **Part(s) Used:** Flower, leaf / Fresh. **Geographic distribution:** Australia & cultivated.
Reference(s): Bharatan *et al.* 2002; Clarke, 2008; Müntz, n.d.

Padus avium see *Prunus padus*

Paeonia officinalis

Scientific Name(s) / [Botanical Family]: *Paeonia officinalis* L. [Ranunculaceae, Paeoniaceae].
Common Name(s): Common peony, double peony [English]. Pivoine [French]. Erva de Santa Rosa, rosa albardeira [Portuguese].
Life form: Herb. **Part(s) Used:** Root / Fresh; flowers / Dried.
Geographic distribution: Europe (France-Albania).
Reference(s): Bharatan *et al.* 2002; Dorta Soares, n.d.; Remedia/at, 2010; Tiwari *et al.* 2013.

Papaver orientale

Scientific Name(s) / [Botanical Family]: *Papaver orientale* L. = *Papaver grandiflorum* Moench. = *Papaver orientale* var. *paucifoliatum* Trautv. = *Papaver bracteatum* Lindl. = *Papaver paucifoliatum* (Trautv.) Fedde [Papaveraceae].

Common Name(s): Oriental poppy [English]. Pavot d'Orient [French]. Papoula orinetal [Portuguese]. Amapola oriental [Spanish].
Life form: Herb. **Part(s) Used:** seeds / Fresh. **Geographic distribution:** Temperate-Asia. Naturalized in North America.
Reference(s): Bharatan *et al.* 2002; Müntz, n.d.; American Institute of Homeopathy, 1979.

Papaver rhoeas

Scientific Name(s) / [Botanical Family]: *Papaver rhoeas* L. [Papaveraceae].
Common Name(s): Corn poppy, field poppy, Flanders poppy [English]. Coquelicot [French]. Ababol, adormidera, amapola, amapola de China [Spanish]. Borboleta, dormideira, papoula [Portuguese].
Life form: Herb. **Part(s) Used:** Flower, leaf / Fresh; flower / Dried. **Geographic distribution:** Africa. Temperate-Asia. Europe. Naturalized in North America.
Reference(s): Dorta Soares, n.d.; Müntz, n.d.; Remedia/at, 2010; Tiwari *et al.* 2013.

Parietaria

Scientific Name(s) / [Botanical Family]: *Parietaria officinalis* L. [Urticaceae].
Common Name(s): Pellitory-of-the-wall, wall pellitory [English]. Alfavaca de obra, erva de Santa Ana [Portuguese].
Life form: Herb. **Part(s) Used:** Aerial part in bloom / Fresh.
Geographic distribution: Temperate-Asia. Europe.
Reference(s): Bharatan *et al.* 2002; Bolte *et al.* 1997; Dorta Soares, n.d.; Müntz, n.d.; Seror, 2000.

Paris

Scientific Name(s) / [Botanical Family]: *Paris quadrifolia* L.

[Melanthiaceae, Liliaceae, Trilliaceae].

Common Name(s): Four-leaf ed grass, fox grape, herb Paris [English]. Parisette, raisin de renard [French]. Uva lupulina [Portuguese].

Life form: Herb. **Part(s) Used:** Complete plant / Fresh collected during fruits ripening; Complete plant in bloom / Fresh.

Geographic distribution: Europe, England.

Reference(s): Bharatan *et al.* 2002; Dorta Soares, n.d.; Müntz, n.d.

Paronichia illecebrum (Paronychia)

Scientific Name(s) / [Botanical Family]: *Alternanthera repens* (L.) Kuntze = *Alternanthera repens* Steud. = *Achyranthes repens* L. = *Achyranthes repens* Ell. = *Achyranthes repens* Heyne = *Peronichia illecebrum?*) [Amaranthaceae].

Common Name(s): Algerian tea, sanguinaria of Cuba, silvery paronychia [English]. Amara, cabalxtez, tiangüis pepetla [Spanish].

Life form: Herb. **Part(s) Used:** Complete plant / Fresh.

Geographic distribution: Mexico. Turkey.

Reference(s): Bharatan *et al.* 2002; Dorta Soares, n.d.; Müntz, n.d.; Plants for a future, 2009; Tiwari *et al.* 2013; American Institute of Homeopathy, 1979.

Parthenium

Scientific Name(s) / [Botanical Family]: *Parthenium hysterophorus* L. = *Parthenium lobatum* Buckley = *Parthenium pinnatifidum* Stokes = *Echetrosis pentasperma* Phil. = *Argyrochaeta parviflora* Cav. [Asteraceae, Compositae].

Common Name(s): Bitterweed, carrot-grass, false ragweed, feverfew, parthenium-weed, ragweed parthenium, Santa Maria, Santa Maria feverfew, whitetop [English]. Altamisa, amargo, amargosa, arrocillo, chaile, cicutilla, confitilla, escoba amarga,

hauay, hierba amarga, hierba amargosa, hierba del burro, hierba del gusano, huachochole, jihuite amargo, tzaile, tzail-cuet, zacate amargo [Spanish].
Life form: Herb. **Part(s) Used:** Complete plant / Dried.
Geographic distribution: Africa. Asia. North America (North & Central Mexico). Caribe. Central & South America. Madagascar. Extensively naturalized in several places.
Reference(s): Bharatan *et al.* 2002; De Legarreta, 1961; Müntz, n.d.; Tiwari *et al.* 2013; American Institute of Homeopathy, 1979.

Passiflora incarnata

Scientific Name(s) / [Botanical Family]: *Passiflora incarnata* L. = *Passiflora incarnata* Ker.-Gawl = *Passiflora incarnata* Gaul. = *Passiflora edulis* Sims. [Passifloraceae].
Common Name(s): Apricot-vine, granadilla, maypop, maypop passionflower, passionflower [English]. Barbadine [French]. Clavos del Señor, Flor de la pasión, granada china, granadita de China, granadilla, pasionaria, túnica de Cristo [Spanish]. Maracujá, passiflora [Portuguese].
Life form: Herb. **Part(s) Used:** Aerial part / Fresh; flower, leaves / Dried. **Geographic distribution:** East North America. Central America. Cultivated.
Reference(s): Bharatan *et al.* 2002; Dorta Soares, n.d.; Müntz, n.d.; Tiwari *et al.* 2013; Zandvoort, 2006.

Pastinaca sativa

Scientific Name(s) / [Botanical Family]: *Pastinaca sativa* L. = *Pastinaca urens* Req. ex Godr. [Apiaceae, Umbelliferae].
Common Name(s): Parsnip, wild parsnip [English]. Panais [French]. Chirivi, pastinaca [Spanish]. Cenoura branca, chirivia, pastinaca [Portuguese].
Life form: Herb. **Part(s) Used:** Root / Fresh collected during the

second year of the plant life. **Geographic distribution:** Temperate-Asia. Europe. Naturalized in Africa, Australia, Canada, South America & United States of America.
Reference(s): Bharatan *et al.* 2002; Comisión Editora de la Farmacopea Homeopática de los Estados Unidos Mexicanos, 1988; Dorta Soares, n.d.; Müntz, n.d.; Plants for a future, 2009; Tiwari *et al.* 2013; American Institute of Homeopathy, 1979.

Peganum harmala

Scientific Name(s) / [Botanical Family]: *Peganum harmala* L. [Nitrariaceae, Peganaceae, Zygophyllaceae].
Common Name(s): African-rue, Syrian-rue, wild rue [English]. Rue sauvage [French]. Harmel [Indian]. Alharma, gamarza, ruda Siria [Spanish].
Life form: Shrub. **Part(s) Used:** seeds / Dried. **Geographic distribution:** Temperate-Asia. Europe. Naturalized in several places.
Reference(s): Bharatan *et al.* 2002; Müntz, n.d.; American Institute of Homeopathy, 1979.

Pelargonium odoratissimum

Scientific Name(s) / [Botanical Family]: *Pelargonium odoratissimum* Ait. = *Pelargonium odoratissimum* Soland. = *Pelargonium odoratissimum* (L.) L'Hér. = *Geranium odoratissimum* L. [Geraniaceae].
Common Name(s): Apple geranium, sweet-scent pelargonium [English]. Géranium, geranium rosat [French]. Geranio. Geranio de olor, geranio rosa, malva, malva de olor, malvón [Spanish]. Gerânio, jardineira [Portuguese].
Life form: Herb. **Part(s) Used:** Complete plant, flower / Fresh.
Geographic distribution: Africa. Mexico. Cultivated.
Reference(s): Dorta Soares, n.d.; Müntz, n.d.; Rowe, 2006.

Penthorum sedoides

Scientific Name(s) / [Botanical Family]: *Penthorum sedoides* L. [Crassulaceae, Penthoraceae, Saxifragaceae].

Common Name(s): Ditch stonecrop, Virginia penthorum, Virginia stonecrop [English]. Pinhão de rato [Portuguese].

Life form: Herb. **Part(s) Used:** Complete plant / Fresh.

Geographic distribution: North America (East & West Canada. United States of America).

Reference(s): Bharatan *et al.* 2002; Dorta Soares, n.d.; Seror, 2000; Tiwari *et al.* 2013.

Perilla frutescens

Scientific Name(s) / [Botanical Family]: *Perilla frutescens* (L.) Britton = *Perilla ocymoides* L. [Lamiaceae, Labiatae].

Common Name(s): Beefsteak-mint, beefsteakplant, perilla. Périlla [French]. Shiso-zoku [Japanese]. Perilla [Spanish].

Life form: Herb. **Part(s) Used:** Aerial part / Fresh. **Geographic distribution:** Temperate-Asia. Extensively cultivated & naturalized.

Reference(s): Bharatan *et al.* 2002; Bolte *et al.* 1997; Dorta Soares, n.d.; Müntz, n.d.; Tiwari *et al.* 2013; American Institute of Homeopathy, 1979.

Periploca graeca

Scientific Name(s) / [Botanical Family]: *Periploca graeca* (L.) Schult. [Asclepiadaceae].

Common Name(s): Silkvine [English]. Periploca [Spanish].

Life form: Herb. **Part(s) Used:** Stem. **Geographic distribution:** Temperate-Asia. South Europe. Naturalized in Mediterranean region.

Reference(s): Bharatan *et al.* 2002; Müntz, n.d.; Remedia/at, 2010.

Persea americana

Scientific Name(s) / [Botanical Family]: *Persea americana* Mill = *Persea gratissima* Gaertn. = *Persea leiogyna* S.F. Blake = *Persea persea* (L.) Cockerell = *Laurus persea* L. [Lauraceae].

Common Name(s): Avocado, avocado pear, alligator pear, butter pear, trapp avocado, west-indian avocado [English]. Avocat, avocatier [French]. Aguacate, ahuacate, aguacatillo, ahoacaquáhuitl, ahuacaquáhuitl, cupanda, cupandram pagua, palta, palto, tonalahuate [Spanish]. Abacate, abacateriro [Portuguese].

Life form: Tree. **Part(s) Used:** Fruit complete seeds included; seed-bark or also epicarp. **Geographic distribution:** cultivated through Mexico & in several regions.

Reference(s): Bharatan *et al.* 2002; Bolte *et al.* 1997; Dorta Soares, n.d.; Tiwari *et al.* 2013.

Petiveria

Scientific Name(s) / [Botanical Family]: *Petiveria tetrandra* B. A. Gomes = *Petiveria alliacea* L. var. *tetrandra* (B.A. Gomes) Hauman = *Petiveria hexaglochin* Fisch. & C. A. Mey [Phytolaccaceae].

Common Name(s): Congo root, garlic leed, Guinea hen-plant, gully root [English]. Apacina, hierba de las gallinitas, hierba del zorrillo, anamú [Spanish]. Amansa senhor, ecoembp, embiaembo [Portuguese].

Life form: Herb. **Part(s) Used:** Root / Fresh / Dried; leaf / Dried collected during bloom. **Geographic distribution:** South & South Central United States of America. North & Central Mexico. Caribe. Central & South America.

Reference(s): Bharatan *et al.* 2002; Bolte *et al.* 1997; American Institute of Homeopathy, 1979.

Petroselinum

Scientific Name(s) / [Botanical Family]: *Petroselinum crispum* (Mill.) Nym. ex A. W. Hill = *Apium petroselinum* L. = *Apium crispum* Mill. = *Petroselinum sativum* Hoefn. = *Carum petroselinum* (L.) Benth. & Hook. f. [Apiaceae, Umbelliferae].
Common Name(s): Common parsley, parsley [English]. Persil commun [French]. Perejil [Spanish].
Life form: Herb. **Part(s) Used:** Complete plant / Fresh.
Geographic distribution: Extensively cultivated & naturalized.
Reference(s): Allen, 2006-2010; Bharatan *et al.* 2002; Clarke, 2008; Fuentes, 1996; Müntz, n.d.; Tiwari *et al.* 2013; Zandvoort, 2006.

Petroselinum sativum see *Petroselinum*

Peumus boldus

Scientific Name(s) / [Botanical Family]: *Peumus boldus* (L.) Molina = *Boldea fragrans* (Ruiz & Pav.) Gay = *Peumus fragrans* Ruiz & Pavón [Monimiaceae, Nyctaginaceae].
Common Name(s): Boldo, Boldo tree, boldu [English]. Boldo [Spanish, French]. Boldo, boldo do Chile [Portuguese].
Life form: Tree. **Part(s) Used:** Leaf / Dried; leaves collected during the bloom. **Geographic distribution:** South America (Chile).
Reference(s): Allen, 2006-2010; Bharatan *et al.* 2002; Dorta Soares, n.d.; American Institute of Homeopathy, 1979.

Phaseolus

Scientific Name(s) / [Botanical Family]: *Phaseolus vulgaris* L. = *Phaseolus compressus* DC. = *Phaseolus ellipticus* Schur = *Phaseolus gonospermus* Savi = *Phaseolus nanus* L. = *Phaseolus oblongus* Savi = *Phaseolus sphaericus* Savi = *Phaseolus zebra* Fingerh.; all the species with different varieties. [Fabaceae,

Leguminosae].
Common Name(s): Bean, common bean, French bean [English]. Haricot [French]. Feijão [Portuguese]. Frijol, frijol blanco, frijol colorado, frijol colorado de bolita, frijol negro, frijol prieto, habichuela, judía, poroto, thatzin [Spanish]. Feijão [Portuguese].
Life form: Herb. **Part(s) Used:** Complete plant in bloom / Fresh; fruit & seeds / Dried. **Geographic distribution:** cultivated & naturalized around the world.
Reference(s): Bharatan *et al.* 2002; Bolte *et al.* 1997; Dorta Soares, n.d.; Müntz, n.d.; Tiwari *et al.* 2013.

Phaseolus lunatus

Scientific Name(s) / [Botanical Family]: *Phaseolus lunatus* L. (wih different varieties) = *Phaseolus falcatus* Benth. ex Hemsl. = *Phaseolus inamoenus* L. = *Phaseolus limensis* Macfad. = *Phaseolus macrocarpus* Moench = *Phaseolus tunkinensis* Lour. = *Phaseolus viridis* Piper [Fabaceae, Leguminosae].
Common Name(s): Haba bean, Lima bean, pallar bean, Burma bean, sugar bean [English]. Haricot de Lima. haricot du Cap, pois du Cap [French]. Feijão-de-Lima, fava-Belém [Portuguese]. Frijol blanco, frijol de luna, haba lima, judía de Lima, pallar. [Spanish].
Life form: Herb. **Part(s) Used:** Seeds. **Geographic distribution:** America. Extensively cultivated & naturalized.
Reference(s): Bharatan *et al.* 2002; Clarke, 2008; Plants for a future, 2009; Vithoulkas, n.d.

Phaseolus nanus see *Phaseolus vulgaris*

Phellandrium

Scientific Name(s) / [Botanical Family]: *Oenanthe aquatica* (L.) Poir. = *Oenanthe phellandrium* Lam. = *Phellandrium aquaticum* L. [Apiaceae, Umbelliferae].
Common Name(s): Fine-leaf ewater-dropwort, water-fennel, water-hemlock [English]. Cicuta aquática, erva pombinha,

felandrio [Portuguese].
Life form: Herb. **Part(s) Used:** Fruit mature / Fresh / Dried; root / Fresh; seeds / Dried. **Geographic distribution:** Temperate-Asia. Europe.
Reference(s): Bharatan *et al.* 2002; Dorta Soares, n.d.; Müntz, n.d.; Tiwari *et al.* 2013.

Philadelphus coronarius

Scientific Name(s) / [Botanical Family]: *Philadelphus coronarius* L. [Hydrangeaceae, Philadelphaceae].
Common Name(s): Sweet mockorange [English]. Seringat [French]. Celinda, filadelfo, jeringuilla, falso jazmín, falso naranjo, jazmín mosqueta, mosqueta [Spanish]. Filadelfo [Portuguese].
Life form: Shrub. **Part(s) Used:** Flower / Fresh. **Geographic distribution:** Europe. Russia. Cultivated & naturalized in several places.
Reference(s): Bharatan *et al.* 2002; Dorta Soares, n.d.; Plants for a future, 2009; American Institute of Homeopathy, 1979.

Phleum

Scientific Name(s) / [Botanical Family]: *Phleum pratense* L. [Gramineae, Poaceae].
Common Name(s): Meadow cat's-tail, timothy [English]. Fléole des prés [French]. Capim-timóteo, rabo-de-gato [Portuguese]. Cola de topo, fleo, timoti [Spanish].
Life form: Herb. **Part(s) Used:** Aerial part / Fresh. **Geographic distribution:** North Africa. Temperate & tropical Asia. Europe. Australia.
Reference(s): Müntz, n.d.

Phragmites vulgaris

Scientific Name(s) / [Botanical Family]: *Phragmites vulgaris*

(Lam.) Crép. = *Phragmites australis* (Cav.) Trin. ex Steud. = *Arundo vulgaris* Lam. [Gramineae, Poaceae].
Common Name(s): Common reed, ditch reed, giant reed, phragmites, reed grass [English]. Phragmite commun, roseau commun [French]. Caniço [Portuguese]. Carrizo común [Spanish].
Life form: Herb. **Part(s) Used:** Roots. **Geographic distribution:** Europe. Extensively naturalized.
Reference(s): Bharatan *et al.* 2002; Seror, 2000; Müntz, n.d.

Phyla scaberrima see *Lippia mexicana*

Phyllitis scolopendrium
Scientific Name(s) / [Botanical Family]: *Asplenium scolopendrium* L. = *Phyllitis scolopendrium* (L.) Newman [Aspleniaceae].
Common Name(s): Hart's-tongue fern [English]. Helecho [Spanish]. Escolopendra [Portuguese].
Life form: Herb. **Part(s) Used:** Complete plant / Fresh.
Geographic distribution: Africa. Temperate-Asia. Europe. Cultivated in several places.
Reference(s): Dorta Soares, n.d.; Müntz, n.d.

Physalis
Scientific Name(s) / [Botanical Family]: *Physalis alkekengi* L. = *Physalis bunyardii* hort. = *Physalis alkekengi* var. *franchetii* = *Physalis franchetii* Mast. [Solanaceae].
Common Name(s): Alkekengi, bladderherb, cape gooseberry, chinese-lantern, japanese-lantern, lantern, strawberry groundcherry, strawberry tomato, winter-cherry [English]. Alkékenge, coqueret, lanterne, lanterne chinoise [French]. Alkekengi, alquequenje, cereja de invierno [Portuguese]. Alicacabí, alquequenje, capulí, farolito, tomate de culebra, tomate inglés, vejiga de perro [Spanish].

Life form: Herb. **Part(s) Used:** Fruit mature / Fresh. **Geographic distribution:** Temperate & tropical Asia. Europe. Extensively naturalized in temperate regions.
Reference(s): Bharatan *et al.* 2002; Dorta Soares, n.d.; Gotfredsen, 2009; Müntz, n.d.

Physalis peruviana

Scientific Name(s) / [Botanical Family]: *Physalis peruviana* L. [Solanaceae].
Common Name(s): Cape-gooseberry, golden berry, gooseberry-tomato, Peruvian ground-cherry, Peruvian-cherry. Capuli, coqueret du Peru [French]. Groselha-do-Peru, bate-testa [Portuguese]. Alquequenje, capulí, cereza del Peru, tomate, tomatl, uvilla [Spanish].
Life form: Shrub. **Part(s) Used:** Complete plant. **Geographic distribution:** Extensively cultivated.
Reference(s): Bharatan *et al.* 2002; Fuentes, 1996; Müntz, n.d.; Plants for a future, 2009; Remedia/at, 2010.

Phytolacca decandra

Scientific Name(s) / [Botanical Family]: *Phytolacca decandra* L. = *Phytolacca americana* L. [Phytolaccaceae].
Common Name(s): American nightshade, clakum, chougras, garget-weed, poke, pokeweed [English]. Morellař grppes, raisin d'Amerique, teinturière [French]. Cóngora, hierba carmín, namole [Spanish]. Carurú bravo, erva da America, erva de laca [Portuguese].
Life form: Liana. **Part(s) Used:** Fruit, leaf, root / Fresh; complete plant with mature fruits / Fresh. **Geographic distribution:** North & Central North America. Mediterranean. Cultivated in several places.
Reference(s): Bharatan *et al.* 2002; Dorta Soares, n.d.; Remedia/at, 2010; Tiwari *et al.* 2013.

Pichi pichi

Scientific Name(s) / [Botanical Family]: *Fabiana imbricata* Ruiz & Pavón [Solanaceae].

Common Name(s): Pichi pichi [Spanish]. Fabiana, pichi pichi [Portuguese].

Life form: Herb. **Part(s) Used:** Branch with leaves / Dried.

Geographic distribution: South America (Argentine, Chile).

Reference(s): Allen, 2006-2010; Bharatan *et al.* 2002; Clarke, 2008; Dorta Soares, n.d.; Müntz, n.d.; Plants for a future, 2009; Tiwari *et al.* 2013; American Institute of Homeopathy, 1979.

Pimpinella anisum

Scientific Name(s) / [Botanical Family]: *Pimpinella anisum* L. [Apiaceae, Umbelliferae].

Common Name(s): Anise, sweet-cumin [English]. Anis vert, anis [French]. Erva-doce [Portuguese]. Anís [Spanish].

Life form: Herb. **Part(s) Used:** Root / Fresh. **Geographic distribution:** Extensively cultivated in temperate regions.

Reference(s): Dorta Soares, n.d.; Müntz, n.d.; Tiwari *et al.* 2013.

Pimpinella saxifraga

Scientific Name(s) / [Botanical Family]: *Pimpinella saxifraga* L. = *Pimpinella alba* Gueldenst [Apiaceae].

Common Name(s): Bibermell, Burneo saxifrage, pimpinel, saxifrage [English]. Grand boucage [French]. Pimpinella [Spanish]. Saxifraga minor [Portuguese].

Life form: Herb. **Part(s) Used:** Root / Fresh. **Geographic distribution:** North Europe. Temperate-Asia (Iraq, Iran, Turkey, Siberia, etc.).

Reference(s): Bharatan *et al.* 2002; Bolte *et al.* 1997; Dorta Soares, n.d.; Fuentes, 1996; Müntz, n.d.; Remedia/at, 2010; Tiwari *et al.* 2013.

Pinguicula vulgaris

Scientific Name(s) / [Botanical Family]: *Pinguicula vulgaris* L. [Lentibulariaceae].

Common Name(s): Butterwort, common butterwort, marsh violet, Yorkshire sanicle [English]. Grassette vulgaire, grassette commune [French]. Grasilla, tieraña [Spanish].

Life form: Herb. **Part(s) Used:** Complete plant. **Geographic distribution:** Europe, North America (Canada. United States of America). North Asia.

Reference(s): Bharatan *et al.* 2002; Clarke, 2008; Remedia/at, 2010; American Institute of Homeopathy, 1979.

Pinus abies

Scientific Name(s) / [Botanical Family]: *Pinus abies* Mill. = *Picea abies* (L.) H. Karst [Pinaceae].

Common Name(s): Norway spruce, white spruce [English]. Épicéa [French].

Life form: Tree. **Part(s) Used:** Tiller / Fresh. **Geographic distribution:** Europe. Naturalized in several regions.

Reference(s): Gotfredsen, 2009; Plants for a future, 2009.

Pinus cembra

Scientific Name(s) / [Botanical Family]: *Pinus cembra* L. = *Pinus cembra* Thunb. [Pinaceae].

Common Name(s): Swiss pine, Arolla pine [English]. Pin [French].

Life form: Tree. **Part(s) Used:** Seeds. **Geographic distribution:** Europe, Asia.

Reference: Müntz, n.d.

Pinus lambertiana

Scientific Name(s) / [Botanical Family]: *Pinus lambertiana*

Douglas [Pinaceae].
Common Name(s): Sugar pine [English]. Pinheiro doce [Portuguese].
Life form: Tree. **Part(s) Used:** Bud, sap / Fresh. **Geographic distribution:** North, West & Southwest of United States of America. North Mexico (Baja California).
Reference(s): Bharatan *et al.* 2002; Dorta Soares, n.d.; Remedia, at/, 2010; USA 1979.

Pinus palustres

Scientific Name(s) / [Botanical Family]: *Pinus palustris* L. [Pinaceae].
Common Name(s): Longleaf pine, longleaf yellow pine, pitch pine, southern pine, southern yellow pine [English]. Chang ye song [Chinese]. Pitchpin du Sud [French].
Life form: Tree. **Part(s) Used:** The resin from the trunk of the tree? / Fresh. **Geographic distribution:** North America (South United States of America).
Reference(s): Bharatan *et al.* 2002; Clarke, 2008.

Pinus pumillionis

Scientific Name(s) / [Botanical Family]: *Pinus montana* Mill. = *Pinus pumilio* (Haenke in Jirazek, *et al.*) Franco [Pinaceae].
Common Name(s): Dwarf pine, mountain pine [English].
Life form: Shrub. **Part(s) Used:** Root resin / Fresh. **Geographic distribution:** Europe.
Reference: Müntz, n.d.

Pinus silvestris

Scientific Name(s) / [Botanical Family]: *Pinus sylvestris* L. = *Pinus sylvestris* Baumg. = *Pinus sylvestris* Lour. = *Pinus sylvestris* Mill. = *Pinus laricio* Poir = *Pinus pinaster* Bess. [Pinaceae].
Common Name(s): Scotch pine, Scots pine [English]. Pin

sylvestre [French]. Pino silvestre [Italian]. Pino silvestris [Spanish]. Pinheiro comum, pinheiro de Genebra, pinheiro da Rússia [Portuguese].
Life form: Tree. **Part(s) Used:** Bud, young branches & leaves, mature fruits / Fresh. **Geographic distribution:** Europe, Temperate-Asia. Cultivated in several places.
Reference(s): Bharatan *et al.* 2002; Dorta Soares, n.d.; Remedia/at, 2010; Tiwari *et al.* 2013.

Pinus teocote

Scientific Name(s) / [Botanical Family]: *Pinus teocote* Schiede ex Schltdl. [Pinaceae].
Common Name(s): Jalocote, ocote, ocotl, pino, pino real, pino colorado, teocote, teocotl, tos'arza, tzal'adi, xalocotl [Spanish].
Life form: Tree. **Part(s) Used:** Sap. / Fresh, the resin from the trunk of the tree. **Geographic distribution:** North America (Mexico).
Reference(s): Bharatan *et al.* 2002; Müntz, n.d.; Provings, 2008-2009; Remedia/at, 2010; American Institute of Homeopathy, 1979; Zandvoort, 2006.

Pistacia lentiscus

Scientific Name(s) / [Botanical Family]: *Pistacia lentiscus* L. [Anacardiaceae].
Common Name(s): Chios mastictree, mastic, mastictree [English]. Arbre au mastic, lentisque [French]. Almecegueira [Portuguese]. Lentisco [Spanish].
Life form: Tree. **Part(s) Used:** Root resin / Fresh. **Geographic distribution:** Africa & Mediterranean.
Reference: American Institute of Homeopathy, 1979.

Plantago lanceolata

Scientific Name(s) / [Botanical Family]: *Plantago lanceolata* L.

[Plantaginaceae].
Common Name(s): Buckhorn, buckhorn plantain, English plantain, ribgrass, ribwort, ribwort plantain [English]. Petit plantain [French]. Tanchagem-Minor [Portuguese]. Llantén Minor [Spanish].
Life form: Herb. **Part(s) Used:** Complete plant / Fresh.
Geographic distribution: North America, Asia, Europe, naturalized in several places.
Reference(s): Dorta Soares, n.d.; Müntz, n.d.

Plantago major

Scientific Name(s) / [Botanical Family]: *Plantago major* L. = *Plantago major* Bert. ex Barnéoud = *Plantago major* Ell. = *Plantago major* Lour. = *Plantago berteroi* Steinh ex Decne. = *Plantago major* ssp. *intermedia* (DC.) Arcangeli [Plantaginaceae].
Common Name(s): Broadleaf plantain, common plantain, greater plantain, plantain [English]. Grand plantain, plantain majeur [French]. Tanchagem-maior [Portuguese]. Lanté, lantén, llantén, uitzuaqua sipiati [Spanish].
Life form: Herb. **Part(s) Used:** Complete plant in bloom / Fresh; leaf / Dried. **Geographic distribution:** Cosmopolitan, wickedness considered around the world.
Reference(s): Bharatan *et al.* 2002; Dorta Soares, n.d.; Remedia/at, 2010; Tiwari *et al.* 2013.

Plantago minor

Scientific Name(s) / [Botanical Family]: *Plantago minor* Garsault = *Plantago minor* Gilib. *Plantago minor* Fries = *Plantago tenuiflora* Waldst. & Kit. [Plantaginaceae].
Common Name(s): Common plantain [English]. Llantén menor [Spanish].
Life form: Herb. **Part(s) Used:** Complete plant, root? / Fresh.
Geographic distribution: Europe.

Reference(s): Bharatan *et al.* 2002; Müntz, n.d.; Remedia/at, 2010; American Institute of Homeopathy, 1979. Zandvoort, 2006.

Platanus acerifolia

Scientific Name(s) / [Botanical Family]: *Platanus x acerifolia* (Aiton) Willd. [Platanaceae].
Common Name(s): Platan, sycamore butterwood, sycamore-buttonwood, London planetree [English]. Fa guo wu tong [Chinese]. Plátano de paseo [Spanish].
Life form: Tree. **Part(s) Used:** Bark rama, tillers (buds) / Fresh.
Geographic distribution: cultivated.
Reference(s): Bharatan *et al.* 2002; Zandvoort, 2006.

Platanus acerifolia see *Platanus occidentalis*

Platanus occidentalis

Scientific Name(s) / [Botanical Family]: *Platanus x hispanica* Mill. ex Münch. = *Platanus occidentalis* L. = *Platanus lobata* Moench = *Platanus vulgaris* var. *angulosa* Spach = *Platanus densicoma* Dode = *Platanus escelsa* Salisb. = *Platanus glabrata* Fernald = *Platanus integrifolia* Hort. ex C. Koch [Platanaceae].
Common Name(s): American plane, American sycamore, buttonball, button-weed, sycamore [English]. Álamo, plátano de occidente, sicamoro [Spanish]. Plátano americano, sicômoro [Portuguese].
Life form: Tree. **Part(s) Used:** Buds, bark / Fresh. **Geographic distribution:** North America (East Canada. North East, North Central, Southeast & South Central United States of America). Cultivated in other regions.
Reference(s): Bharatan *et al.* 2002; Boericke, 1927, 1927b.; Bolte *et al.* 1997; Clarke, 2008; Dorta Soares, n.d.; Müntz, n.d.; Remedia/at, 2010.

Platanus orientalis see *Platanus occidentalis*

Platycerium bifurcatum

Scientific Name(s) / [Botanical Family]: *Platycerium bifurcatum* (Cav.) C. Chr. [Polypodiaceae].
Common Name(s): Common staghorn fern, elkhorn fern [English].
Life form: Herb. **Part(s) Used:** Complete plant. **Geographic distribution:** Australia.
Reference: Bharatan *et al.* 2002.

Plumbago capensis

Scientific Name(s) / [Botanical Family]: *Plumbago capensis* Thunb. = *Plumbago auriculata* Lam. [Plumbaginaceae].
Common Name(s): Cape plumbago [English]. Belesa, embelesa, jazmín azul, jazmín del cielo, plúmbago [Spanish].
Life form: Herb. **Part(s) Used:** Leaf. **Geographic distribution:** cultivated.
Reference(s): Müntz, n.d.; Remedia/at, 2010.

Plumeria celinus

Scientific Name(s) / [Botanical Family]: *Plumeria rubra* L. [Apocynaceae].
Common Name(s): Plume, frangipani, pagoda-tree, red paucipan, red-jasmine, templetree [English]. Hong ji dan hua [Chinese]. Frangipanier [French]. Flor-de-Santo-Antônio, jasmim-do-Pará [Portuguese]. Alhelí, alhelí cimarrón, cacajoyó, cacalosúchil, campechana, cundá, chak-nikté, chak-sabak-nikté, Flor de mayo, jacaloshúchil rojo, lengua de toro, nopinjoyó, suche, súchil [Spanish].
Life form: Tree. **Part(s) Used:** Flower / Fresh. **Geographic distribution:** North America (Central Mexico). Central & South America. Cultivated.

Reference: François-Flores, 2007.

Podophyllum peltatum

Scientific Name(s) / [Botanical Family]: *Podophyllum peltatum* L. [Berberidaceae].
Common Name(s): American mandrake, may apple, wild mandrake, wild lemon [English]. Podophylle peltracute, pomme de mai [French]. Manzana de mayo, podofilo [Spanish]. Limão silvestre, mandrágora, podófilo [Portuguese].
Life form: Herb. **Part(s) Used:** Subterraneous parts / Fresh; complete plant. **Geographic distribution:** North America (East Canada. North East, North Central, Southeast & South Central United States of America).
Reference(s): Bharatan *et al.* 2002; Boericke, 1927, 1927b.; Bolte *et al.* 1997; Dorta Soares, n.d.; Remedia/at, 2010; Tiwari *et al.* 2013; Zandvoort, 2006.

Poinsettia see *Euphorbia pulcherrima*

Polei see *Mentha pulegium*

Polygala amara

Scientific Name(s) / [Botanical Family]: *Polygala amara* L. = *Polygala amarella* Crtz. = *Polygala ulginosa* Rchb. = *Polygala amarum* L. = *Polygala austriaca* Crantz [Polygalaceae].
Common Name(s): Milkwort [English]. Polygale amer [French]. Polígala amarga, polígala oficinal [Spanish]. Polígala [Portuguese].
Life form: Herb. **Part(s) Used:** Complete plant in bloom / Fresh.
Geographic distribution: Europe.
Reference(s): Dorta Soares, n.d.; Müntz, n.d.; Remedia/at, 2010.

Polygala senega see *Senega*

Polygonatum officinale

Scientific Name(s) / [Botanical Family]: *Polygonatum odoratum* (Mill.) Druce = *Polygonatum japonicum* C. Morren & Decne. = *Polygonatum officinale* All. = *Convallaria odorata* Mill. [Ruscaceae, Convallariaceae, Liliaceae].
Common Name(s): Angular Solomon's-seal, aromatic Solomon's-seal, Solomon's-seal [English]. Yu zhu [Chinese]. Sceau de Salomon [French]. Beata María, poligonato, sello de Salomón, soldaconsolda [Spanish].
Life form: Herb. **Part(s) Used:** Complete plant - Flower? / Fresh.
Geographic distribution: Temperate-Asia. Europe.
Reference(s): Bharatan *et al.* 2002; Bolte *et al.* 1997; Müntz, n.d.; Plants for a future, 2009; American Institute of Homeopathy, 1979; Zandvoort, 2006.

Polygonum aviculare

Scientific Name(s) / [Botanical Family]: *Polygonum aviculare* L. = *Polygonum calcatum* Lindm. = *Polygonum heterophyllum* Lindm. = *Polygonum neglectum* Bess. [Polygonaceae].
Common Name(s): Knotgrass, knotweed, goose-grass, doorweed [English]. Renouée des oiseaux [French]. Centinodia, ciennudos, correhuela of caminos, hierba de las calenturas, lengua de pájaro, pico de gorrión, sanguinaria mayor [Spanish]. Sanguinária [Portuguese]. **Life form:** Herb. **Part(s) Used:** Complete plant / Fresh. Complete plant in bloom. **Geographic distribution:** Mexico. United States of America. Cosmopolitan, wickedness considered within farmings (cultivars) around the world.
Reference(s): Bharatan *et al.* 2002; Dorta Soares, n.d.; Müntz, n.d.; Remedia/at, 2010.

Polygonum hydropiperoides

Scientific Name(s) / [Botanical Family]: *Polygonum punctatum* Elliot = *Polygonum hydropiperoides* Pursh = *Polygonum hydropiper* L. = *Polygonum acre* Kunth = *Persicaria punctata* (Elliot) Small [Polygonaceae].

Common Name(s): Dotted smartweed, hydropiper smartweed, water smart wee [English]. Renouée ponctuée [French]. Acataia, erva de bicho-pontuada [Portuguese]. Chilillo [Spanish].

Life form: Herb. **Part(s) Used:** Complete plant in bloom, leaf / Fresh; leaves / Dried collected before bloom. **Geographic distribution:** Europe (Mediterranean). North Africa. Temperate-Asia. United States of America. Considered wickedness.

Reference(s): Allen, 2006-2010; Bharatan *et al.* 2002; Dorta Soares, n.d.; Guermonprez *et al.* 1989; Müntz, n.d.; Tiwari *et al.* 2013.

Polygonum persicaria

Scientific Name(s) / [Botanical Family]: *Polygonum persicaria* L. = *Persicaria maculosa* S.F. Gray [Polygonaceae].

Common Name(s): Lady's-thumb, redshank, spotted lady's-thumb [English]. Renouée persicaire [French]. Erva-de-bicho, erva-de-pessegueiro [Portuguese]. Altabaquillo, duraznillo, hierba pejiguera, moco de guajolote, persicaria, pimentillo [Spanish].

Life form: Herb. **Part(s) Used:** Complete plant / Fresh. **Geographic distribution:** North America. Europe & Asia.

Reference(s): Allen, 2006-2010; Bharatan *et al.* 2002; Boericke, 1927, 1927b.; Plants for a future, 2009; Remedia/at, 2010; American Institute of Homeopathy, 1979.

Polygonum sagittatum

Scientific Name(s) / [Botanical Family]: *Polygonum sagittatum* L. [Polygonaceae].

Common Name(s): Arrow leaf tear-thumb, false buckwheat [English].
Life form: Herb. **Part(s) Used:** Complete plant / Fresh.
Geographic distribution: North America, United States of America.
Reference: Bharatan *et al*. 2002.

Polygonum viviparum

Scientific Name(s) / [Botanical Family]: *Polygonum viviparum* L. = *Bistorta vivipara* (L.) Delarbre [Polygonaceae].
Common Name(s): Alpine bistort, viviparous knotweed [English].
Life form: Herb. **Part(s) Used:** Complete plant / Fresh.
Geographic distribution: North America (United States of America). Europe, Southwest Asia, Thailand, Russia, India, Japan.
Reference: Bharatan *et al*. 2002.

Polymnia

Scientific Name(s) / [Botanical Family]: *Polymnia uvedalia* (L.) L. = *Smallanthus uvedalia* (L.) Mack. ex Small [Asteraceae, Compositae].
Common Name(s): Bear's-foot, yellow bear's-foot, yellow leaf-cup, yellow-flowered leaf-cup [English]. Polimnia [Spanish].
Life form: Herb. **Part(s) Used:** Aerial part?. **Geographic distribution:** North America (United States of America).
Reference: Bharatan *et al*. 2002.

Polyporus pinicola see *Polyporus pinicolus*

Polyporus pinicolus

Scientific Name(s) / [Botanical Family]: *Polyporus pinicola* Sw. Fr. = *Fomitopsis pinicola* (Sw. = Fr.) P. Karst. = *Boletus pinicola* Sw. = *Fomes pinicola* (Sw.) Fr. [Coriolaceae = Polyporaceae].

Common Name(s): Pine agaric, red-belted polypore, root rot conifers [English]. Pourridie des racines du pin [French]. Tsugasaruno-hoshikake [Japanese]. Podredumbre de las raíces del pino [Spanish]. Agárico pinheiro [Portuguese].
Life form: Fungi. **Part(s) Used:** Complete mushroom / Dried-Fresh. **Geographic distribution:** United States of America. Europe (Polonia).
Reference(s): Bharatan *et al.* 2002; Dorta Soares, n.d.

Populus alba

Scientific Name(s) / [Botanical Family]: *Populus alba* L. [Salicaceae].
Common Name(s): Abele, silver leaf poplar, white poplar [English]. Peuplier blanc [French]. Álamo blanco [Spanish].
Life form: Tree. **Part(s) Used:** Branch, leaf, root / Fresh.
Africa, Temperate-Asia. Europe. **Geographic distribution:** cultivated.
Reference(s): Bharatan *et al.* 2002; Müntz, n.d.; Provings, 2008-2009; Remedia/at, 2010; American Institute of Homeopathy, 1979.

Populus balsamifera see *Populus x jackii*

Populus candicans

Scientific Name(s) / [Botanical Family]: *Populus candicans* Aiton = *Populus candicans* F. Michx. auct. non L. = *Populus balsamifera* L. subsp. *balsamifera* = *Populus gileandensis* Rouleau = *Populus x jackii* Sarg. [Salicaceae].
Common Name(s): Balm-of-Gilead, balm-of-Gilead-buds, jack's popular, Ontario poplar Balsam poplar, hackmatack, tacamahac poplar [English]. Peuplier baumier [French]. Álamo branco [Portuguese]. Álamo balsámico [Spanish].
Life form: Tree. **Part(s) Used:** Bark gum or resin from stem or bud, leaf, bud / Fresh. **Geographic distribution:** North America

(Alaska. Canada. United States of America). China. Europe. Extensively cultivated in several places.
Reference(s): Bharatan *et al.* 2002; Dorta Soares, n.d.; Müntz, n.d.; Remedia/at, 2010; Tiwari *et al.* 2013.

Populus gileadensis see *Populus x jackii*

Populus tremula

Scientific Name(s) / [Botanical Family]: *Populus tremula* L. = *Populus pseudotremula* N.I. Rubtzov [Salicaceae].
Common Name(s): Ou zhou shan yang [Chinese]. Aspen, Eurasian aspen, European aspen, quaking aspen [English]. Peuplier tremble [French]. Choupo [Portuguese]. Álamo temblón, álamo tembloroso, chopo temblón, lamparilla [Spanish].
Life form: Tree. **Part(s) Used:** Inner bark & leaf or also branch / Fresh. **Geographic distribution:** Africa. North America. Temperate-Asia (China). Europe.
Reference(s): Bharatan *et al.* 2002; Dorta Soares, n.d.; Plants for a future, 2009; Remedia/at, 2010; Vithoulkas, n.d.

Populus tremuloides

Scientific Name(s) / [Botanical Family]: *Populus tremuloides* Michx. [Salicaceae].
Common Name(s): American aspen, american poplar, quaking aspen, trembling aspen [English]. Peuplier faux-tremble, tremble [French]. Choupo [Portuguese]. Álamo [Spanish].
Life form: Tree. **Part(s) Used:** Complete plant, leaf / Fresh.
Geographic distribution: North America (Canada. United States of America. Mexico).
Reference(s): Dorta Soares, n.d.; Müntz, n.d.; Remedia/at, 2010; Tiwari *et al.* 2013.

Portulaca grandiflora

Scientific Name(s) / [Botanical Family]: *Portulaca grandiflora* Hook.f. = *Portulaca caryophylloides* Hort. ex Vilm. = *Portulaca gilliesii* Hook. = *Portulaca gilliesii* Speg. = *Portulaca hilaireana* G. Don = *Portulaca immersostellulata* Poelln. = *Portulaca megalantha* Steud. = *Portulaca mendocinensis* Gillies ex Hook. = *Portulaca mendocinensis* Gillies ex Rohrb. = *Portulaca multistaminata* Poellin = *Portulaca pilosa* subsp. *cisplatina* D. Legrand [Portulaceae].

Common Name(s): Eleven-or also 'clock, mexican-rose, moss rose, rose-moss, portu, sun-plant [English]. Pourpier à grandes fleurs [French]. Portelaca, portulaca [Spanish].

Life form: Herb. **Part(s) Used:** Complete plant / Dried.
Geographic distribution: America. (Argentine. Mexico. Peru).
Reference(s): Allen, 2006-2010; Bharatan *et al.* 2002; Remedia/at, 2010; American Institute of Homeopathy, 1979. Zandvoort, 2006.

Potentilla anserina

Scientific Name(s) / [Botanical Family]: *Potentilla anserina* L. = *Argentine anserina* (L.) Rydb. [Rosaceae].

Common Name(s): Anserina, goose-grass, goose-tansy, silverweed, silverweed cinquefoil, wild tansy [English]. Anserine, potentille ansérine [French]. Potentilha Argentine [Portuguese]. Anserina, Argentine, plateada [Spanish].

Life form: Herb. **Part(s) Used:** Aerial part in bloom / Fresh; branches bark collected before bloom / Dried. **Geographic distribution:** Temperate-Asia & tropical. Europe. North America. Naturalized in temperate regions.

Reference(s): Bharatan *et al.* 2002; Dorta Soares, n.d.; Remedia/at, 2010; Tiwari *et al.* 2013.

Potentilla erecta see *Potentilla tomentilla*

Potentilla tomentilla

Scientific Name(s) / [Botanical Family]: *Potentilla tormentilla* Neck. = *Potentilla erecta* (L.) Raeusch = *Tormentilla erecta* L. [Rosaceae].
Common Name(s): Tormentil. Erect cinquefoil [English]. Potentille tormentille [French]. Consólida vermelha, tomentilla [Portuguese]. Consuelda roja, loranca, siete in rama, sietenrama, tormentilla, zazpitoso [Spanish].
Life form: Herb. Part(s) Used **Part(s) Used:** Complete plant in bloom / Fresh; Subterraneous parts / Dried. **Geographic distribution:** Europe. West Asia. North East United States of America.
Reference(s): Bharatan *et al.* 2002; Dorta Soares, n.d.; Fuentes, 1996; Müntz, n.d.; Plants for a future, 2009; Provings, 2008-2009; Tiwari *et al.* 2013.

Pothos foetidus see *Ictodes foetida*

Primula farinosa

Scientific Name(s) / [Botanical Family]: *Primula farinosa* L. = *Primula laurentiana* Fern. [Primulaceae].
Common Name(s): Bird-eye primrose [English]. Primevère farineuse [French]. Primavera [Spanish].
Life form: Herb. **Part(s) Used:** Leaf?. **Geographic distribution:** Temperate-Asia (Siberia, Mongolia, China). Europe. United States of America.
Reference(s): Bharatan *et al.* 2002; Plants for a future, 2009.

Primula obconca see *Primula obconica*

Primula obconica

Scientific Name(s) / [Botanical Family]: *Primula obconica* Hance [Primulaceae].
Common Name(s): E bao chun [Chinese]. German primrose, poison primrose [English]. Primevère de Chine [French]. Primavera [Portuguese].
Life form: Herb. **Part(s) Used:** Complete plant in bloom / Fresh; flower / Dried. **Geographic distribution:** Temperate-Asia (China) & Tropical-Asia
Reference(s): Bharatan *et al.* 2002; Dorta Soares, n.d.; Plants for a future, 2009.

Primula veris

Scientific Name(s) / [Botanical Family]: Primula veris L. = Primula columnae Ten. = Primula macrocalyx Bunge = Primula officinalis (L.) Hill = Primula suaveolens Bertol. = Primula uralensis Fisch. ex Rchb. [Primulaceae].
Common Name(s): Primevère officinale, primevère du printemps, primevère vraie [French]. Cowslip primerose [English]. Primavera, prímula [Portuguese]. Hierba de San Pablo mayor, hierba de San Pedro, Manguitos, Primavera, prímula, vellorita [Spanish].
Life form: Herb. **Part(s) Used:** Complete plant / Fresh.
Geographic distribution: West Temperate-Asia (Iran, Turkey, Caucasus). Europe central. Cultivated in West United States of America.
Reference(s): Bharatan *et al.* 2002; Clarke, 2008; Dorta Soares, n.d.; Guermonprez *et al.* 1989; Müntz, n.d.

Primula vulgaris see *Primula veris*

Prunus armeniaca

Scientific Name(s) / [Botanical Family]: *Prunus armeniaca* L. [Rosaceae].
Common Name(s): Apricot [English]. Abricoter [French]. Albaricoque, chabacano, Damasco, damasquino [Spanish].
Life form: Tree. **Part(s) Used:** Fruit. **Geographic distribution:** Temperate-Asia (China). Extensively cultivated.
Reference(s): Bharatan *et al.* 2002; Clarke, 2008; Vithoulkas, n.d.

Prunus cerasifera

Scientific Name(s) / [Botanical Family]: *Prunus cerasifera* Ehrh. [Rosaceae].
Common Name(s): Cherry plum, myrobalan plum [English]. Bacarinier, cerisette, prunier cerise [French]. Arañon, ciruela chabacana, ciruelo mirobalan, guindo [Spanish].
Life form: Tree. **Part(s) Used:** Flower. **Geographic distribution:** Extensively cultivated.
Reference(s): Bharatan *et al.* 2002; Remedia/at, 2010.

Prunus cerasus

Scientific Name(s) / [Botanical Family]: *Prunus cerasus* L. = *Prunus acida* (Dum.) K. Koch = *Cerasus vulgaris* Miller = , *432 acida* Gaertn. = *Cerasus caproniana* DC. [Rosaceae].
Common Name(s): Cherry plum, cherry tree, pie cherry, sour cherry [English]. Ceisier acide, cerisier, griottier [French]. Ginjeira [Portuguese]. Cerezo ácido, cereza común, guindo [Spanish].
Life form: Shrub, Tree. **Part(s) Used:** Bark seeds?. **Geographic distribution:** Only cultivated and introduced in North, Central & East United States of America.
Reference(s): Bharatan *et al.* 2002; Remedia/at, 2010.

Prunus domestica

Scientific Name(s) / [Botanical Family]: *Prunus domestica* L. = *Prunus domestica* ssp. *domestica* = *Prunus domestica* var. *damascena* L. [Rosaceae].

Common Name(s): Common plum, European plum, garden plum, plum [English]. Prunier [French]. Abrunheiro manso, ameixeira, ameixeira preta [Portuguese]. Almendra, almendro, ciruela, ciruelo, ciruelo de España [Spanish].

Life form: Tree. **Part(s) Used:** Bark / Fresh; Fruit. **Geographic distribution:** Europe to West Asia. Russia (Caucasus). Naturalized in Great Britain. West & North East & Texas State in United States of America.

Reference(s): Dorta Soares, n.d.; Zandvoort, 2006.

Prunus mahaleb

Scientific Name(s) / [Botanical Family]: *Prunus mahaleb* L. = *Cerasus mahaleb* (L.) Mill. [Rosaceae].

Common Name(s): Mahaleb cherry, perfumed cherry, St. Lucie cherry, St. Lucie's cherry [English]. Bois-de-Sainte-Lucie, cerisier de Mahaleb [French]. Árbol de Santa Lucia, cerecino [Spanish].

Life form: Tree. **Part(s) Used:** Bark with young branches / Fresh.
Geographic distribution: Central & South Europe. West, North & East United States of America. Orient proximal.

Reference(s): Dorta Soares, n.d.; Zandvoort, 2006.

Prunus padus

Scientific Name(s) / [Botanical Family]: *Cerasus padus* (L.) Delarbre = *Prunus padus* L. = *Prunus racemosa* (Lam.) C. K. Schneid. = *Prunus racemosa* Lam. = *Prunus seoulensis* H. Lév. [Rosaceae].

Common Name(s): Bird cherry, European bird cherry [English]. Cerisier putiet [French]. Cerejeira [Portuguese]. Árbol de Santa

Lucia, cerecino, cerezo aliso, cerezo de Mahoma, cerezo de racimo, cerezo de Santa Lucía, ciruelo de Bahama, pudriera [Spanish].
Life form: Tree. **Part(s) Used:** Bark & leaf / Fresh; young leaves collected at initial bloom. **Geographic distribution:** Asia Minor & North Europe. Escocia, North Inglaterra & Gales. North Russia. Alaska & East United States of America. Naturalized in several places.
Reference(s): Dorta Soares, n.d.; Tiwari *et al*. 2013; Zandvoort, 2006.

Prunus persica see *Amygdalus persica*.

Prunus spinosa

Scientific Name(s) / [Botanical Family]: *Prunus spinosa* L. [Rosaceae].
Common Name(s): Blackthorn, blackthron tree, sloe [English]. Epine noire [French]. Abrunheiro, ameixeira brava [Portuguese]. Ciruelo silvestre, espino negro [Spanish].
Life form: Shrub. **Part(s) Used:** Bud at begining of bloom; flowers / Fresh. **Geographic distribution:** North Africa. Great Britain, Europe, America. (Northwest & West United States of America). Proximal Orient.
Reference(s): Allen, 2006-2010; Bharatan *et al.* 2002; Clarke, 2008; Dorta Soares, n.d.; Müntz, n.d.; Remedia/at, 2010; Tiwari *et al*. 2013; American Institute of Homeopathy, 1979.

Prunus virginiana

Scientific Name(s) / [Botanical Family]: *Prunus virginiana* L. = *Prunus serotina* Poir. = *Cerasus virginiana* (L.) Michx. = *Cerasus serotina* Hook. [Rosaceae].
Common Name(s): Chokecherry, common chokecherry, Virginian bird cherry, western choke cherry, wild cherry [English]. Cerisier de Virginie [French]. Cerejeira da Virgínia

[Portuguese]. Cerezo de Virginia, ciruelo virginiano [Spanish].
Life form: Tree. **Part(s) Used:** Bark / Fresh / Dried. **Geographic distribution:** North America (Canada-United States of America).
Reference(s): Bharatan *et al.* 2002; Dorta Soares, n.d.; Schumacher, 2009; Tiwari *et al.* 2013.

Pseudotsuga menziesii

Scientific Name(s) / [Botanical Family]: *Pseudotsuga menziesii* (Mirbel.) Franco = *Abies menziezzi* Mirbel [Abietaceae, Pinaceae].
Common Name(s): Coast Douglas fir, Douglas fir, Oregon-pine [English]. Sapin de Douglas [French]. Pinabete, pino oregón [Spanish].
Life form: Tree. **Part(s) Used:** Bark leaf, root-resin?. **Geographic distribution:** North America (West Canada, Mexico. United States of America).
Reference(s): Bharatan *et al.* 2002; Müntz, n.d.; Remedia/at, 2010; American Institute of Homeopathy, 1979; Zandvoort, 2006.

Psilocybe

Scientific Name(s) / [Botanical Family]: *Psilocybe caerulescens* Murrill. et Sing. [Agaricaceae, Strophariaceae].
Common Name(s): Landslide mushroom [English]. Di-chi-te-ki-sho, derrumbes, hongo, nanacate, razón-bei [Spanish].
Life form: Fungi. **Part(s) Used:** Complete mushroom.
Geographic distribution: North America (Mexico). Central & South America (Guatemala. Venezuela & Brazil).
Reference(s): Bharatan *et al.* 2002; Plants for a future, 2009.

Psoralea

Scientific Name(s) / [Botanical Family]: *Psoralea bituminosa* L. = *Bituminaria bituminosa* (L.) Stirton [Fabaceae, Leguminosae].

Common Name(s): Arabian pea, arabian scurfpea, pitch trfoil, scurfy pea [English]. Psoralée bitumeuse [French]. Treo dos jardins [Portuguese]. Cabrilla, herba bruna, hierba cabrera, trébol bastardo, trébol de mal olor [Spanish].
Life form: Herb, Shrub. **Part(s) Used:** Complete plant / Fresh; complete plant in bloom / Fresh. **Geographic distribution:** Europe (Mediterranean). United States of America.
Reference(s): Bharatan *et al.* 2002; Dorta Soares, n.d.; Müntz, n.d.

Psoralea corylifolia

Scientific Name(s) / [Botanical Family]: *Psoralea corylifolia* L. = *Cullen corylifolium* (L.) Medik. [Fabaceae, Leguminosae].
Common Name(s): Babchi, babchi seeds s, black dot, bu gu zhi, Malay tea, Malaya tea, Malaysian scurf pea, psoralea fruit, scurf pea fruit, scurfy pea [English]. Psoraléa [French]. Trébol hediondo [Spanish].
Life form: Herb. **Part(s) Used:** Leaf, stem?. **Geographic distribution:** West Asia-Iran.
Reference(s): Bharatan *et al.* 2002; Plants for a future, 2009; Tiwari *et al.* 2013; Zandvoort, 2006.

Ptelea trifoliata

Scientific Name(s) / [Botanical Family]: *Ptelea trifoliata* L. = *Ptelea trifoliata* Bol. = *Ptelea angustifolia* Benth. = *Ptelea baldwinii* Torr. & A. Gray = *Ptelea viticifolia* Salisb. [Rutaceae].
Common Name(s): Hop tree, shruby treefoil, stinking ash, three leaf ed hop tree, wafer ash [English]. Orme de Samarie [French]. Olmo da Samária, olmo de três folhas, trevo arbusto [Portuguese]. Olmo de tres hojas [Spanish].
Life form: Tree. **Part(s) Used:** Root-bark / Fresh; leaf collected in bloom / Dried; root-bark / Fresh. **Geographic distribution:** North America (East Canada. United States of America. North Mexico).

Reference(s): Bharatan *et al.* 2002; Dorta Soares, n.d.; Plants for a future, 2009; Tiwari *et al.* 2013; Zandvoort, 2006.

Pulmonaria officinalis

Scientific Name(s) / [Botanical Family]: *Pulmonaria officinalis* L. = *Pulmonaria maculata* Dietr. [Boraginaceae].

Common Name(s): Dage of Jerusalem, lungwort, common lungwort, suffolk lungwort [English]. Pulmonaire officinale [French]. Pulmonaria [Spanish]. Pulmonaria manchada [Portuguese].

Life form: Herb. **Part(s) Used:** Buds, leaf / Fresh; Aerial part / Fresh; leaf collected in bloom / Dried. **Geographic distribution:** Europe. Naturalized in Great Britain.

Reference(s): Bharatan *et al.* 2002; Clarke, 2008; Dorta Soares, n.d.; Guermonprez *et al.* 1989; American Institute of Homeopathy, 1979.

Pulsatilla

Scientific Name(s) / [Botanical Family]: *Anemone pratensis* L. = *Anemone nigricans* (Störck) A. Kern = *Pulsatilla nigricans* Störck = *Pulsatilla pratensis* (L.) Mill. [Ranunculaceae].

Common Name(s): Pasque flower, small pasque flower, meadow anemone [English]. Anémone pulsatille [French]. Anêmonas [Portuguese].

Life form: Herb. **Part(s) Used:** Complete plant, flower / Fresh. **Geographic distribution:** Europe.

Reference(s): Allen, 2006-2010; Bharatan *et al.* 2002; Bolte *et al.* 1997; Dorta Soares, n.d.; Müntz, n.d.; Plants for a future, 2009; Remedia/at, 2010; Tiwari *et al.* 2013; American Institute of Homeopathy, 1979; Zandvoort, 2006.

Pulsatilla nuttalliana

Scientific Name(s) / [Botanical Family]: *Pulsatilla nuttalliana*

Spreng = *Pulsatilla patens* (L.) Mill. = *Anemone flavescens* Zucc. = *Anemone patens* L. = *Anemone nuttaliana* DC. [Ranunculaceae].
Common Name(s): American pasque flower, american pulsatilla, eastern pasque flower, pasque flower, wind flower [English]. Pulsatilla americana [Portuguese].
Life form: Herb. **Part(s) Used:** Complete plant / Fresh.
Geographic distribution: Temperate-Asia. Europe. North America (Canada. United States of America).
Reference(s): Bharatan *et al.* 2002; Dorta Soares, n.d.; Guermonprez *et al.* 1989; Remedia/at, 2010; Plants for a future, 2009; American Institute of Homeopathy, 1979.

Pulsatilla vulgaris see *Pulsatilla* or also *Anemone pratensis*

Punica granatum

Scientific Name(s) / [Botanical Family]: *Punica granatum* L. [Lytraceae, Punicaceae].
Common Name(s): Pomegranate [English]. Grenadier [French]. Milgreira, romã, romeira [Portuguese]. Granada, granado, granado dulce, raíz de granada [Spanish].
Life form: Tree. **Part(s) Used:** Bark-root, stem / Fresh.
Geographic distribution: North Africa. South Europe. Also cultivated in many regions.
Reference(s): Bharatan *et al.* 2002; Dorta Soares, n.d.; Gotfredsen, 2009; Tiwari *et al.* 2013.

Pyracantha coccinea

Scientific Name(s) / [Botanical Family]: *Pyracantha coccinea* Middle Roem [Rosaceae].
Common Name(s): Buisson, firethorn, pyracanth, scarlet firethorn [English]. Espino de fuego, piracanta, piracanto [Spanish].
Life form: Shrub. **Part(s) Used:** Flower, Leaf, spine / Fresh.
Geographic distribution: Naturalized in several places.

Reference(s): Bharatan *et al.* 2002; Remedia/at, 2010.

Pyrethrum

Scientific Name(s) / [Botanical Family]: *Anacyclus officinarum* Hayne [Asteraceae].
Common Name(s): German pellitory, pellitory [English]. Pyrèthre d'Allemagne [French]. Piretro, pó da Pérsia [Portuguese].
Life form: Herb. **Part(s) Used:** Root / Dried. **Geographic distribution:** South Europe & cultivated in other regions.
Reference(s): Dorta Soares, n.d.; Remedia/at, 2010.

Pyrethrum parthenium

Scientific Name(s) / [Botanical Family]: *Chrysanthemum parthenium* (L.) Bernh. = *Aphanostephus pinulensis* J. M. Coult. = *Matricaria parthenium* L. = *Tanacetum parthenium* (L.) Schultz-Bip. [Asteraceae, Compositae].
Common Name(s): Feverfew [English]. Grande camomille, matricaire [French]. Altamisa, hierba de Santa María, magarza [Spanish].
Life form: Herb. **Part(s) Used:** Complete plant?. **Geographic distribution:** North America (Canada. United States of America. Mexico). Central & South America. Naturalized in several places.
Reference(s): Bharatan *et al.* 2002; Remedia/at, 2010.

Pyrola rotundifolia

Scientific Name(s) / [Botanical Family]: *Pyrola rotundifolia* Oed. = *Pyrola americana* Sweet [Pyrolaceae].
Common Name(s): American wintergreen, round-leaf ed wintergreen, wild lily-of the-valley [English]. Pyrole ŕ feuilles rondes [French]. Pirola [Spanish].
Life form: Herb. **Part(s) Used:** Leaf. **Geographic distribution:** Temperate-Asia. Europe. North America.

Reference(s): Dorta Soares, n.d.; Remedia/at, 2010.

Pyrus americana

Scientific Name(s) / [Botanical Family]: *Sorbus americana* Marshall = *Sorbus decora* (Sarg.) C. K. Schneid. = *Pyrus americana* Gray = *Pyrus americana* (Marshall) DC. [Rosaceae].

Common Name(s): American mountain ash, mountain ash, northern mountain-ash, pear fertility [English].

Life form: Shrub, Tree. **Part(s) Used:** Bark / Fresh. **Geographic distribution:** North America (Canada. North & North Central United States of America).

Reference(s): Bharatan *et al.* 2002; Dorta Soares, n.d.; Plants for a future, 2009; Tiwari *et al.* 2013; Zandvoort, 2006.

Pyrus communis

Scientific Name(s) / [Botanical Family]: *Pyrus communis* L. [Rosaceae].

Common Name(s): Graden pear, pear, pear fertility, pear tree, wild pear [English]. Poirier [French]. Pera, peral [Spanish].

Life form: Tree. **Part(s) Used:** Fruit / Fresh?. **Geographic distribution:** Extensively cultivated & naturalized.

Reference(s): Bharatan *et al.* 2002; Clarke, 2008; Remedia/at, 2010; American Institute of Homeopathy, 1979; Zandvoort, 2006.

Pyrus malus

Scientific Name(s) / [Botanical Family]: *Pyrus malus* L. = *Malus domestica* Borkh. = *Malus pumila* Mill. = *Malus sylvestris* Miller = *Malus acerba* Mérat. = *Malus communis* = *Malus communis* ssp. *acerba* [Rosaceae].

Common Name(s): Apple, apple-tree, bad or rotten apple [English]. Pommier commun [French]. Manzana, manzano, perón [Spanish].

Life form: Tree. **Part(s) Used:** Bark fruit, root / Fresh. **Geographic distribution:** Cultivated in many temperate regions.
Reference(s): Bharatan *et al.* 2002; Müntz, n.d.; Plants for a future, 2009.

Quebracho
Scientific Name(s) / [Botanical Family]: *Macaglia quebracho-blanco* (Schltdl.) A. Lyons = *Macaglia* quebracho Rich. = *Aspidosperma quebracho-blanco* Schltdl. = *Aspidosperma quebracho* Schltdl. [Apocynaceae].
Common Name(s): White quebracho [English]. Quebracho blanco, quebracho [Spanish].
Life form: Tree. **Part(s) Used:** Branch-bark / Dried. **Geographic distribution:** South America (Argentine, Bolivia, Paraguay, Uruguay).
Reference(s): Bharatan *et al.* 2002; Müntz, n.d.; Plants for a future, 2009; Tiwari *et al.* 2013.

Quercus
Scientific Name(s) / [Botanical Family]: *Quercus ilex* L. = *Quercus ilex* Lour = *Quercus avellaniformis* Colmeiro & Boutelou = *Quercus avellaeformis* Colmeiro & Boutelou = *Quercus sempervirens* Mill. = *Quercus gracilis* Lange = *Quercus smilax* L. [Fagaceae].
Common Name(s): Evergreen oak, holly oak [English]. Chęne vert, yeuse [French]. Acebo, alsina, carrasca, chaparra, coscoja, encina, encino [Spanish].
Life form: Tree. **Part(s) Used:** Bark, fruit / Fresh. **Geographic distribution:** Europe (England, Mediterranean). United States of America. Cultivated in several european countries.
Reference(s): Bharatan *et al.* 2002; Bolte *et al.* 1997;

Remedia/at, 2010.

Quercus robur

Scientific Name(s) / [Botanical Family]: *Quercus robur* L. = *Quercus pedunculata* Ehrh. [Fagaceae].

Common Name(s): Common oak, english oak, French oak, oak, pedunculate oak [English]. Chęne pédonculé [French]. Carvalho [Portuguese]. Roble albar, roble carvallo, roble europeo [Spanish].

Life form: Tree. **Part(s) Used:** Fruit / Fresh; bark branches & rhizome / Dried; leaves collected in bloom time / Dried; fruit.

Geographic distribution: England, Asia, Europe (except North East Mediterranean). Russia. Also cultivated.

Reference(s): Bharatan *et al.* 2002; Bolte *et al.* 1997; Dorta Soares, n.d.; Müntz, n.d.; Remedia/at, 2010.

Quillaia (Quillaja) saponaria

Scientific Name(s) / [Botanical Family]: *Quillaja saponaria* Molina = *Quillaya saponaria* Molina = *Quillaja smegmadermos* D. C. [Quillajaceae, Rosaceae].

Common Name(s): Murrillo's-bark, Panama, Panama bark, quillaja, soap tree, soap-bark tree, soapbark [English]. Quillaia [French]. Àrvore de Sabão, casca do Panamá [Portuguese]. Jabón de palo, Leño de Panamá, palo de jabón, quillaya [Spanish].

Life form: Tree. **Part(s) Used:** Bark / Dried. **Geographic distribution:** South America (Brazil, Chile, Peru).

Reference(s): Bharatan *et al.* 2002; Bolte *et al.* 1997; Dorta Soares, n.d.; Remedia/at, 2010; Tiwari *et al.* 2013.

Quillaja see *Quillaia*

Quillaya saponaria see *Quillaia*

Rajania subsamarata

Scientific Name(s) / [Botanical Family]: *Amphipterygium adstringens* (Schltdl.) Schiede ex Standl. = *Juliania adstringens* (Schldtdl.) Schldtdl. = *Hypopterygium adstringens* Schldtdl. [Anacardiaceae, Julianaceae].
Common Name(s): Cuachalala, cuachalalate, cuauchalotl [Spanish].
Life form: Tree. **Part(s) Used:** Bark / Dried. **Geographic distribution:** North America (Mexico). Central America (Guatemala).
Reference(s): Bharatan *et al.* 2002; Dorta Soares, n.d.; Müntz, n.d.; Remedia/at, 2010; American Institute of Homeopathy, 1979; Zandvoort, 2006.

Ranunculus acris

Scientific Name(s) / [Botanical Family]: *Ranunculus acris* L. = *Ranunculus acer* L. = *Ranunculus dissectus* sensu not Hook. & Arn. = *Ranunculus acris* var. *latisectus* Beck [Ranunculaceae].
Common Name(s): Buttercup, goldcup, upright meadow crowfoot, meadow buttercup, tall buttercup [English]. Bouton d'or, renoncule âcre [French]. Botão de ouro, ranúnculo alto [Portuguese]. Botón de oro, francesilla, hierba belida [Spanish].
Life form: Herb. **Part(s) Used:** Complete plant / Fresh.
Geographic distribution: Europe. North Asia. United States of America & Canada. Greenland. Introduced in Caribe.
Reference(s): Bharatan *et al.* 2002; Dorta Soares, n.d.; Müntz,

n.d.; Remedia/at, 2010; Tiwari *et al*. 2013; American Institute of Homeopathy, 1979; Zandvoort, 2006.

Ranunculus bulbosus

Scientific Name(s) / [Botanical Family]: *Ranunculus bulbosus* L. [Ranunculaceae].

Common Name(s): Bulbous buttercup, bulbous crowfoot, buttercup [English]. Renoncule bulbeuse [French]. Botão-de-ouro, pé de galo [Portuguese]. Botón de oro, hierba velluda, ranúnculo [Spanish].

Life form: Herb. **Part(s) Used:** Complete plant in bloom or also whitout flower / Fresh. **Geographic distribution:** Europe. Introduced & naturalized in United States of America.

Reference(s): Bharatan *et al*. 2002; Bolte *et al*. 1997; Dorta Soares, n.d.; Remedia/at, 2010; Tiwari *et al*. 2013; American Institute of Homeopathy, 1979.

Ranunculus ficaria

Scientific Name(s) / [Botanical Family]: *Ranunculus ficaria* L. = *Ficaria ranunculoides* Roth. = *Ficaria verna* Hudson [Ranunculaceae].

Common Name(s): Fieg buttercup, figroot buttercup, lesser celandine, pileworth [English]. Renoncule ficaire, ficaire fausse renoncule [French]. Botão de ouro, celidonia menor, ficaria [Portuguese]. Celidonia menor [Spanish].

Life form: Herb. **Part(s) Used:** Complete plant / Fresh. **Geographic distribution:** North Africa. Europe. Naturalized in several places.

Reference(s): Bharatan *et al*. 2002; Bolte *et al*. 1997; Dorta Soares, n.d.; Remedia/at, 2010; American Institute of Homeopathy, 1979; Zandvoort, 2006.

Ranunculus flammula

Scientific Name(s) / [Botanical Family]: *Ranunculus flammula* L. [Ranunculaceae].
Common Name(s): Lesser spearwort, spearwort [English].
Life form: Herb. **Part(s) Used:** Complete plant / Fresh.
Geographic distribution: Africa. Temperate-Asia. Europe. North America (Canada. United States of America). Naturalized in Australia & North New Zealand.
Reference(s): Bharatan *et al.* 2002; Bolte *et al.* 1997; Dorta Soares, n.d.; Müntz, n.d.; Remedia/at, 2010; Plants for a future, 2009; Zandvoort, 2006.

Ranunculus glacialis

Scientific Name(s) / [Botanical Family]: *Ranunculus glacialis* L. [Ranunculaceae].
Common Name(s): Glacier buttercup, reindeer flower [English].
Life form: Herb. **Part(s) Used:** Complete plant / Fresh.
Geographic distribution: Temperate-Asia. North & East Europe. North America (Alaska, Greenland).
Reference(s): Bharatan *et al.* 2002; Dorta Soares, n.d.; Müntz, n.d.; Plants for a future, 2009.

Ranunculus repens

Scientific Name(s) / [Botanical Family]: *Ranunculus repens* L. [Ranunculaceae].
Common Name(s): Creeping buttercup, gold-balls [English]. Renoncule rampante [French]. Botão de ouro, celidonia minor, ficaria, ranúnculo-rasteiro [Portuguese].
Life form: Herb. **Part(s) Used:** Complete plant / Fresh.
Geographic distribution: Africa. Temperate-Asia. Europe. Naturalized in several regions.
Reference(s): Bharatan *et al.* 2002; Bolte *et al.* 1997; Dorta Soares, n.d.; Müntz, n.d.; Remedia/at, 2010; Tiwari *et al.* 2013;

Zandvoort, 2006

Ranunculus sceleratus

Scientific Name(s) / [Botanical Family]: *Ranunculus sceleratus* L. [Ranunculaceae].
Common Name(s): Blister buttercup, blister plant, celery-leaf ed crowfoot, marsh buttercup, marsh crowfoot [English]. Renoncule scélérate [French]. Ranúnculo d'água [Portuguese]. Hierba sardóncica, sardonia [Spanish].
Life form: Herb. **Part(s) Used:** Complete plant / Fresh.
Geographic distribution: Africa. Temperate-Asia. Europe. United States of America. Extensively naturalized
Reference(s): Bharatan *et al.* 2002; Dorta Soares, n.d.; Müntz, n.d.; Tiwari *et al.* 2013; American Institute of Homeopathy, 1979; Zandvoort, 2006.

Raphanistrum arvense

Scientific Name(s) / [Botanical Family]: *Raphanistrum arvense* Wallr. = *Raphanus raphanistrum* L. [Brassicaceae, Cruciferae].
Common Name(s): Jointed-podded charlock, runch, wild radish, white charlock [English]. Raifort sauvage, raveluche [French]. Cabresto, rabanete de cavalo, saramago [Portuguese]. Rabanillo, rabanillo blanco [Spanish].
Life form: Herb. **Part(s) Used:** Complete plant / Fresh.
Geographic distribution: Africa. Temperate-Asia. Europe. Extensively naturalized in several places.
Reference(s): Bharatan *et al.* 2002; Bolte *et al.* 1997; Dorta Soares, n.d.; Müntz, n.d.; Remedia/at, 2010; American Institute of Homeopathy, 1979.

Raphanus sativus

Scientific Name(s) / [Botanical Family]: *Raphanus sativus* L. = *Raphanus nigrum* Mill. [Brassicaceae, Cruciferae].

Common Name(s): Black or garden radish, cultivated radish [English]. Radis cultivé, rave [French]. Coo-guiña-nagali, gu-gilaztilla, rábanillo, rabanillo blanco, rabanito, rábano, rábano silvestre [Spanish].
Life form: Herb. **Part(s) Used:** Root / Fresh. **Geographic distribution:** cultivated in several places.
Reference(s): Bharatan *et al.* 2002; Dorta Soares, n.d.; Plants for a future, 2009; Tiwari *et al.* 2013; Zandvoort, 2006.

Ratanhia see *Ratanhia peruviana*

Ratanhia peruviana

Scientific Name(s) / [Botanical Family]: *Krameria lappacea* (Dombey) Burdet & Simpson. = *Krameria triandra* Ruiz & Pavón = *Krameria iluca* Phil. = *Landia lappacea* Dombey [Krameriaceae].
Common Name(s): Rhatany, rhatany root [English]. Ratanhia du Pérou [French]. Mapato [Spanish].
Life form: Shrub. **Part(s) Used:** Root / Dried. **Geographic distribution:** South America (Argentine, Bolivia, Chile, Ecuador, Peru).
Reference(s): Bharatan *et al.* 2002; Fuentes, 1996; Guermonprez *et al.* 1989; Müntz, n.d.; Remedia/at, 2010; Tiwari *et al.* 2013; American Institute of Homeopathy, 1979.

Rauwolfia

Scientific Name(s) / [Botanical Family]: *Rauvolfia serpentina* (L.) Benth. ex Kurz = *Rauwolfia serpentina* (L.) Benth. & Kurz = *Ophioxylon serpentinum* L. = *Ophioxylon majus* Hassk. [Apocynaceae].
Common Name(s): Ajmaline, rauwolfia, serpentine-wood, snakewood [English]. She gen mu [Chinese]. Rauwolfia [Portuguese]. Boboró, rauwolfia, serpentina, sarna de perro, sarpagandha de la India [Spanish].

Life form: Shrub. **Part(s) Used:** Root / Dried; bark collected in bloom / Dried. **Geographic distribution:** Temperate-Asia (China, India, Sri-Lanka, Tailandia).
Reference(s): Bharatan *et al.* 2002; Dorta Soares, n.d.; Guermonprez *et al.* 1989; Tiwari *et al.* 2013; American Institute of Homeopathy, 1979; Zandvoort, 2006.

Rhamnus californica

Scientific Name(s) / [Botanical Family]: *Rhamnus californica* Eschsch. = *Frangula californica* (Eschsch.) A. Gray [Rhamnaceae].
Common Name(s): California buchthorn, buckthorn, California coffeeberry [English]. Prunier de Californie [French]. Café da Califórnia [Portuguese].
Life form: Shrub, Tree. **Part(s) Used:** Bark-branch / Dried; fruit recently mature. **Geographic distribution:** North America (Northwest, South Central & Southwest United States of America. North Mexico).
Reference(s): Bharatan *et al.* 2002; Dorta Soares, n.d.; Remedia/at, 2010; Tiwari *et al.* 2013; American Institute of Homeopathy, 1979.

Rhamnus cathartica

Scientific Name(s) / [Botanical Family]: *Rhamnus cathartica* L. = *Rhamnus catharticus* L. = *Frangula caroliniana* A. Gray. [Rhamnaceae].
Common Name(s): Buckthorn, common buckthorn, European buckthorn, purging buckthorn. [English]. Nerprun purgatif [French]. Espino cerval [Spanish].
Life form: Tree. **Part(s) Used:** Fruit mature / Fresh / Dried.
Geographic distribution: North Asia. South Europe. North Africa.
Reference(s): Bharatan *et al.* 2002; Dorta Soares, n.d.; Remedia/at, 2010; Tiwari *et al.* 2013; American Institute of

Homeopathy, 1979; Zandvoort, 2006.

Rhamnus frangula

Scientific Name(s) / [Botanical Family]: *Rhamnus frangula* L. = *Frangula vulgaris* Hill. = *Frangula vulgaris* Rchb. = *Frangula alnus* Mill. [Rhamnaceae].
Common Name(s): Alder buckthorn, berry-bearing buckthorn, clack alder [English]. Bourdaine [French]. Amieiro preto, amieiro negro [Portuguese]. Alno baccífero, arraclán, avellanillo, frángula, hediondo, pudio, rabiacán, sangueño [Spanish].
Life form: Shrub. **Part(s) Used:** Bark-branch / Fresh. **Geographic distribution:** North Africa. Asia. Europe. United States of America.
Reference(s): Bharatan *et al.* 2002; Dorta Soares, n.d.; Tiwari *et al.* 2013; American Institute of Homeopathy, 1979; Zandvoort, 2006.

Rheum

Scientific Name(s) / [Botanical Family]: *Rheum emodi* Wall. ex Meisn. = *Rheum australe* D. Don [Polygonaceae].
Common Name(s): Zang bian da huang [Chinese]. Himalayan rhubarb, Indian rhubarb [English]. Ruibarbo [Spanish].
Life form: Herb. **Part(s) Used:** Root, rhizome. **Geographic distribution:** Temperate-Asia. India. China. Pakistan.
Reference(s): Bharatan *et al.* 2002; Müntz, n.d.; Tiwari *et al.* 2013; American Institute of Homeopathy, 1979.

Rheum

Scientific Name(s) / [Botanical Family]: *Rheum officinale* Baill. [Polygonaceae].
Common Name(s): Chinese rhubarb, Indian rhubarb, turkey rhubarb [English]. Rhubarbe officinale [French]. Ruibarbo da China [Portuguese]. Ruibarbo, ruibarbo chino [Spanish].

Life form: Herb. **Part(s) Used:** Subterraneous parts / Fresh; Root / Dried. **Geographic distribution:** Temperate-Asia. India, China, Europe.
Reference(s): Remedia/at, 2010; Tiwari *et al*. 2013.

Rheum

Scientific Name(s) / [Botanical Family]: *Rheum palmatum* L. [Polygonaceae].
Common Name(s): Chinese (Indian) rhubarb [English]. Rhubarbe [French]. Ruibarbo, ruibarbo de Levante [Spanish].
Life form: Herb. **Part(s) Used:** Root / Dried. **Geographic distribution:** India. China. Europe.
Reference(s): Bharatan *et al*. 2002; Dorta Soares, n.d.; Guermonprez *et al*. 1989; Remedia/at, 2010; Tiwari *et al*. 2013; American Institute of Homeopathy, 1979.

Rheum

Scientific Name(s) / [Botanical Family]: *Rheum x cultorum* Thorsrud. & Reis. = *Rheum undulatum* L. [Polygonaceae].
Common Name(s): Rhubarb [English]. Ruibarbo [Spanish].
Life form: Herb. **Part(s) Used:** Root / Dried. **Geographic distribution:** East Asia-Siberia.
Reference(s): Bharatan *et al*. 2002; Plants for a future, 2009; Remedia/at, 2010; American Institute of Homeopathy, 1979.

Rhododendron

Scientific Name(s) / [Botanical Family]: *Rhododendron aureum* Georgi = *Rhododendron officinale* Salisb. = *Rhododendron chrysanthum* Pall. [Ericaceae].
Common Name(s): Golden flower rhododendron, rosebay, yellow snow rose [English]. Rose de Sibérie [French]. Azalea [Spanish]. Alecrim selvagem, rosa da Siberia [Portuguese].
Life form: Shrub. **Part(s) Used:** Flower's buds, leaves & branches

/ Dried; leaves / Fresh. **Geographic distribution:** Temperate-Asia (Siberia, Kamtschatka, China, Japan). Alpes.
Reference(s): Bharatan *et al.* 2002; Dorta Soares, n.d.; Guermonprez *et al.* 1989; Plants for a future, 2009; Remedia/at, 2010; Tiwari *et al.* 2013.

Rhododendron campylocarpum see *Rhododendron*

Rhododendron chrysanthemum see *Rhododendron*

Rhododendron chrysanthum see *Rhododendron*

Rhododendron ferrugineum see *Rhododendron*

Rhus aromatica

Scientific Name(s) / [Botanical Family]: *Rhus aromatica* Aiton = *Rhus suaveolens* Aiton. = *Rhus canadense* Marshall = *Rhus canadensis* Marshall = *Schmalzia serotina* Greene [Anacardiaceae].
Common Name(s): Zumaque aromático, zumaque oloroso [Spanish]. Aromatic sumac, fragrant sumac, polecatbush, skunkbrush, squawbush, sweet sumac [English]. Sumagre cheiroso [Portuguese].
Life form: Shrub. **Part(s) Used:** Root-bark / Fresh; Bark collected in bloom / Dried. **Geographic distribution:** North America (Canada, United States of America, Mexico).
Reference(s): Bharatan *et al.* 2002; Dorta Soares, n.d.; Remedia/at, 2010; American Institute of Homeopathy, 1979.

Rhus coriaria see *Rhus typhina*

Rhus diversiloba see *Rhus diversilobum*

Rhus diversilobum
Scientific Name(s) / [Botanical Family]: *Toxicodendron*

diversilobum (Torr. & A. Gray) Greene = *Toxicodendron radicans* subsp. *diversiloba* (Torr. & A. Gray) Thorne = *Rhus diversiloba* Torr. & A. Gray [Anacardiaceae].
Common Name(s): California poison oak, Pacific poison-oak, western poison-oak [English]. Sumac plurilobaire [French].
Life form: Shrub. **Part(s) Used:** Leaf / Fresh. **Geographic distribution:** North America (Canada. Northwest & Southwest United States of America. North Mexico).
Reference(s): Bharatan *et al.* 2002; Remedia/at, 2010.

Rhus glabra

Scientific Name(s) / [Botanical Family]: *Rhus glabra* L. = *Rhus elgans* Aiton = *Rhus carolinense* Marshall = *Toxicodendron glabrum* Kuntze = *Toxicodendron glabrum* Kuntze = *Schmaltzia glabra* Small. [Anacardiaceae].
Common Name(s): Smooth sumac, smooth sumach [English]. Sumac des corroyeurs [French]. Zumaque lampiño [Spanish].
Life form: Shrub. **Part(s) Used:** Bark, leaf / Fresh. **Geographic distribution:** North America.
Reference(s): Bharatan *et al.* 2002; Clarke, 2008; Dorta Soares, n.d.; Remedia/at, 2010.

Rhus lentii

Scientific Name(s) / [Botanical Family]: *Rhus lentii* Kellogg [Anacardiaceae].
Common Name(s): Pink flowering sumac, sugar bush [English]. Lentisco [Spanish].
Life form: Shrub. **Part(s) Used:** Leaf / Fresh. **Geographic distribution:** North America (Mexico).
Reference(s): Bharatan *et al.* 2002; American Institute of Homeopathy, 1979.

Rhus ovata

Scientific Name(s) / [Botanical Family]: *Rhus ovata* S. Watson [Anacardiaceae].
Common Name(s): Sugar sumac, sugar bush [English].
Life form: Shrub. **Part(s) Used:** Leaf / Fresh. **Geographic distribution:** North America (Southwest United States of America. North Mexico).
Reference(s): Remedia/at, 2010.

Rhus radicans

Scientific Name(s) / [Botanical Family]: *Rhus radicans* L. = *Toxicodendron radicans* (L.) Kuntze [Anacardiaceae].
Common Name(s): Poison ivy [English]. Sumax vénéneux [French]. Bembérecua, huembéreua, chechén, dominguilla, guadalagua, guau, hiedra, hiedra mala, hiedra venenosa, hincha huevos, lachi-golilla, lachicobilla, yaga-beche-topa, yaga-peche-topa, mala mujer, mexie, meye, zumaque, sumaque, fuego, betz-tzaj [Spanish].
Life form: Shrub, Tree. **Part(s) Used:** Bark, leaf, root / Fresh; leaves collected before bloom / Fresh. **Geographic distribution:** Temperate-Asia. North America (Canada. United States of America. Mexico). Central America.
Reference(s): Dorta Soares, n.d.; Remedia/at, 2010.

Rhus toxicodendron

Scientific Name(s) / [Botanical Family]: *Toxicodendron pubescens* Mill. = *Toxicodendron radicans* (L.) Kuntze subsp. *verrucosum* (Scheele) Gillis = *Rhus verrucosa* Scheele = *Rhus toxicodendron* L. = *Rhus radicans* var. *verrucosum* (Scheele) Fernald [Anacardiaceae].
Common Name(s): Atlantic poison-oak, poison ash, oak or vine, Mercury vine, three-leaf ed ivy [English]. Arbre à poison, sumac, sumax vénéneux [French]. Árbol de las pulgas, hiedra venenosa,

toxíguero, zumaque venenoso [Spanish]. Árvore da sarna, árvore das pulhas, árvore venenosa [Portuguese].
Life form: Herb, Shrub. **Part(s) Used:** Leaf / Fresh. **Geographic distribution:** North America (North, Central & South Central United States of America. North Mexico). Japan.
Reference(s): Bharatan *et al.* 2002; Dorta Soares, n.d.; Remedia/at, 2010.

Rhus typhina

Scientific Name(s) / [Botanical Family]: *Rhus coriaria* L. [Anacardiaceae].
Common Name(s): Sicilian sumac, tanner's sumac, Tanner's sumach [English]. Sumac des corroyeurs [French]. Zumaque [Spanish].
Life form: Shrub. **Part(s) Used:** Root-bark?. / Fresh. **Geographic distribution:** North Africa. Temperate-Asia. Europe.
Reference(s): Bharatan *et al.* 2002; Guermonprez *et al.* 1989; Plants for a future, 2009; Remedia/at, 2010; American Institute of Homeopathy, 1979.

Rhus venenata see *Rhus vermix*

Rhus vernix

Scientific Name(s) / [Botanical Family]: *Toxicodendron vernix* (L.) Kuntze = *Rhus vernix* L. = *Rhus venenata* DC. [Anacardiaceae].
Common Name(s): Dog wood, elder, sumach, poison-ash, poison-sumach, poison elder, poison dogwood, poison tree, poison wood, varnish tree [English]. Sumaque venenoso, hiedra venenosa, zumaque venenoso [Spanish].
Verniz da China [Portuguese].
Life form: Shrub, Tree. **Part(s) Used:** Bark, leaf, stem / Fresh; leaves collected before bloom / Dried. **Geographic distribution:** North America (Canada. United States of America).
Reference(s): Bharatan *et al.* 2002; Dorta Soares, n.d.;

Remedia/at, 2010; Tiwari *et al.* 2013.

Ribes nigrum

Scientific Name(s) / [Botanical Family]: *Ribes nigrum* L. = *Ribes cyathiforme* Pojark = *Botrycarpum nigrum* (L.) A. Rich. = *Grossularia nigra* (L.) Rupr. = *Ribes olidum* Moench. = *Ribes pauciflorum* Turcz. ex Ledeb. [Grossulariaceae].

Common Name(s): Black currant, european currant, garden black currant [English]. Cassis, cassissier, groseillier ŕfruits noirs, groseillier noir [French]. Ribes nero [Italian]. Casis, grosella negra, grosellero negro [Spanish]. Hei cha biao zi [Chinese]. Casis, groselha negra [Portuguese].

Life form: Shrub. **Part(s) Used:** Leaf, fruit / Fresh. **Geographic distribution:** Temperate-Asia. Europe. United States of America. Naturalized in several places.

Reference(s): Bharatan *et al.* 2002; Dorta Soares, n.d.; Remedia/at, 2010; American Institute of Homeopathy, 1979.

Ribes rubrum

Scientific Name(s) / [Botanical Family]: *Ribes rubrum* L. *sensu lato* = *Ribes sativum* (Reichenb.) Syme = *Ribes sylvestre* (Lam.) Mert. & W.D. J. Koch = *Ribes vulgare* Lam. [Grossulariaceae].

Common Name(s): Common currant, garden currant, redcurrant, white currant [English]. Groseillier rouge, groseillier commun [French]. Grosella colorada, grosella común, grosella roja, zarzaparrilla roja [Spanish].

Life form: Shrub. **Part(s) Used:** Fruit / Fresh. **Geographic distribution:** Europe. Extensively cultivated & naturalized in temperate regions.

Reference(s): Bolte *et al.* 1997; Müntz, n.d.; Plants for a future, 2009; Remedia/at, 2010.

Ribes uva-crispa

Scientific Name(s) / [Botanical Family]: *Ribes uva-crispa* L. = *Ribes grossularia* L. = *Ribes reclinatum* L. = *Grossularia reclinata* (L.) Mill. [Grossulariaceae].
Common Name(s): European gooseberry, goosebery [English]. Groseillier épineux, groseillier à maquereau [French]. Agrazón, grosellero espinoso, grosellero silvestre, uva espina [Spanish].
Life form: Shrub. **Part(s) Used:** Fruit, leaf. **Geographic distribution:** North Africa. Temperate-Asia. Europe. Cultivated.
Reference: Bolte *et al.* 1997.

Ricinus communis

Scientific Name(s) / [Botanical Family]: *Ricinus communis* L. [Euphorbiaceae].
Common Name(s): Castor, castor bean, castor oil plant [English]. Févé castor, grand ricin, ricin [French]. Al-pai-ue, cashilandacui, cashtilenque, k'ooch, x-kooch, degha, guechi-beyo, quechi-peyo-Castilla, yaga-bilape, yaga-higo, higuera infernal, higuera del diablo, higuerilla, ricino, thiquela, tapólotl, québe'enogua, xoxopajtzi [Spanish]. Carrapateira, figueira-do-inferno, mamona [Portuguese].
Life form: Shrub. **Part(s) Used:** seeds / Dried; squeezed oil seed's.
Geographic distribution: Africa, Asia (India). Cosmopolitan & naturalized in tropical & subtropical regions.
Reference(s): Bharatan *et al.* 2002; Bolte *et al.* 1997; Dorta Soares, n.d.; Müntz, n.d.; Plants for a future, 2009; Remedia/at, 2010; Tiwari *et al.* 2013.

Robinia

Scientific Name(s) / [Botanical Family]: *Robinia pseudoacacia* L. = *Robinia fragilis* Salisb. = *Robinia bessoniana* Hort. ex K. Koch [Fabaceae, Leguminosae].
Common Name(s): Black locust, false or yellow locust, false

acacia, locust tree [English]. Robinier, robinier faux-acacia [French]. Acacia blanca, acacia espinosa, falsa acacia, langosta negra, lobo, robinia [Spanish]. Acácia amarela, acácia bastarda [Portuguese].
Life form: Tree. **Part(s) Used:** Bark & branches young, bark Root / Fresh; seeds / Fresh. **Geographic distribution:** North America (United States of America). Extensively cultivated & naturalized in Europe, Australia & South America.
Reference(s): Bharatan *et al.* 2002; Dorta Soares, n.d.; Guermonprez *et al.* 1989; Remedia/at, 2010; Tiwari *et al.* 2013; American Institute of Homeopathy, 1979.

Robinia bessoniana see *Robinia*

Robinia pseudoacacia see *Robinia*

Rosa canina

Scientific Name(s) / [Botanical Family]: *Rosa canina* L. = *Rosa bakeri* Déségl. = *Rosa lutetiana* Léman = *Rosa montivaga* Déségl. [Rosaceae].
Common Name(s): Common briar, dog rose, dogbrier, wild rose [English]. Eglantier commun, rosier des chiens [French]. Escaramujo, galabardera, rosal, rosal montés, rosal silvestre [Spanish]. Rosa, rosa bandalha, roseira silvestre [Portuguese].
Life form: Shrub. **Part(s) Used:** Leaves & flower / Fresh; fresh petals; fruit mature. **Geographic distribution:** Africa. Asia. Europe. Naturalized in America & Australia.
Reference(s): Dorta Soares, n.d.; Remedia/at, 2010.

Rosa centifolia

Scientific Name(s) / [Botanical Family]: *Rosa x centifolia* L. = *Rosa centifolia* Lour. [Rosaceae].
Common Name(s): Cabbage rose, pale rose, provence rose [English]. Rose á cent feuilles, rose pâle [French]. Guia-be-cohua, rosa de Castilla, rosa común [Spanish]. Rosa branca, roseira

branca [Portuguese].
Life form: Shrub. **Part(s) Used:** Flower / Fresh. **Geographic distribution:** Caucasic region, or also cultivated in different regions.
Reference(s): Dorta Soares, n.d.; Remedia/at, 2010;

Rosa damascena

Scientific Name(s) / [Botanical Family]: *Rosa x damascena* Mill. = *Rosa gallica* f. *trigintipetala* Dieck.
Common Name(s): Damask rose, four-seasons rose, Portland rose, York-and-Lancaster rose [English]. Rosier de Damas [French]. Rosa-pálida, rose-de-Damasco [Portuguese]. Rosa de Alejandría, rosa de las cuatro estaciones, rosa francesa, rosal castellano [Spanish]. Rosa de Damasco [Portuguese].
Life form: Shrub. **Part(s) Used:** Flower / Fresh / Dried.
Geographic distribution: Orient or also cultivated.
Reference(s): Dorta Soares, n.d.; Fuentes, 1996; Müntz, n.d.; Remedia/at, 2010.

Rosmarinus

Scientific Name(s) / [Botanical Family]: *Rosmarinus officinalis* L. [Lamiaceae, Labiatae].
Common Name(s): Rosemary, rosmarin [English]. Romarin [French]. Osmarini, rosmarino [Italian]. Alecrim [Portuguese]. Guixu-cicanaca, romero [Spanish].
Life form: Shrub. **Part(s) Used:** Complete plant / Fresh. leaves collected before bloom / Dried; leaves & flowers recently collected / Dried. **Geographic distribution:** Africa. Temperate-Asia. Europe (Mediterranean). Extensively world's cultivated.
Reference(s): Bharatan *et al.* 2002; Dorta Soares, n.d.; Müntz, n.d.

Rubia tinctorum

Scientific Name(s) / [Botanical Family]: *Rubia tinctorum* L. [Rubiaceae].

Common Name(s): Alizarin, common madder, dyer's madder, European madder, madder [English]. Garance des teinturiers, garance [French]. Granza, royuela, ribia, rubia de tintes [Spanish]. Amo de Hortelã, granda, rubia [Portuguese].

Life form: Herb. **Part(s) Used:** Root collected before bloom / Dried. **Geographic distribution:** Temperate-Asia. Europe (Mediterranean). Extensively cultivated.

Reference(s): Allen, 2006-2010; Bharatan *et al.* 2002; Dorta Soares, n.d.; Remedia/at, 2010.

Rubus fruticosus

Scientific Name(s) / [Botanical Family]: *Rubus fruticosus* L. = *Rubus bergii* Eckl. & Zeyh. = *Rubus fruticosus* Eckl. & Zeyh. = *Rubus myrianthus* Baker [Rosaceae].

Common Name(s): Blackberry, European blackberry [English]. Brombeere [French]. Zarza, zarzamora [Spanish].

Life form: Shrub. **Part(s) Used:** Leaf / Fresh. **Geographic distribution:** Europe. Naturalized in South Africa, Asia. United States of America.

Reference(s): Bharatan *et al.* 2002; Bolte *et al.* 1997; Plants for a future, 2009.

Rubus idaeus

Scientific Name(s) / [Botanical Family]: *Rubus idaeus* L. [Rosaceae].

Common Name(s): European red raspberry, raspberry, red raspberry [English]. Fu pen zi [Chinese]. Framboise, framboisier [French]. Ezo-ichigo [Japanese]. Framboeseira, framboesa [Portuguese]. Chordón, frambuesa, frambueso [Spanish].

Life form: Shrub. **Part(s) Used:** Leaf / Fresh. **Geographic**

distribution: naturalized & cultivated in several places.
Reference: Remedia/at, 2010.

Rumex

Scientific Name(s) / [Botanical Family]: *Rumex crispus* L. [Polygonaceae].
Common Name(s): Curled dock, curly dock, garden patience, narrow, sour dock, yaller dock, yellow dock, winter dock [English]. Patience frisée, reguette [French]. Azeda crespa, língua-de-vaca, labaça-crespa [Portuguese]. Acedera, acedera de culebra, acedera de perro, bandana, canagria, lampazo, lengua de vaca, paniega, romaza rizada, ruibarbo silvestre, rumaza, tabaco, tabaquera, vinagrera, yerba mulata [Spanish].
Life form: Herb. **Part(s) Used:** Root / Fresh; seeds / Dried.
Geographic distribution: Africa. Temperate-Asia. Europe. Naturalized in several places.
Reference: Bharatan *et al.* 2002; Dorta Soares, n.d.; Remedia/at, 2010; Tiwari *et al.* 2013.

Rumex acetosa

Scientific Name(s) / [Botanical Family]: *Rumex acetosa* L. [Polygonaceae].
Common Name(s): Common sorrel, garden sorrel, sorrel [English]. Oseille des prés, oseille, oseille sauvage [French]. Azeda-brava [Portuguese]. Acedera, acedera común, vinagrera [Spanish].
Life form: Herb. **Part(s) Used:** Bulb, leaf, root / Fresh.
Geographic distribution: Africa. Temperate-Asia. Australia. Europe. United States of America. Naturalized in several places.
Reference(s): Allen, 2006-2010; Bharatan *et al.* 2002; Dorta Soares, n.d.; Guermonprez *et al.* 1989; Plants for a future, 2009; Remedia/at, 2010; Tiwari *et al.* 2013; American Institute of Homeopathy, 1979.

Ruscus aculeatus

Scientific Name(s) / [Botanical Family]: *Ruscus aculeatus* L. [Asparagaceae, Liliaceae, Ruscaceae].

Common Name(s): Box-holly, butcher's-broom [English]. Fragon épineux, fragon piquant, petit houx [French]. Silbarda [Portuguese]. Acebo menor, albernera, brusco, escoba de carnicero, rusco [Spanish].

Life form: Shrub. **Part(s) Used:** Rhizome, root. **Geographic distribution:** Temperate-Asia. Europe (Mediterranean).

Reference(s): Allen, 2006-2010; Bharatan *et al.* 2002; Plants for a future, 2009; Remedia/at, 2010; American Institute of Homeopathy, 1979.

Russula

Scientific Name(s) / [Botanical Family]: *Russula foetens* (Persoon) Fr. = *Russula foetens* (Pers.) Pers. = *Agaricus foetens* Pers. [Russulaceae].

Common Name(s): Fetid russula, stinking brittlegill [English]. Russule fetide [French]. Champiñón amarilleante, seta [Spanish].

Life form: Fungi. **Part(s) Used:** Complete mushroom / Fresh. **Geographic distribution:** North America (United States of America. Mexico.). Europe.

Reference: Bharatan *et al.* 2002; Remedia/at, 2010.

Ruta chalepensis

Scientific Name(s) / [Botanical Family]: *Ruta chalepensis* L. = *Ruta chalepensis* Wall. = *Ruta hortensis* Mill. = *Ruta graveolens* L. = *Ruta bracteosa* DC. [Rutaceae].

Common Name(s): Aleppo rue, Egyptian rue, fringed rue [English]. Rue fétide [French]. Acuitze-uaricua, ruda, ruda común, ruta [Spanish].

Life form: Herb. **Part(s) Used:** Complete plant / Fresh.
Geographic distribution: Africa. Temperate-Asia. Europe (Mediterranean). Extensively world's cultivated.
Reference(s): Bharatan *et al.* 2002; Clarke, 2008; Dorta Soares, n.d.; Tiwari *et al.* 2013.

Sabina

Scientific Name(s) / [Botanical Family]: *Juniperus sabina* L. = *Sabina officinalis* Garcke. [Cupressaceae].
Common Name(s): Juniper, sabina, savin, savin juniper [English]. Cha zi yuan bai [Chinese]. Sabine [French]. Sabino, sabina [Spanish].
Life form: Shrub, Tree. **Part(s) Used:** Leaf, branch / Fresh.
Geographic distribution: Europe. North America. North Africa. Russia. Temperate-Asia.
Reference(s): Bharatan *et al.* 2002; Dorta Soares, n.d.; Fuentes, 1996; Plants for a future, 2009; American Institute of Homeopathy, 1979.

Salix alba

Scientific Name(s) / [Botanical Family]: *Salix alba* L. [Salicaceae].
Common Name(s): Blue willow, criclet-bat willow, willow white, white willow [English]. Saule blanc [French]. Salgueiro, salgueiro branco, sinceiro [Portuguese]. Sauce, sauce blanco, sauz [Spanish].
Life form: Tree. **Part(s) Used:** Bark / Fresh. **Geographic distribution:** Asia, Europe. Cultivated in several places.
Reference(s): Bharatan *et al.* 2002; Dorta Soares, n.d.; Guermonprez *et al.* 1989; Müntz, n.d.

Salix fragilis

Scientific Name(s) / [Botanical Family]: *Salix fragilis* L. = *Salix decipiens* Hoffm. [Salicaceae].

Common Name(s): Brittle willow, crack willow [English]. Saule fragile, saule cassant [French]. Bardaguera, mimbrera, mimbrera frágil, Sauce [Spanish].

Life form: Tree. **Part(s) Used:** Bark / Fresh. **Geographic distribution:** Africa. Australia. Europe. Temperate-Asia. North America.

Reference: Remedia/at, 2010.

Salix mollissima

Scientific Name(s) / [Botanical Family]: *Salix mollissima* Hoffm. = *Salix x mollissima* Ehrh. = *Salix hippophaeifolia* Thuill. [Salicaceae].

Common Name(s): Sharp-stipule willow [English].

Life form: Shrub. **Part(s) Used:** Bark / Fresh. **Geographic distribution:** Only cultivated.

Reference: Remedia/at, 2010.

Salix nigra

Scientific Name(s) / [Botanical Family]: *Salix nigra* Marshall = *Salix falcata* Pursh = *Salix purshiana* Spreng [Salicaceae].

Common Name(s): Black willow [English]. salgueiro negro [Portuguese]. Sauce negro, sauz [Spanish].

Life form: Tree. **Part(s) Used:** Bark / Fresh. **Geographic distribution:** North America (East Canada. United States of America).

Reference(s): Bharatan *et al.* 2002; Dorta Soares, n.d.; Tiwari *et al.* 2013.

Salix purpurea

Scientific Name(s) / [Botanical Family]: *Salix purpurea* L. = *Salix monandra* Hoffm. = *Salix monandra* Ard. = *Salix helix* L. [Salicaceae].

Common Name(s): Basket willow, purple osier, purple willow [English]. Purpur pil [Danés]. Osier rouge, saule pourpre [French]. Salcio da vimini, salcio rosso wierzba. Purpurowa [Polaco]. Salgueiro, salgueiro-de-casca-roxa [Portuguese] Sargatillo, sauce colorado [Spanish].

Life form: Tree. **Part(s) Used:** Bark / Fresh. **Geographic distribution:** North Africa. Temperate-Asia. Europe. Extensively cultivated.

Reference(s): Bharatan *et al.* 2002; Dorta Soares, n.d.; Müntz, n.d.; Remedia/at, 2010; Tiwari *et al.* 2013; American Institute of Homeopathy, 1979.

Salvia

Scientific Name(s) / [Botanical Family]: *Salvia officinalis* L. [Lamiaceae, Labiatae].

Common Name(s): Common sage, garden sage, sage [English]. Sauge, sauge officinale [French]. Salva das boticas, salva dos jardins, sálvia [Portuguese]. Salvia, salvia oficinal, salvia real [Spanish].

Life form: Herb. **Part(s) Used:** Leaf / Fresh; Aerial parts in bloom / Fresh; leaves collected during the bloom / Dried. **Geographic distribution:** Europe (Mediterranean). Cultivated & naturalized in several places.

Reference(s): Bharatan *et al.* 2002; Dorta Soares, n.d.; Tiwari *et al.* 2013; American Institute of Homeopathy, 1979.

Salvia sclarea

Scientific Name(s) / [Botanical Family]: *Salvia sclarea* L. [Lamiaceae, Labiatae].

Common Name(s): Clary, clary sage, sage clary [English]. Sauge sclarée, sclarée [French]. Esalarea, salvia romana [Spanish].
Life form: Herb. **Part(s) Used:** Flower, leaf / Fresh. **Geographic distribution:** Europe. Temperate-Asia. Tropical Asia (India, Pakistan).
Reference(s): Bharatan *et al.* 2002; Remedia/at, 2010; American Institute of Homeopathy, 1979.

Sambucus canadensis

Scientific Name(s) / [Botanical Family]: *Sambucus canadensis* L. = *Sambucus nigra* subsp. *canadensis* = *Sambucus simpsonii* Rehder = *Sambucus humilis* Raf. = *Sambucus glauca* Nutt. ex Torr. & Gray [Adoxaceae, Caprifoliaceae, Sambucaceae].
Common Name(s): American elder, American elderberry, Canadian elder, elder-bush, Mexican elder, sweet elder [English]. Southeau du Canada [French]. Sabugueiro do Canada [Portuguese]. Sauco [Spanish].
Life form: Tree. **Part(s) Used:** Flower / Fresh; equal parts of leaves & flowers / Fresh. **Geographic distribution:** North America (Canada. United States of America. Central Mexico). Central America. Cultivated & naturalized in several places.
Reference(s): Bharatan *et al.* 2002; Dorta Soares, n.d.; Remedia/at, 2010; Tiwari *et al.* 2013.

Sambucus ebulus

Scientific Name(s) / [Botanical Family]: *Sambucus ebulus* L. = *Sambucus humilis* [Adoxaceae, Caprifoliaceae, Sambucaceae].
Common Name(s): Danewort, dwarf-elder [English]. Pertit Southeau [French]. Ébulo [Portuguese]. Sauco, sauco enano, sauco menor, sauquillo, yezgo [Spanish].
Life form: Tree. **Part(s) Used:** Flower, fruit / Fresh; flower / Dried. **Geographic distribution:** North Africa. Temperate-Asia (Himalaya). Europe.

Reference(s): Bharatan *et al.* 2002; Bolte *et al.* 1997; Dorta Soares, n.d.; Remedia/at, 2010; American Institute of Homeopathy, 1979.

Sambucus nigra

Scientific Name(s) / [Botanical Family]: *Sambucus nigra* L. [Adoxaceae, Caprifoliaceae, Sambucaceae].
Common Name(s): Black elder, borte tree, boul tree, common or European elder [English]. Grand Southeau, Southeau, Southeau noir [French]. Sabugueiro [Portuguese]. Sabuco, sambugo, saúco, cañilero, canillero, cauco negro [Spanish].
Life form: Tree. **Part(s) Used:** Flower, fruit / Fresh; young inner bark branche's / Fresh; flower / Dried. **Geographic distribution:** Temperate-Asia. Europe central & southern. Naturalized in North Africa, Asia & North New Zealand.
Reference(s): Bharatan *et al.* 2002; Bolte *et al.* 1997; Dorta Soares, n.d.; Plants for a future, 2009.

Sanguinaria canadensis

Scientific Name(s) / [Botanical Family]: *Sanguinaria canadensis* L. [Papaveraceae].
Common Name(s): Blood root, bloodwort, indian pait, puccoon, red root, tetterwort [English]. Sanguinaire du Canada [French]. Raiz sanguinária, tinta indiana [Portuguese]. Sanguinaria del Canadá [Spanish].
Life form: Herb. **Part(s) Used:** Subterraneous parts / Fresh; Root / Fresh / Dried. Leaf collected before bloom / Dried. **Geographic distribution:** North America (Canada. United States of America).
Reference(s): Bharatan *et al.* 2002; Bolte *et al.* 1997; Dorta Soares, n.d.; Guermonprez *et al.* 1989; Müntz, n.d.; Remedia/at, 2010; Tiwari *et al.* 2013; American Institute of Homeopathy, 1979.

Sanguisorba officinalis

Scientific Name(s) / [Botanical Family]: *Sanguisorba officinalis* L. = *Sanguisorba carnea* Fisch. ex Link = *Sanguisorba polygama* F. Nyl. = *Poterium officinale* (L.) A. Gray [Rosaceae].

Common Name(s): Di yu [Chinese]. Burnet bloodwort, common, great or salad burnet, sanguisorba [English]. Grande pimprenelle [French]. Pimpinela mayor [Spanish].

Life form: Herb. **Part(s) Used:** Complete plant in bloom / Fresh.

Geographic distribution: Temperate-Asia. Europe. North America (Canada. Northwest & Southwest United States of America). Naturalized in several places.

Reference(s): Allen, 2006-2010; Bharatan *et al.* 2002; Bolte *et al.* 1997; Dorta Soares, n.d.; Plants for a future, 2009; Remedia/at, 2010; American Institute of Homeopathy, 1979.

Sanicula europaea

Scientific Name(s) / [Botanical Family]: *Sanicula europaea* L. [Apiaceae, Umbelliferae].

Common Name(s): Butterwort, european sanicle, sanicle, wood sanicle [English]. Sanicle d'Europe [French]. Sanícula [Portuguese]. Hierba de la estocada, hierba de San Lorenzo, sanícula, sanícula macho [Spanish].

Life form: Herb. **Part(s) Used:** Complete plant in bloom / Fresh.

Geographic distribution: South Africa. Temperate-Asia. Europe.

Reference(s): Bharatan *et al.* 2002; Dorta Soares, n.d.; Müntz, n.d.; Plants for a future, 2009; Remedia/at, 2010; Zandvoort, 2006.

Saponaria

Scientific Name(s) / [Botanical Family]: *Saponaria officinalis* L. [Caryophyllaceae].

Common Name(s): Bouncing-bet, common soapwort [English]. Saponaire [French]. Erva saboneira, saboeira, saponária

[Portuguese]. Saponaria, jabonera [Spanish].
Life form: Herb. **Part(s) Used:** Complete plant in bloom / Fresh; fruit mature / Dried. **Geographic distribution:** Temperate-Asia. Europe. Cultivated & extensively naturalized in several places.
Reference(s): Bharatan *et al.* 2002; Dorta Soares, n.d.; Remedia/at, 2010.

Sarracenia purpurea

Scientific Name(s) / [Botanical Family]: *Sarracenia purpurea* L. [Rosaceae, Sarraceniaceae].
Common Name(s): Eve's cup, fly trap, Huntsman's cup, pitcher plant [English]. Sarracenie pourpre [French]. Copo de caçador, xícara de Eva [Portuguese]. Sarracenia [Spanish].
Life form: Herb. **Part(s) Used:** Complete plant / Fresh.
Geographic distribution: North America (Canada. North East, North, Central & Southeast United States of America).
Reference(s): Bharatan *et al.* 2002; Dorta Soares, n.d.; Fuentes, 1996; Guermonprez *et al.* 1989; Remedia/at, 2010.

Sarsaparilla

Scientific Name(s) / [Botanical Family]: *Smilax regelli* Killip & C. V. Morton = *Smilax medica* Schlecht. & Cham. = *Smilax sarsaparilla* L. = *Smilax officinalis* Kunth [Smilacaceae, Liliaceae].
Common Name(s): Gray, Mexican sarsaparilla, sarsaparilla, Veracruz sarsaparilla. Salsepareille du Mexique [French]. Sarzaparrilla, Zarzaparilla [Spanish].
Life form: Herb. **Part(s) Used:** Root / Dried. **Geographic distribution:** North America (Central Mexico). Central America.
Reference(s): Bharatan *et al.* 2002; Remedia/at, 2010; Tiwari *et al.* 2013; American Institute of Homeopathy, 1979.

Sassafras

Scientific Name(s) / [Botanical Family]: *Sassafras albidum*

(Nutal) Ness = *Sassafras officinalis* T. Ness & C. H. Eberm. = *Sassafras officinale* T. Ness = *Laurus sassafras* L. = *Laurus albida* Nutt. [Lauraceae].
Common Name(s): Sassafras, white sassafras [English]. Sassafras [French]. Canela sassafrás, sassafás [Portuguese]. Sasafrás [Spanish].
Life form: Tree. **Part(s) Used:** Wood / Dried; bark root, bark wood / Dried. **Geographic distribution:** North America (East Canada. North East, North Central, Southeast & South Central United States of America).
Reference(s): Bharatan *et al.* 2002; Dorta Soares, n.d.; Guermonprez *et al.* 1989; Remedia/at, 2010; Tiwari *et al.* 2013.

Satureja

Scientific Name(s) / [Botanical Family]: *Satureja hortensis* L. [Lamiaceae, Labiatae].
Common Name(s): Savory, summer savory [English]. Sarriette des jardins, savourée [French]. Sergurelha [Portuguese]. Ajedrea blanca, ajedrea común, saborida, tomillo real [Spanish].
Life form: Herb. **Part(s) Used:** Leaf / Dried. **Geographic distribution:** Temperate-Asia (Turkey). East Southeast & Southwest Europe. Cultivated United States of America.
Reference(s): Bharatan *et al.* 2002; Bolte *et al.* 1997; Remedia/at, 2010; American Institute of Homeopathy, 1979.

Saxifraga granulata

Scientific Name(s) / [Botanical Family]: *Saxifraga granulata* L. [Grossulariaceae, Saxifragaceae].
Common Name(s): Saxi, Saxifraga, meadox saxifrage [English]. Saxifrage granulée [French]. Quebra-pedra, saxifraga [Portuguese]. Saxífraga, cañivano, uvas de gato [Spanish].
Life form: Herb. **Part(s) Used:** Aerial part in bloom / Fresh. **Geographic distribution:** North Africa. Europe.

Reference(s): Bharatan *et al.* 2002; Dorta Soares, n.d.; Müntz, n.d.; Remedia/at, 2010.

Scabiosa arvensis

Scientific Name(s) / [Botanical Family]: *Knautia arvensis* (L.) Coult. = *Scabiosa arvensis* L. = *Trichera arvensis* (L.) Schrad. [Dipsacaceae].

Common Name(s): Egyptian rose, field scabious, gypsies rose [English]. Knautie des champs, scabieuse des prés [French]. Escabiosa dos campos, erva-dos-prados [Portuguese]. Escabiosa [Spanish].

Life form: Herb. **Part(s) Used:** Aerial part in bloom / Fresh; flower or also root / Dried. **Geographic distribution:** Temperate-Asia. Central Europe. Great Britain. Asia. Naturalized in several places.

Reference(s): Dorta Soares, n.d.; Remedia/at, 2010.

Scabiosa succisa

Scientific Name(s) / [Botanical Family]: *Scabiosa pratensis* Moench. = *Scabiosa praemorsa* Gilib. = *Scabiosa succisa* L. = *Succisa praemorsa* Asch. = *Succisa pratensis* Moench = *Asterocephalus succisa* (L.) Wallr. [Dipsacaceae].

Common Name(s): Blue buttons, devil's bit scabious, devlsbit scabious [English]. Scabieuse de prés, scabieuse succise, succise des prés [French]. Morso del diavolo [Italian]. Escabiosa mordida, lengua de vaca, viuda silvestre [Spanish].

Life form: Herb. **Part(s) Used:** Complete plant; root / Fresh. **Geographic distribution:** Asia. Europe. North Africa. North America (United States of America) introduced.

Reference(s): Bolte *et al.* 1997; Dorta Soares, n.d.; Müntz, n.d.; Plants for a future, 2009; Remedia/at, 2010.

Scammonium

Scientific Name(s) / [Botanical Family]: *Convolvulus scammonia* L. = *Convolvulus pseudo-scammonia* C. Koch = *Convolvulus elongatus* Salisb. = *Scammonia syriaca* Bauh. [Convolvulaceae].
Common Name(s): Scammony, Syrian Bindweed [English]. Scammonée [French]. Sak munia [India]. Escamônia [Portuguese]. Escamonia [Spanish].
Life form: Herb. **Part(s) Used:** Latex (resin) root / Dried.
Geographic distribution: Temperate-Asia (West Asia). East Europe.
Reference(s): Bharatan *et al.* 2002; Bolte *et al.* 1997; Dorta Soares, n.d.; Müntz, n.d.; Remedia/at, 2010.

Schinus

Scientific Name(s) / [Botanical Family]: *Schinus molle* L. = *Schinus areira* L. = *Schinus huygan* Molina [Anacardiaceae].
Common Name(s): California pepper tree, pepper tree, peruvian mastictree [English]. Faux poivrier, molée des jardins, poivrier d'Amérique [French]. Aroeira-do-Amazonas, aroeira-folha-de-salso, aroeiro-mole, corneíba, pimenteira bastarda [Portuguese]. Árbol del Perú, pimienta de America, pimentero falso, peloncuáhuitl, pirú, pirul, tsactumi, tzantumi, xasa, xaza, yaga-cica, yaga-lache [Spanish].
Life form: Tree. **Part(s) Used:** Fruit mature, leaf / Dried.
Geographic distribution: Mexico. Naturalized in several places.
Reference(s): Bharatan *et al.* 2002; Dorta Soares, n.d.

Scilla see *Squilla*

Scleranthus annus

Scientific Name(s) / [Botanical Family]: *Scleranthus annuus* L. [Caryophyllaceae, Illecebraceae].
Common Name(s): Annual knawel, German-knotweed, knawel,

Knotgrass [English]. Scléranthe annuel [French]. Escleranto [Spanish].
Life form: Herb. **Part(s) Used:** Flower?. **Geographic distribution:** Africa. Temperate-Asia. Europe. Naturalized in several parts in temperate regions.
Reference: Bharatan *et al.* 2002.

Scolopendrium see *Phyllitis scolopendrium*

Scorzonera hispanica

Scientific Name(s) / [Botanical Family]: *Scorzonera hispanica* L. [Asteraceae, Compositae].
Common Name(s): Black salsify, common viper's-grass, salsify black oysterplant, scorzonera, Spanish-salsify [English]. Salsifis noir, scorsonère [French]. Escorcioneira [Portuguese]. Escorzonera, escurzo, salsifí negro [Spanish].
Life form: Herb. **Part(s) Used:** Complete plant / Fresh.
Geographic distribution: Temperate-Asia Europe. Naturalized & cultivated in several places.
Reference(s): Bharatan *et al.* 2002; Remedia/at, 2010.

Scrofularia nodosa

Scientific Name(s) / [Botanical Family]: *Scrophularia nodosa* L. = *Scrophularia foetida* Garsault [Scrophulariaceae].
Common Name(s): Figwort [English]. Scrofularie noureuse [French]. Erva de São Pedro, pimpinela azul [Portuguese]. Escrofularia, Escrophularia, hierba de lamparones, hierba de San Pedro [Spanish].
Life form: Herb. **Part(s) Used:** Complete plant / Fresh; Aerial parts collected in early bloom / Fresh. **Geographic distribution:** Temperate-Asia. Europe. Naturalized in several parts of the temperate region of the North Hemisphere.
Reference(s): Bharatan *et al.* 2002; Dorta Soares, n.d.;

Remedia/at, 2010; Tiwari *et al.* 2013.

Scutellaria

Scientific Name(s) / [Botanical Family]: *Scutellaria lateriflora* L. [Lamiaceae, Labiatae].

Common Name(s): Blue skullcap, mad-dog scullcap, scullcap [English]. Scutellaire d'America ique [French]. Gorra de cráneo [Spanish].

Life form: Herb. **Part(s) Used:** Complete plant, leaf, stem / Fresh.

Geographic distribution: North America (Canada. United States of America).

Reference(s): Bharatan *et al.* 2002; Dorta Soares, n.d.; Guermonprez *et al.* 1989; Remedia/at, 2010; Seror, 2000; Tiwari *et al.* 2013.

Scutellaria galericulata

Scientific Name(s) / [Botanical Family]: *Scutellaria galericulata* L. = *Scutellaria epilobiifolia* A. Ham. [Lamiaceae, Labiatae].

Common Name(s): Common skullcap, mad-dog skullcap, marsh scullcap, skullcap. [English]. Scutellaire casquée [French]. Cráneo gorra, hierba de la celada, tercianaria [Spanish].

Life form: Herb. **Part(s) Used:** seeds / Dried. **Geographic distribution:** Temperate-Asia. Europe. North America.

Reference(s): Bharatan *et al.* 2002; Dorta Soares, n.d.

Scutellaria laterifolia see *Scutellaria*

Secale cornutum see *Claviceps purpurea*

Selaginella lepidophylla

Scientific Name(s) / [Botanical Family]: *Selaginella lepidophylla* (Hook. & Grev.) Spring [Selaginellaceae].

Common Name(s): Resurrection-plant, rose-of-Jericho [English].

Doradilla, flor de piedra, Flor de resurrección, siempreviva, tequequetzal [Spanish].
Life form: Herb. **Part(s) Used:** Complete plant. **Geographic distribution:** North America (Mexico. United States of America). Central America.
Reference(s): Bharatan *et al.* 2002; Remedia/at, 2010.

Semecarpus anacardium

Scientific Name(s) / [Botanical Family]: *Semecarpus anacardium* L. f. = *Anacardium offixinarum* Gaertn. [Anacardiaceae].
Common Name(s): Cashew [English]. Anacardier [French]. Cajú, cajú-da-India, cajueiro [Portuguese]. Anacardo, marañón, nuez de caoba, nuez del pantano [Spanish].
Life form: Tree. **Part(s) Used:** Fruit / Dried; fruit juice & seeds.
Geographic distribution: India, Tropical Asia. America (North South & West South America). Cultivated.
Reference(s): Bharatan *et al.* 2002; Dorta Soares, n.d.; Remedia/at, 2010.

Senecio aureus

Scientific Name(s) / [Botanical Family]: *Senecio aureus* L. = *Packera aurea* (L.) Á. Löve & D. Löve [Asteraceae, Compositae].
Common Name(s): Golden ragwort, golden squaw-weed, heart-leaf groundsel, liferoot [English]. Sénéçon doré [French]. Valeriana falsa [Portuguese]. Senecio americano [Spanish].
Life form: Herb. **Part(s) Used:** Complete plant / Fresh / Dried; leaves collected during the bloom / Dried. **Geographic distribution:** East & West Canada. North, West & Southeast United States of America.
Reference(s): Bharatan *et al.* 2002; Boericke, 1927, 1927b.; Clarke, 2008; Dorta Soares, n.d.; Remedia/at, 2010; Tiwari *et al.* 2013.

Senecio hieracifolia see *Erechtites hieracifolia*

Senecio jacobaea
Scientific Name(s) / [Botanical Family]: *Senecio jacobaea* L. = *Jacobaea vulgaris* Gaertn. [Asteraceae, Compositae].
Common Name(s): St. James'-wort, stinking Willie, ragwort, tansy ragwort [English]. Erva de Santiago, erva lanceta do Canada [Portuguese]. Hierba cana, hierba de Santiago [Spanish].
Life form: Herb. **Part(s) Used:** Complete plant / Fresh / Dried.
Geographic distribution: Europe. North Africa. West Asia. Naturalized in several places.
Reference(s): Bharatan *et al.* 2002; Dorta Soares, n.d.

Senecio vulgaris
Scientific Name(s) / [Botanical Family]: *Senecio vulgaris* L.
Common Name(s): Common groundsel [English]. Cardo-morto, tasneirinha [Portuguese]. Senecio lechugilla [Spanish].
Life form: Herb. **Part(s) Used:** Complete plant or also flower / Dried. **Geographic distribution:** Europe, North Africa. Temperate-Asia.
Reference(s): Bharatan *et al.* 2002; Dorta Soares, n.d.; Plants for a future, 2009.

Senega
Scientific Name(s) / [Botanical Family]: *Polygala senega* L. and other species of *Polygala* genus [Polygalaceae].
Common Name(s): Milkwort, mountain flag, Polygala virginiana, Snake root, seneca [English]. Polygala de Virginie [French]. Polígala da Virgínia, senega [Portuguese]. Serpentaria senegalesa [Spanish].
Life form: Herb. **Part(s) Used:** Root / Dried; root collected when the leaves are dried / Dried. **Geographic distribution:** North

America (East & West Canada. North East, North, Central & Southeast United States of America).
Reference(s): Bolte *et al.* 1997; Dorta Soares, n.d.; Müntz, n.d.; Plants for a future, 2009; Remedia/at, 2010; Tiwari *et al.* 2013.

Sequoiadendron giganteum

Scientific Name(s) / [Botanical Family]: *Sequoiadendron giganteum* (Lindl.) J. Buchholz [Cupressaceae, Taxodiaceae].
Common Name(s): Big tree, giant redwood, giant-sequoia, Indian redwood, sequoia, sierra redwood, wellingtonia [English]. Séquoia [French].
Life form: Tree. **Part(s) Used:** seeds / Fresh. **Geographic distribution:** North America (Southwest United States of America).
Reference(s): Bharatan *et al.* 2002; Guermonprez *et al.* 1989; Müntz, n.d.; Remedia/at, 2010.

Serpentaria

Scientific Name(s) / [Botanical Family]: *Aristolochia serpentaria* L. = *Aristolochia convolvulacea* Small = *Aristolochia hastata* Nutt. = *Aristolochia nashii* Kearney [Aristolochiaceae].
Common Name(s): Red river snake root, sangrel, serpentaria, Texas snake-root, Virginia snake-root, Virginia dutchmanspipe, Virginia snakeroot [English]. Raiz de cobra da Virgínia, serpentaria [Portuguese]. Serpentaria de Virginia [Spanish].
Life form: Herb. **Part(s) Used:** Root / Dried. **Geographic distribution:** North America (North East, Southwest & South Central United States of America. Texas state).
Reference(s): Dorta Soares, n.d.; Remedia/at, 2010.

Siegesbeckia

Scientific Name(s) / [Botanical Family]: *Siegesbeckia orientalis* L. = *Siegesbeckia brachiata* Roxb. = *Siegesbeckia gracilis* DC. =

Siegesbeckia microcephala DC. = *Siegesbeckia orientalis* var. *angustifolia* Makino = *Sigesbeckia humilis* Koidz. = *Sigesbeckia iberica* Willd. [Asteraceae, Compositae].
Common Name(s): Xi xian cao [Chinese]. Eastern Saint Paul wort, siegesbeckia, the holy herb [English]. Erva santa [Portuguese].
Life form: Herb. **Part(s) Used:** Complete plant. **Geographic distribution:** Africa. Temperate-Asia (China, India). Australia. Madagascar.
Reference(s): Bharatan *et al.* 2002; Bolte *et al.* 1997; Clarke, 2008; Dorta Soares, n.d.; Remedia/at, 2010; Tiwari *et al.* 2013; American Institute of Homeopathy, 1979.

Siegesbeckia orientalis see *Siegesbeckia*

Sigesbeckia see *Siegesbeckia*

Siliqua dulcis see *Ceratonia siliqua*

Silphion

Scientific Name(s) / [Botanical Family]: *Thapsia silphium* Viv. = *Thapsia garganica* L. var. *silphium* [Apiaceae = Umbelliferae].
Common Name(s): Deadly carrot?, laser, silphion [English].
Life form: Herb. **Part(s) Used:** Root-bark resin, trunk or also root / Fresh. **Geographic distribution:** Europe (Mediterranean).
Reference(s): Dorta Soares, n.d.; Zandvoort, 2006.

Sinapis alba

Scientific Name(s) / [Botanical Family]: *Brassica alba* (L.) Rabenh = *Brassica hirta* Moench. = *Sinapis alba* L. = *Sinapis alba* subsp. *alba* = *Sinapis alba* var. *melanosperma* Alef. [Brassicaceae, Cruciferae].
Common Name(s): White mustard, wild mustard [English]. Moutarde blanche [French]. Mostarda clara, mostarda branca

[Portuguese]. Mostaza blanca [Spanish].
Life form: Herb. **Part(s) Used:** seeds / Fresh. **Geographic distribution:** Extensively naturalized. Introduced in United States of America.
Reference(s): Bharatan *et al.* 2002; Dorta Soares, n.d.; Remedia/at, 2010; Tiwari *et al.* 2013.

Sinapis nigra

Scientific Name(s) / [Botanical Family]: *Brassica nigra* (L.) W. D. J. Koch [Cruciferae, Brassicaceae].
Common Name(s): Black or brown mustard [English]. Moutarde noire [French]. Mostarda-petra [Portuguese]. Mostaza negra [Spanish].
Life form: Herb. **Part(s) Used:** seeds / Fresh. **Geographic distribution:** Europe. United States of America introduced. Extensively cultivated & naturalized.
Reference(s): Bharatan *et al.* 2002; Remedia/at, 2010; Tiwari *et al.* 2013 , American Institute of Homeopathy, 1979.

Smilax cordifolia

Scientific Name(s) / [Botanical Family]: *Smilax cordifolia* Humb. et Bonp. ex Willd. [Smilacaceae].
Common Name(s): Cocolmeca, cozolmécatl, cuculmeca, raíz de China [Spanish]. China root, greenbrier [English].
Life form: Herb. **Part(s) Used:** Root / Dried. **Geographic distribution:** Mexico. India.
Reference(s): Bharatan *et al.* 2002; Dorta Soares, n.d.; Fuentes, 1996; Remedia/at, 2010; American Institute of Homeopathy, 1979.

Solanum carolinense

Scientific Name(s) / [Botanical Family]: *Solanum carolinense* L. [Solanaceae].

Common Name(s): Apple of Sodome, ball nightshade, ball-nettle, Carolina horse-nettle, horse-nettle [English]. Morelle de Caroline [French]. Urtiga de cavalo [Portuguese].
Life form: Herb. **Part(s) Used:** Fruit mature / Fresh; seeds.
Geographic distribution: North America (Canada. United States of America. Mexico). Naturalized in several places.
Reference(s): De Legarreta, 1961; Dorta Soares, n.d.; Tiwari *et al.* 2013; American Institute of Homeopathy, 1979.

Solanum malacoxylon

Scientific Name(s) / [Botanical Family]: *Solanum malacoxylon* Sendtn. = *Solanum glaucum* Bertoloni = *Solanum glaucum* Dunal = *Solanum glaucophyllum* Desf. [Solanaceae].
Common Name(s): Waxyleaf nightshade [English].
Life form: Herb. **Part(s) Used:** Fruit, leaf?. **Geographic distribution:** South America (Argentine, Bolivia, Brazil, Paraguay, Uruguay).
Reference(s): Bharatan *et al.* 2002; Müntz, n.d.; Plants for a future, 2009; Remedia/at, 2010.

Solanum mammosum

Scientific Name(s) / [Botanical Family]: *Solanum mammosum* L. = *Solanum mammosissium* Ramirez = *Solanum platanifolium* Hook. [Solanaceae].
Common Name(s): Apple of Sodom, macawbush, nipplefruit, pig's-ears, Sodom apple, sodomsapfel [English]. Tétons de jeune fille, morelle à fruit ornemental, morelle molle [French]. Beringela, juá bravo [Portuguese]. Tetilla, berenjena, berenjena de gallina, berenjena de teta, berenjenita peluda, chichigûita, cijón de gato, cuchito, chuuch, pichichio [Spanish].
Life form: Herb. **Part(s) Used:** Fruit mature / Fresh. **Geographic distribution:** North America (Mexico). Central & South America. & cultivated.

Reference(s): Bharatan *et al.* 2002; Dorta Soares, n.d.; Remedia/at, 2010.

Solanum nigrescens

Scientific Name(s) / [Botanical Family]: *Solanum nigrescens* M. Martens et Galeotti = *Solanum aloysiaefolium* Dunal = *Solanum approximatum* Bitter = *Solanum basilobum* Bitter = *Solanum costaricense* Heiser = *Solanum crenato-dentatum* Dunal = *Solanum crenato-dentatum* var. *ramossissium* Dunal = *Solanum deltaicum* Cabrera & 19 scientific synonyms more. [Solanaceae].

Common Name(s): Divine nightshade [English]. Hierba mora [Spanish].

Life form: Herb. **Part(s) Used:** Complete plant, fruit / Fresh.

Geographic distribution: Europe. North America (Mexico. United States of America). Central & South America.

Reference(s): Bharatan *et al.* 2002; Remedia/at, 2010.

Solanum nigrum

Scientific Name(s) / [Botanical Family]: *Solanum nigrum* L. [Solanaceae].

Common Name(s): Black nightshade, common nightshade, poisonberry [English]. Morelle noire [French]. Aguaraquía, carachichu, erva moura, pimenta-de-galinha [Portuguese]. Bahab-kan, bahalkan, bi-tache, hierba mora, ich-kan, la-bithoxi, pak'al-kan, pettoxe, pitoxe, pitoxi, vishate, chichiquelite, chichiquelitl, chuchilitas, mambia, maniliche, mutztututi, tonchichi [Spanish].

Life form: Herb. **Part(s) Used:** Complete plant / Fresh.

Geographic distribution: Africa. Temperate-Asia (Australasia). Europe. North, Central & South America. Naturalized in several places.

Reference(s): Bharatan *et al.* 2002; Dorta Soares, n.d.; Fuentes,

1996; Tiwari *et al.* 2013.

Solanum oleraceum

Scientific Name(s) / [Botanical Family]: *Solanum americanum* Mill. = *Solanum oleraceum* Dunal ex Poir. = *Solanum nigrum* auct. non L. [Solanaceae].
Common Name(s): American or glossy nightshade, black nightshade [English]. Herbe à calalou [French]. Hierba mora negra, yerba mora [Spanish].
Life form: Herb. **Part(s) Used:** Fruit, leaf?. **Geographic distribution:** Naturalized in several places.
Reference(s): Bharatan *et al.* 2002; Remedia/at, 2010.

Solanum pseudocapsicum

Scientific Name(s) / [Botanical Family]: *Solanum pseudocapsicum* L. [Solanaceae].
Common Name(s): Jerusalemkersie [African]. False Jerusalem-cherry, Jerusalem-cherry, Madeira winter-cherry, Madeira-cherry, winter-cherry [English]. Ginjeira da tierra [Portuguese]. Cereza de Jerusalén [Spanish].
Life form: Herb. **Part(s) Used:** Complete plant in bloom / Fresh.
Geographic distribution: Mexico. South America (Argentine, Bolivia, Brazil, Ecuador, Peru).
Reference(s): Bharatan *et al.* 2002; Dorta Soares, n.d.; Fuentes, 1996; Plants for a future, 2009; Tiwari *et al.* 2013.

Solanum tuberosum

Scientific Name(s) / [Botanical Family]: *Solanum tuberosum* L. = Poepp. ex Walp. = *Solanum maglia* Schltdl. [Solanaceae].
Common Name(s): Irish potato, potato, potatoes, white potato [English]. Patate, pommes de terre [French]. Batata inglesa, batatinha [Portuguese]. Jroca, nyami-tecuinti, papa, papa correlona, papa común, patata, rerohue, rerogûe, rirohui,

[Spanish].
Life form: Herb. **Part(s) Used:** Fruit, tuber, complete plant / Fresh; tuber whitout bark / Dried. **Geographic distribution:** Peru (Andes). Cultivated cosmopolitan.
Reference(s): Bharatan *et al.* 2002; Dorta Soares, n.d.

Solanum xanthocarpum

Scientific Name(s) / [Botanical Family]: *Solanum virginianum* L. = *Solanum xanthocarpum* Schrad. et H. Wendl. [Solanaceae].
Common Name(s): Yellow-fruit nightshade [English].
Life form: Herb. **Part(s) Used:** Leaf?, fruit. **Geographic distribution:** Temperate-Asia. Tropical Asia. Naturalized in several places.
Reference(s): Bharatan *et al.* 2002; Müntz, n.d.; Remedia/at, 2010; Tiwari *et al.* 2013.

Solanum xanthocarpus see *Solanum xanthocarpum*

Solidago

Scientific Name(s) / [Botanical Family]: *Solidago virgaurea* L. [Asteraceae, Compositae].
Common Name(s): European goldenrod [English]. Verge d'or [French]. Mao gao yi zhi huang hua [Chinese]. Arnica silvestre, erva lanceta, vara de ouro [Portuguese]. Consuelda sarracénica, hierba of indios, plumeros amarillos, solidago virgaurea, vara de oro, vara de San José [Spanish].
Life form: Herb. **Part(s) Used:** Flower (inflorescence) / Fresh / Dried; complete plant / Fresh. **Geographic distribution:** Temperate-Asia (China, Mongolia, Nepal, Pakistan, Russia). Europe. Naturalized in several places.
Reference(s): Bharatan *et al.* 2002; Dorta Soares, n.d.; Tiwari *et al.* 2013.

Sophora japonica

Scientific Name(s) / [Botanical Family]: *Sophora japonica* L. = *Styphnolobium japonicum* (L.) Schott [Fabaceae, Leguminosae].
Common Name(s): Chinese scholartree, Japanese pagoda-tree, pagoda-tree [English]. Acácia do Japão, àrvore dos pagodes [Portuguese]. Acacia del Japón, árbol de las pagodas, sófora [Spanish].
Life form: Tree. **Part(s) Used:** Leaf / Fresh; mature seeds / Dried.
Geographic distribution: Temperate-Asia (China, Japan). Cultivated in several places.
Reference(s): Bharatan *et al.* 2002; Dorta Soares, n.d.; Guermonprez *et al.* 1989; Müntz, n.d.; Remedia/at, 2010.

Sorbus aucuparia

Scientific Name(s) / [Botanical Family]: *Pyrus aucuparia* (L.) Gaertn. = *Pyrus americana* DC. = *Sorbus aucuparia* L. subsp. *aucuparia* = *Sorbus lanuginosa* Kit. = *Sorbus maderensis* (Lowe) Dode = *Sorbus aucuparia* subsp. *maderensis* = *Sorbus pohuashanensis* (Hance) Hedl. = *Sorbus aucuparia* subsp. *pohuashanensis* = *Sorbus sibirica* Hedl. [Rosaceae].
Common Name(s): European mountain-ash, mountain-ash, quick beam, rowan, rowantree [English]. Sorbier des oiseleurs [French]. Capudre, capudrio, serbal de cazadores, serbal silvestre, sorbito [Spanish].
Life form: Shrub, Tree. **Part(s) Used:** Bark, fruit / Fresh.
Geographic distribution: Asia. Europe. North America (Canada. United States of America) naturalized.
Reference(s): Dorta Soares, n.d.; Remedia/at, 2010.

Soya blüte

Scientific Name(s) / [Botanical Family]: *Glycine max* (L.) Merr. [Fabaceae, Leguminosae].
Common Name(s): Soy bean, soya bean [English]. Soja [French].

Soja [Portuguese]. Frijol de soya, soja, soya [Spanish].
Life form: Herb. **Part(s) Used:** Seeds. **Geographic distribution:** North America (Mexico, United States of America). Cultivated.
Reference(s): Remedia/at, 2010.

Soya fluor see *Soya blüte*

Spartium scoparium see *Cytisus scoparius*

Spigelia

Scientific Name(s) / [Botanical Family]: *Spigelia anthelmia* L. [Loganiaceae].
Common Name(s): East Indian-pink; worm-grass [English]. Spigélie vermifuge [French]. Arapabaca, erva lombrigueira [Portuguese]. Hierba de la lombricera, lombricera, ocolintequitcua, tequitcua [Spanish].
Life form: Herb. **Part(s) Used:** Aerial part / Fresh-Dried; Complete plant recently collected during the fructifying including flowers & seeds / Dried. **Geographic distribution:** North, Central & South America. Naturalized in several places.
Reference(s): Bharatan *et al.* 2002; Dorta Soares, n.d.; Tiwari *et al.* 2013.

Spigelia marilandica

Scientific Name(s) / [Botanical Family]: *Spigelia marilandica* (L.) L. = *Lonicera marilandica* L. [Loganiaceae].
Common Name(s): Indian pink, indian pink root, pinkroot, woodland pinkroot [English]. Eillet de la Caroline [French]. Cravo da carolina, espigelia de Maryland [Portuguese].
Life form: Herb. **Part(s) Used:** Complete plant; Root / Dried. **Geographic distribution:** North America (United States of America).
Reference(s): Bharatan *et al.* 2002; Dorta Soares, n.d.; Remedia/at, 2010.

Spilanthes acmella

Scientific Name(s) / [Botanical Family]: *Spilanthes acmella* (L.) L. = *Spilanthes acmella* (L.) Murr. = *Blainvillea acmella* (L.) Philipson = *Bidens acmella* (L.) Lam. = *Blainvillea latifolia* (L. f.) DC. = *Blainvillea rhomboidea* Cass. = *Coreopsis acmella* (L.) K. Krause = *Pyrethrum acmella* (L.) Medik. = *Spilanthes acmella* (L.) Dalz. & Gibs. = *Spilanthes acmella* (L.) L. = *Spilanthes acmella* (L.) Murr. = *Spilanthes arrayana* Gardn. = *Verbesina acmella* L. [Asteraceae, Compositae].
Common Name(s): Annual paracress, paracress, Paraguay cress, Pellitary spotflower, toothache plant [English]. Cresson de para [French]. Akarkara [Indio]. Abecedaria, canela-de-urubú, erva-palha, picão-grande [Portuguese]. Jambu [Spanish].
Life form: Herb. **Part(s) Used:** Flower / Fresh / Dried. **Geographic distribution:** South America. Temperate-Asia (China-India). Naturalized in tropics.
Reference(s): Bharatan *et al.* 2002; Bolte *et al.* 1997; Dorta Soares, n.d.

Spiraea

Scientific Name(s) / [Botanical Family]: *Filipendula ulmaria* (L.) Maxim. = *Spiraea ulmaria* L. = *Ulmaria pentapetala* Gilb. [Rosaceae].
Common Name(s): Xuan guo wen zi cao [Chinese]. Queen of the meadow, meadowsweet [English]. Erva das abelhas, rainha dos prados [Portuguese]. Barba de cabra, filipendula ulmaria, ulmaria [Spanish].
Life form: Herb. **Part(s) Used:** Inflorescences, root / Fresh. **Geographic distribution:** Temperate-Asia. Europe. North America (East United States of America).
Reference(s): Bharatan *et al.* 2002; Dorta Soares, n.d.; Remedia/at, 2010.

Spiranthes

Scientific Name(s) / [Botanical Family]: *Spiranthes spiralis* (L.) Chevall. = *Ophrys spiralis* L. = *Ophrys autumnalis* Balb. [Orchidaceae].
Common Name(s): Autumn Lady's tresses. [English]. Spiranthe d'automne [French]. Trança de mulher [Portuguese].
Life form: Herb. **Part(s) Used:** Complete plant in bloom, root / Fresh. **Geographic distribution:** Europe. West Asia.
Reference(s): Bharatan *et al.* 2002; Bolte *et al.* 1997; Dorta Soares, n.d.; Müntz, n.d.; Plants for a future, 2009; Remedia/at, 2010.

Spiranthes autumnalis see *Spiranthes*

Spiritus glandium Quercus

Scientific Name(s) / [Botanical Family]: *Quercus robur* L.
Common Name(s): Common oak, english oak, french oak, oak, pedunculate oak [English]. Chęne pédonculé, chéne rouvre [French]. Roble común, roble fresnal [Spanish].
Life form: Tree. **Part(s) Used:** Bark, fruit / Fresh. **Geographic distribution:** England. Asia. Europe (except North East Mediterranean). Russia cultivated.
Reference: Bharatan *et al.* 2002.

Squilla

Scientific Name(s) / [Botanical Family]: *Urginea maritima* (L.) Baker = *Urginea scilla* Steinh. = *Scilla maritima* (L.) Stein. = *Drimia maritima* (L.) Stearn [Hyacinthaceae, Liliaceae].
Common Name(s): European squill, red-squill, sea-onion, sea-squill, squill [English]. Scille maritime [French]. Escila [Spanish].
Life form: Herb. **Part(s) Used:** Bulb, bud / Fresh. **Geographic distribution:** Southeast & Southwest Europe (Mediterranean).

Temperate-Asia.
Reference(s): Bharatan *et al.* 2002; Dorta Soares, n.d.; Guermonprez *et al.* 1989; Müntz, n.d.; Tiwari *et al.* 2013.

Stachys betonica

Scientific Name(s) / [Botanical Family]: *Betonica officinalis* L. = *Stachys betonica* Benth. = *Stachys betonica* Crantz = *Stachys betonica* Scop. = *Stachys annua* L. = *Stachys annua* Walter = *Stachys annua* Sibth & Sm. = *Stachys officinalis* Franch. = *Stachys officinalis* (L.) Trevisan = *Stachys recta* L. = *Stachys recta* d'Urv. = *Stachys recta* Parol ex Vis [Lamiaceae, Labiatae].
Common Name(s): Betony, Bishop's wort, purple betony, wood betony [English]. Bétoine officinale [French]. Betônica [Portuguese]. Betónica [Spanish].
Life form: Herb. **Part(s) Used:** Complete plant / Fresh.
Geographic distribution: Europe. Asia Minor. Cosmopolitan.
Reference(s): Bharatan *et al.* 2002; Dorta Soares, n.d.; Guermonprez *et al.* 1989; Müntz, n.d.; Remedia/at, 2010; Tiwari *et al.* 2013.

Staphisagria

Scientific Name(s) / [Botanical Family]: *Delphinium staphisagria* L. = *Delphinium staphysagria* L. [Ranunculaceae].
Common Name(s): Louse wort, Staphisagria, stavesacre [English]. Herbe aux poux, staphysaigre, staphisagria, staphisaigre [French]. Erva de pioho [Portuguese]. Estafisagria [Spanish].
Life form: Herb. **Part(s) Used:** seeds / Dried. **Geographic distribution:** Southeast & Southwest Europe (Italy, Greece, Asia Mediterranean). Temperate-Asia.
Reference(s): Bharatan *et al.* 2002; Bolte *et al.* 1997; Dorta Soares, n.d.; Guermonprez *et al.* 1989; Müntz, n.d.; Plants for a future, 2009; Remedia/at, 2010; Tiwari *et al.* 2013.

Staphysagria see *Staphisagria*

Sticta pulmonaria

Scientific Name(s) / [Botanical Family]: *Lobaria pulmonaria* (L.) Hoffm. = *Lichen pulmonarius* L. = *Sticta pulmonaria* Hook. = *Sticta pulmonacea* Ach. = *Parmelia pulmonacea* (L.) Biroli [Lobariaceae, Stictaceae].
Common Name(s): Lungwort lichen, oak lungs [English]. Lichen pulmonaire [French]. Lobaria, pulmonaria de árbol, pulmonaria arbórea [Spanish].
Life form: Herb (Lichen). **Part(s) Used:** Complete plant / Dried or Fresh. **Geographic distribution:** Central & North Europe. North America (West United States of America [Oregon]. Canada & Mexico).
Reference(s): Bharatan *et al.* 2002; Dorta Soares, n.d.; Tiwari *et al.* 2013.

Stillingia

Scientific Name(s) / [Botanical Family]: *Stillingia sylvatica* Garden ex L. = *Stillingia sylvatica* (L.) Muell. Arg. [Euphorbiaceae].
Common Name(s): Queen's-delight, queen's-root, stillingia, yawroot [English]. Racine royale [French]. Encanto da rainha, raiz da rainha [Portuguese].
Life form: Herb. **Part(s) Used:** Root / Dried. **Geographic distribution:** North America (North Central, Northwest, Southeast & South Central United States of America).
Reference(s): Allen, 2006-2010; Bharatan *et al.* 2002; Dorta Soares, n.d.; Guermonprez *et al.* 1989; Müntz, n.d.; Remedia/at, 2010; Tiwari *et al.* 2013.

Stramonium

Scientific Name(s) / [Botanical Family]: *Datura stramonium* L. = *Datura lurida* Salisb. = *Stramoniun foetidum* Scop. [Solanaceae].
Common Name(s): Jimson weed, stink-weed, Jamestown-weed, Simpson weed, thornapple [English]. Stramoine, datura [French]. Estramonio, erva do diabo, erva dos feiticeiros, erva dos mágicos, figueira brava, figueira do inferno [Portuguese]. Chamico, flor de muerto, hierba del diablo, hierba hedionda, mehen-x-toh-k'u, nacazcul, tapat, tapate, tlapa, tepate, tlapatl, toloatzin, toloache, torescua, xholo [Spanish].
Life form: Herb. **Part(s) Used:** Aerial part in bloom / Fresh; complete plant collected in bloom / Fresh; complete plant with flower & fruit. **Geographic distribution:** Cosmopolitan, naturalized in several parts of the world.
Reference(s): Bharatan *et al.* 2002; Dorta Soares, n.d.; Guermonprez *et al.* 1989; Remedia/at, 2010; Tiwari *et al.* 2013.

Sumbul

Scientific Name(s) / [Botanical Family]: *Ferula sumbul* Hook. f. = *Ferula sumbul* (Kauffm.) Hook. f. = *Ferula moschata* (Reinsch.) K.Pol. = *Euryangium sumbul* Kauffm. [Apiaceae, Umbelliferae].
Common Name(s): Sumbul [English]. Racine de Musc [French]. Sumbul [Spanish-Portugués].
Life form: Herb. **Part(s) Used:** Flower, root, rhizome / Dried.
Geographic distribution: Ex-Soviet Union (West Asia-Turkestan-Tibet).
Reference(s): Bharatan *et al.* 2002; Bolte *et al.* 1997; Dorta Soares, n.d.; Guermonprez et al. 1989; Müntz, n.d.; Tiwari *et al.* 2013.

Sumbul plant see *Sumbul*

Symphoricarpos albus

Scientific Name(s) / [Botanical Family]: *Symphoricarpos albus* (L.) S. F. Blake = *Vaccinum album* L. [Caprifoliaceae].

Common Name(s): Snowberry [English]. Symphorine [French]. Baya de nieve, bonita de nieve [Spanish].

Life form: Tree. **Part(s) Used:** Fruit / Fresh. **Geographic distribution:** North America (United States of America).

Reference(s): Bharatan *et al.* 2002; Gotfredsen, 2009; Guermonprez *et al.* 1989; Müntz, n.d.; Plants for a future, 2009.

Symphoricarpos racemosus

Scientific Name(s) / [Botanical Family]: *Symphoricarpos racemosus* Michx. = *Symphoricarpos albus* (L.) Blake [Caprifoliaceae].

Common Name(s): Common snowberry, St. Peter´s wort [English]. Arbousier d'Amérique [French]. Bola de neve, medronheiro da America [Portuguese].

Life form: Shrub. **Part(s) Used:** Fruit / Fresh; root / Dried. **Geographic distribution:** Canada & West North America. Mexico. Naturalized in Great Britain.

Reference(s): Bharatan *et al.* 2002; Bolte *et al.* 1997; Dorta Soares, n.d.; Plants for a future, 2009; Remedia/at, 2010; Tiwari *et al.* 2013.

Symphytum

Scientific Name(s) / [Botanical Family]: *Symphytum officinale* L. [Boraginaceae].

Common Name(s): Ass ear, blackwort, boneset, bruisewort, comfrey, comfry, common comfrey [English]. Consonde officinale, consoude [French]. Confrei, consolida mayor, erva do cardeal [Portuguese]. Consuelda, suelda consuelda [Spanish].

Life form: Herb. **Part(s) Used:** Leaf, root / Fresh; root collected in bloom / Dried. **Geographic distribution:** Temperate-Asia. Europe.
Reference(s): Bharatan *et al.* 2002; Bolte *et al.* 1997; Dorta Soares, n.d.; Plants for a future, 2009; Remedia/at, 2010; Tiwari *et al.* 2013.

Syringa vulgaris

Scientific Name(s) / [Botanical Family]: *Syringa vulgaris* L. = *Syringa rhodopea* Velen. [Oleaceae].
Common Name(s): Common lilac, lilac [English]. Lila [French, Spanish].
Life form: Herb. **Part(s) Used:** Flower / Fresh. **Geographic distribution:** Europe. Naturalized in several places.
Reference(s): Bharatan *et al.* 2002; Dorta Soares, n.d.; Gotfredsen, 2009; Guermonprez *et al.* 1989; Müntz, n.d.; Plants for a future, 2009; Remedia/at, 2010.

Tabacum

Scientific Name(s) / [Botanical Family]: *Nicotiana tabacum* L. [Solanaceae].
Common Name(s): Taba [Afrikan]. Yan cao [Chinese]. Common tobacco, tobacco, Virginian tobacco [English]. Herbe à l'ambassadeur, herbe à la reine, herbe à Nicot, tabac [French]. Fumo, tabaco [Portuguese]. Hierba el diablo, picietl, tabaco, tabaco de la montaña, tabaco de Virginia, tabaquera [Spanish].
Life form: Herb. **Part(s) Used:** Leaf / Dried. **Geographic distribution:** cultivated & naturalized in many places.
Reference(s): Bharatan *et al.* 2002; Dorta Soares, n.d.; Remedia/at, 2010; Tiwari *et al.* 2013.

Tagetes

Scientific Name(s) / [Botanical Family]: *Tagetes patula* L. = *Tagetes lunulata* Ortega [Asteraceae, Compositae].
Common Name(s): Marigold [English]. French marigold. Ceillet d'Inde [French]. Amapola amarilla, cempaoxóchitl cimarrón, clemole, clemolitos, copetes, copetillo, Flor de muerto, iscoque, zempoala, jacatsnat, molxóchitl, pastora, pastoral, pastorcita, tlemole, tlemolitos, x-puhuk [Spanish].
Life form: Herb. **Part(s) Used:** Aerial part in bloom / Fresh.
North, Central & South America. Naturalized & cultivated in several places.
Reference(s): Bharatan *et al.* 2002; Fuentes, 1996; Guermonprez *et al.* 1989; Müntz, n.d.

Talauma mexicana

Scientific Name(s) / [Botanical Family]: *Talauma mexicana* (DC.) G. Don. [Magnoliaceae].
Common Name(s): Anonillo, cocté, Flor de corazón, guia-lacha-yati, holmashté, hualhua, magnolia, magnolia yolotxóchitl, yo-lachi, yolosóchil, yolosúchil, yoloxóchitl, yolotxóchitl [Spanish].
Life form: Tree. **Part(s) Used:** Flower. **Geographic distribution:** Mexico, cultivated.
Reference: Provings, 2008-2009.

Tanacetum

Scientific Name(s) / [Botanical Family]: *Chrysanthemum vulgare* (L.) Bernh. = *Chrysanthemum tanacetum* Karsch. = *Tanacetum vulgare* L. [Asteraceae, Compositae].
Common Name(s): Tansy [English]. Tanaisie vulgaire [French]. Atanásoa, catinga de mulata, erva lombriguera [Portuguese]. Balsamita menor, hierba lombriguera, palma imperial, palmita de la India, tanaceto [Spanish].

Life form: Herb. **Part(s) Used:** bud-flower, leaf, / Fresh; flower / Dried. **Geographic distribution:** Europe, North Asia. Cultivated in several places.
Reference(s): Bharatan *et al.* 2002; Bolte *et al.* 1997; Tiwari *et al.* 2013.

Tanacetum parthenium see *Pyrethrum parthenium*

Tanacetum vulgare see *Tanacetum*

Taraxacum officinale
Scientific Name(s) / [Botanical Family]: *Taraxacum officinale* (L.) Weber. = *Leontodon taraxacum* L. = *Taraxacum dens-leonis* Desf. = *Taraxacum vulgare* Schrank. [Asteraceae, Compositae].
Common Name(s): Common dandelion, dandelion, lion's-tooth [English]. Dent de lion, pissenlit vulgaire [French]. Alface de cão, amargosa, dente de leão [Portuguese]. Achicoria amarga, amargón, cerraja, diente de león, moraja, nocuana-gueeta [Spanish].
Life form: Herb. **Part(s) Used:** Complete plant in bloom / Fresh; leaf collected in bloom / Dried. **Geographic distribution:** Europe-Asia. Cosmopolitan.
Reference(s): Bharatan *et al.* 2002; Dorta Soares, n.d.; Seror, 2000; Tiwari *et al.* 2013.

Taxus baccata
Scientific Name(s) / [Botanical Family]: *Taxus baccata* L. = *Taxus baccata* Thunb. = *Taxus baccata* Hook. = *Taxus fastigiata* Lindl. [Taxaceae].
Common Name(s): English yew, European yew [English]. If common, if du Pacifique [French]. Teixo [Portuguese]. Tejo [Spanish].
Life form: Tree. **Part(s) Used:** Bud / Fresh; leaf, young branch / Fresh. **Geographic distribution:** North Africa (Algeria, Morocco).

Europe. Temperate-Asia (Japan).

Reference(s): Bharatan *et al.* 2002; Dorta Soares, n.d.; Fuentes, 1996; Guermonprez *et al.* 1989; Tiwari *et al.* 2013.

Taxus brevifolia

Scientific Name(s) / [Botanical Family]: *Taxus brevifolia* Nutt. = *Taxus baccata* subsp. *brevifolia* (Nutt.) Pilg. = *Taxus baccata* var. *brevifolia* (Nutt.) Koehne [Taxaceae].

Common Name(s): Pacific yew, western yew [English]. Tejo [Spanish].

Life form: Tree. **Part(s) Used:** Bud / Fresh. **Geographic distribution:** North America (Alaska. Canada. Northwest & Southwest United States of America).

Reference(s): Bharatan *et al.* 2002; Plants for a future, 2009.

Telopea speciosissima

Scientific Name(s) / [Botanical Family]: *Telopea speciosissima* (Sm.) R. Br. = *Embothrium speciossimum* Sm. [Proteaceae].

Common Name(s): New South Wales waratah, waratah [English].

Life form: Shrub. **Part(s) Used:** Flower?. **Geographic distribution:** Australia.

Reference: Bharatan *et al.* 2002.

Teucrium

Scientific Name(s) / [Botanical Family]: *Teucrium marum* L. [Lamiaceae, Labiatae].

Common Name(s): Cat thyme [English]. Germandée des chats, thym de chat [French]. Carvalhinha do mar [Portuguese]. Hierba del Papa, hierba fuerte, maro, maro de cortusio [Spanish].

Life form: Shrub. **Part(s) Used:** Aerial part collected before or in bloom / Fresh. **Geographic distribution:** Europe (Mediterranean).

Reference(s): Bharatan *et al.* 2002; Dorta Soares, n.d.; Plants for a future, 2009; Provings, 2008-2009; Tiwari *et al.* 2013.

Teucrium scorodonia

Scientific Name(s) / [Botanical Family]: *Teucrium scorodonia* L. [Lamiaceae, Labiatae].
Common Name(s): Germander, wood germander, wood sage [English]. Germandrée scorodoine, sauge-des-bois [French]. Teucrio [Portuguese]. Altamisa real, camedrio de bosque, escorodonia, germandrina de bosque [Spanish].
Life form: Shrub. **Part(s) Used:** Complete plant / Fresh. leaves collected during the bloom / Dried. **Geographic distribution:** Europe.
Reference(s): Bharatan *et al.* 2002; Gotfredsen, 2009; Guermonprez *et al.* 1989; Müntz, n.d.; Tiwari *et al.* 2013.

Thea

Scientific Name(s) / [Botanical Family]: *Camellia sinensis* (L.) Kuntze = *Camellia thea* Link = *Thea sinensis* L. [Theaceae].
Common Name(s): Black tea, green tea, tea, teaplant [English]. Arbreŕ thé, thé, théier [French]. Chá da China, chá-da-Índia, chá prieto [Portuguese]. Árbol del té, té, té negro, té verde [Spanish].
Life form: Shrub. **Part(s) Used:** Flower, leaf / Dried. **Geographic distribution:** Temperate-Asia (China). Extensively cultivated.
Reference(s): Allen, 2006-2010; Bharatan *et al.* 2002; Dorta Soares, n.d.; Fuentes, 1996; Gotfredsen, 2009; Müntz, n.d.; Plants for a future, 2009; Tiwari *et al.* 2013.

Thea chinensis see *Thea*

Thlaspi

Scientific Name(s) / [Botanical Family]: *Capsella bursa-pastoris*

(L.) Medik. = *Thlaspi bursa-pastoris* L. [Brassicaceae, Cruciferae]. **Common Name(s):** Shepherd's purse [English]. Boursef pasteur, Capsellef pasteur [French]. Bolsa-de-pastor, erva-do-bom-pastor [Portuguese]. Bolsa de pastor, zurrón de pastor [Spanish]. **Life form:** Herb. **Part(s) Used:** Aerial part / Fresh. **Geographic distribution:** Cosmopolitan.
Reference(s): Bharatan *et al.* 2002; Dorta Soares, n.d.; Remedia/at, 2010; Tiwari *et al.* 2013.

Thuja

Scientific Name(s) / [Botanical Family]: *Thuja occidentalis* L. [Cupressaceae].
Common Name(s): Arborvitae, eastern arborvitae, northern white-cedar, swamp-cedar, thuya, white-cedar [English]. Arbre de vie, cèdre blanc, thuier cèdre, thuya, thuya du Canada [French]. Cipreste, pinheiro do Canada [Portuguese]. Tuha, tuja, tuya [Spanish].
Life form: Tree. **Part(s) Used:** Branch with leaves/ Fresh; leaves / Fresh collected at begining of bloom; buds / Fresh. **Geographic distribution:** North America (Canada. United States of America). Siberia.
Reference(s): Bharatan *et al.* 2002; Dorta Soares, n.d.; Guermonprez *et al.* 1989; Müntz, n.d.; Plants for a future, 2009; Tiwari *et al.* 2013; Zandvoort, 2006.

Thuja lobbii

Scientific Name(s) / [Botanical Family]: *Thuja plicata* Donn. ex D. Don. = *Thuja gigantea* Nutt. = *Thuja lobbii* Hort. ex Gordon = *Thuja menziesii* Douglas ex Endl. [Cupressaceae].
Common Name(s): Canoe-cedar, giant arborvitae, giant-cedar, pacific red-cedar, shinglewood, western arborvitae, western red-cedar [English]. Thuya de Lobb, thuya géant [French].
Life form: Tree. **Part(s) Used:** branch, leaf / Fresh. **Geographic**

distribution: North America.
Reference(s): Fuentes, 1996; Bharatan *et al.* 2002; Guermonprez et al. 1989; Müntz, n.d.; Plants for a future, 2009.

Thuya see *Thuja*

Thymus

Scientific Name(s) / [Botanical Family]: *Thymus serpyllum* L. [Lamiaceae, Labiatae].
Common Name(s): Breckland garden, Breckland thyme creeping thyme mother-of-thyme, thyme, wild thyme [English]. Serpolet, thym sauvage [French]. Serpão, serpil, serpol, tomilho [Portuguese]. Serpol, tomillo [Spanish].
Life form: Herb. **Part(s) Used:** Aerial part in recently bloom / Fresh. **Geographic distribution:** Temperate-Asia. Europe.
Reference(s): Bharatan *et al.* 2002; Boericke, 1927, 1927b.; Dorta Soares, n.d.; Seror, 2000; Tiwari *et al.* 2013.

Tilia cordata

Scientific Name(s) / [Botanical Family]: *Tilia cordata* Mill. = *Tilia microphylla* Vent. = *Tilia parvifolia* Ehrh. = *Tilia ulmifolia* Scop. [Tiliaceae].
Common Name(s): Linden, little-leaf linden, small-leaf european linden, small-leaf lime, small-leaf linden [English]. Tilleul [French]. Tília [Portuguese]. Tilia [Spanish].
Life form: Tree. **Part(s) Used:** Flower / Fresh; flower buds / Dried. **Geographic distribution:** Temperate-Asia. Europe.
Reference(s): Bharatan *et al.* 2002; Dorta Soares, n.d.; Remedia/at, 2010.

Tilia europaea

Scientific Name(s) / [Botanical Family]: *Tilia x europaea* L. = *Tilia x vulgaris* Hayne [Malvaceae, Tiliaceae].
Common Name(s): European linden, lime [English]. Tilleul

[French].
Life form: Tree. **Part(s) Used:** Flower / Fresh. **Geographic distribution:** Europe. Cultivated in several places.
Reference(s): Bharatan *et al.* 2002; Plants for a future, 2009; Tiwari *et al.* 2013.

Tomentilla see *Potentilla tomentilla*

Torula
Scientific Name(s) / [Botanical Family]: *Saccharomyces cerevisiae* Meyen ex E. C. Hansen = *Torula cerevisiae* Turpin [Saccharomycetaceae].
Common Name(s): Baker's or budding yeast, yeast [English]. Levadura de cerveza [Spanish].
Life form: Unicellular Fungi. **Part(s) Used:** Complete. **Geographic distribution:** Cosmopolitan, cultivated.
Reference(s): Bharatan *et al.* 2002; Boericke, 1927, 1927b.; Seror, 2000.

Trifolium pratense
Scientific Name(s) / [Botanical Family]: *Trifolium pratense* L. = *Trifolium pratense* var. *sativum* Schreb. [Fabaceae, Leguminosae].
Common Name(s): Peavine or purple or red clover [English]. Trèfle rouge, trèfle blanc [French]. Trevo-dos-prados, trevo violeta [Portuguese]. Quie-too-Castilla, trébol común, trébol rojo, trébol violeta [Spanish].
Life form: Herb. **Part(s) Used:** Flower / Fresh. **Geographic distribution:** Europe. Temperate-Asia. United States of America. Cosmopolitan, Extensively naturalized in temperate regions.
Reference(s): Bharatan *et al.* 2002; Dorta Soares, n.d.; Tiwari *et al.* 2013.

Trillium

Scientific Name(s) / [Botanical Family]: *Trillium erectum* L. = *Trillium pendulum* Willd. [Trilliaceae, Convallariaceae].

Common Name(s): Beth root, purpurtreblad [English]. Lirio americano [Spanish].

Life form: Herb. **Part(s) Used:** rhizome, complete plant / Fresh; seeds / Dried. **Geographic distribution:** North America (Canada-United States of America).

Reference(s): Bharatan *et al.* 2002; Dorta Soares, n.d.

Trillium cernuum

Scientific Name(s) / [Botanical Family]: *Trillium cernuum* L. [Trilliaceae, Convallariaceae].

Common Name(s): Nooding trillium seldom, whip-poor-will flower [English].

Life form: Herb. **Part(s) Used:** Rhizome / Fresh-Dried. **Geographic distribution:** North America (East United States of America).

Reference(s): Bharatan *et al.* 2002; Guermonprez *et al.* 1989; Plants for a future, 2009.

Triosteum perfoliatum

Scientific Name(s) / [Botanical Family]: *Triosteum perfoliatum* L. [Caprifoliaceae].

Common Name(s): Feverrot, horse gentian [English]. Ipeca falsa [Portuguese]. Ipecuanha silvestre [Spanish].

Life form: Herb. **Part(s) Used:** Root / Fresh. **Geographic distribution:** North America.

Reference(s): Bharatan *et al.* 2002; Dorta Soares, n.d.; Tiwari *et al.* 2013.

Triticum aestivum

Scientific Name(s) / [Botanical Family]: *Triticum aestivum* L. =

Triticum cereale Schrank = *Triticum cereale* (L.) Salisb. = *Triticum sativum* Lam. = *Triticum vulgare* Vill. = *Zeia vulgaris* var. *aestiva* (L.) Lunell [Gramineae, Poaceae].
Common Name(s): Bread wheat, common wheat, wheat [English]. Blé, blé cultivé, blé ordinaire, blé tendre [French]. Trigo [Portuguese]. Trigo, trigo-blando, trigo de pan [Spanish].
Life form: Herb. **Part(s) Used:** Fruit, seeds, stem / Fresh.
Geographic distribution: Minor Asia. Extensively world cultivated.
Reference(s): Bharatan *et al.* 2002; Bolte *et al.* 1997; Dorta Soares, n.d.

Tropaeolum

Scientific Name(s) / [Botanical Family]: *Tropaeolum majus* L. [[Tropaeolaceae].
Common Name(s): Garden nasturtium, Indian-cress, nasturtium [English]. Cresson d'Inde, grande capucine [French]. Agrião mexicano, capuchina grande, chagas, flor de sangue [Portuguese]. Capuchina, carmelita, cuitziquiendas, curutzuti, marañuela, mastuerzo, pelonchili, pelonmexixquilitl [Spanish].
Life form: Herb. **Part(s) Used:** Complete plant in bloom / Fresh.
Geographic distribution: South America. Extensively cultivated.
Reference(s): Bharatan *et al.* 2002; Dorta Soares, n.d.; Plants for a future, 2009; Provings 2008, 2009.

Tussilago

Scientific Name(s) / [Botanical Family]: *Petasites albus* (L.) Gaertn. = *Tussilago alba* L. [Asteraceae, Compositae].
Common Name(s): Butterbur [English]. Pétasite blanc [French].
Life form: Herb. **Part(s) Used:** Root. **Geographic distribution:** North & Central Europe. Naturalized in Great Britain.
Reference(s): Bharatan *et al.* 2002; Fuentes, 1996; Plants for a future, 2009.

Tussilago fragans

Scientific Name(s) / [Botanical Family]: *Petasites fragans* (Vill.) Central Presl = *Tussilago fragans* Vill. [Asteraceae, Compositae].
Common Name(s): Winter-heliotrope [English].
Life form: Herb. **Part(s) Used:** Root?. **Geographic distribution:** North Africa. South Europe. Cultivated & naturalized in several places.
Reference(s): Bharatan *et al.* 2002; Plants for a future, 2009; Tiwari *et al.* 2013.

Tussilago petasites

Scientific Name(s) / [Botanical Family]: *Petasites hybridus* (L.) G. Gaertn., B. Mey & Scherb. = *Petasites officinalis* Moench. = *Petasites ovatus* Hill. = *Petasites vulgaris* L. = *Tussilago petasites* L. = *Tussilago hybrida* L. [Asteraceae, Compositae].
Common Name(s): Butter bur, butterfly-dock, Colt's foot, pestilente, pestilent wort [English]. Herbe aux teigneux [French]. Petasita, sombrerera, tusilago mayor [Spanish].
Life form: Herb. **Part(s) Used:** Complete plant. **Geographic distribution:** Temperate-Asia (West Asia, Caucasus). Europe. Naturalized in several places.
Reference(s): Bharatan *et al.* 2002; Gotfredsen, 2009; Tiwari *et al.* 2013; American Institute of Homeopathy, 1979.

Ulex europaea

Scientific Name(s) / [Botanical Family]: *Ulex europaea* L. [Fabaceae, Leguminosae].
Common Name(s): Jing dou [Chinese]. Gorse, furze, pricky broom, whin [English]. Abulaga, aulaga, chacay, escajo, espino amarillo, hiniesta espinosa, maticorena, tojo [Spanish].

Life form: Tree. **Part(s) Used:** Seeds. **Geographic distribution:** America. West Europe. Cultivated.
Reference(s): Bharatan *et al.* 2002; Müntz, n.d.; Plants for a future, 2009; American Institute of Homeopathy, 1979.

Ulmus

Scientific Name(s) / [Botanical Family]: *Ulmus glabra* Hudson [Ulmaceae].
Common Name(s): European mountain elm, Scottish elm, wych elm [English]. Orme blanc, orme de montagne [French]. Olmo, olmo montano, olmo de monte [Spanish].
Life form: Tree. **Part(s) Used:** Bark. **Geographic distribution:** Europe. North & West Asia. Naturalized in several regions.
Reference: Remedia/at, 2010.

Ulmus

Scientific Name(s) / [Botanical Family]: *Ulmus rubra* Muhl. = *Ulmus fulva* Michx. [Ulmaceae].
Common Name(s): Red elm, slippery elm [English]. Olmo, olmo americano [Spanish].
Life form: Tree. **Part(s) Used:** Bark?. **Geographic distribution:** North America (Canada-United States of America).
Reference(s): Bharatan *et al.* 2002; Bolte *et al.* 1997; Plants for a future, 2009; Tiwari *et al.* 2013.

Urtica

Scientific Name(s) / [Botanical Family]: *Urtica pilulifera* L. [Urticaceae].
Common Name(s): Roman nettle [English]. Ortiga de pelotilllas [Spanish].
Life form: Herb. **Part(s) Used:** Complete plant / Fresh. **Geographic distribution:** Europe.
Reference: Bharatan *et al.* 2002.

Urtica dioica

Scientific Name(s) / [Botanical Family]: *Urtica dioica* L. = *Urtica dioica* Vell. = *Urtica major* H. P. Fuchs = *Urtica spatulata* Sm. [Urticaceae].

Common Name(s): European nettle, nettle [English]. Grande ortie, ortie [French]. Urtiga [Portuguese]. Achum, achume, ardiga, chichicaste, dominguilla, guechi-bidoo, guichi-bidu, ortiga, ortiga mayor, solimán [Spanish].

Life form: Herb. **Part(s) Used:** Complete plant / Fresh.

Geographic distribution: North America (Canada. United States of America. Mexico). Europe. North Africa.

Reference(s): Dorta Soares, n.d.; Plants for a future, 2009.

Urtica urens

Scientific Name(s) / [Botanical Family]: *Urtica urens* L. = *Urtica urens* Bert. ex Steud. = *Urtica spatulata* Sm. [Urticaceae].

Common Name(s): Burning nettle, lesser nettle, small nettle, stinging-nettle [English]. Ortie, ortie brúlante, petite ortie [French]. Urtiga Minor, utiga branca, urtica queimadeira [Portuguese]. Chichicaste, guechibidoo, ortiga [Spanish].

Life form: Shrub. **Part(s) Used:** Complete plant / Fresh.

Geographic distribution: England. Europe. United States of America. Extensively naturalized.

Reference(s): Allen, 2006-2010; Bharatan *et al.* 2002; Clarke, 2008; Dorta Soares, n.d.; Gotfredsen, 2009; Tiwari *et al.* 2013.

Uva-ursi

Scientific Name(s) / [Botanical Family]: *Arctostaphylos uva-ursi* (L.) Sprengel = *Arbutus uva-ursi* L. = *Arctostaphylos officinalis* Wimm. et Grab. = *Arctostaphylos procumbens* E.Meyer [Ericaceae].

Common Name(s): Common bearberry [English]. Busserole

[French]. Buxilo, búxulo, medronheiro [Portuguese]. Aguarilla, aguavilla, baya del oso, gayuba, manzaneta, manzanilla de pastor, uva de oso, uvaduz [Spanish].
Life form: Liana. **Part(s) Used:** flower's bulbs, fruits & leaf / Fresh; fruits / Dried. **Geographic distribution:** England, Europe. Cold climates of the North Hemisphere.
Reference(s): Bharatan *et al.* 2002; Dorta Soares, n.d.; Plants for a future, 2009; Provings, 2008-2009; Guermonprez *et al.* 1989; Tiwari *et al.* 2013; American Institute of Homeopathy, 1979.

Valeriana officinalis

Scientific Name(s) / [Botanical Family]: *Valeriana officinalis* L. = *Valeriana officinalis* L. & Maillefer [Valerianaceae].
Common Name(s): Common valerian, valerian [English]. Valériane officinale [French]. Erva de gato, valeriana, valeriana oficinal [Portuguese]. Hierba de gatos, valeriana, valeriana menor, valeriana oficinal [Spanish].
Life form: Herb. **Part(s) Used:** Root / Fresh / Dried. **Geographic distribution:** Europe. North Asia. Mexico. Cultivated.
Reference(s): Bharatan *et al.* 2002; Clarke, 2008; Dorta Soares, n.d.; Provings, 2008-2009; Tiwari *et al.* 2013.

Veratrum

Scientific Name(s) / [Botanical Family]: *Veratrum album* L. [Liliaceae, Melanthiaceae].
Common Name(s): European white hellebore, white-hellebore [English]. Flor da verdade, heléboro branco [Portuguese]. Ballestra, ballestra blanca, eléboro blanco, heléboro blanco, hierba de balleastros, rizoma de veratro, Surbia, vedegambre [Spanish].
Life form: Herb. **Part(s) Used:** Root / Fresh; rhizome / Dried;

seeds / Dried. **Geographic distribution:** Temperate-Asia. Europe.
Reference(s): Bolte *et al.* 1997; Dorta Soares, n.d.; Guermonprez *et al.* 1989; Tiwari *et al.* 2013.

Veratrum nigrum

Scientific Name(s) / [Botanical Family]: *Veratrum nigrum* L. [Liliaceae, Melanthiaceae].
Common Name(s): Black false-helleborine, black hellebore [English]. Vérâtre noir [French]. Veratro nero [Italian]. Heléboro negro [Spanish]. **Life form:** Herb. **Part(s) Used:** Rhizome / Dried. **Geographic distribution:** Temperate-Asia. Europe.
Reference(s): Bharatan *et al.* 2002; Dorta Soares, n.d.; American Institute of Homeopathy, 1979.

Veratrum viride

Scientific Name(s) / [Botanical Family]: *Veratrum viride* (Aiton). Ker Gawl. = *Veratrum viride* Aiton [Liliaceae, Melanthiaceae].
Common Name(s): American false hellebore, American white-hellebore, green hellebore, indian-poke, itchweed, white-hellebore [English]. Ellébore vert [French]. Heléboro americano, heléboro verde, veratro [Portuguese]. Eléboro verde [Spanish].
Life form: Herb. **Part(s) Used:** Rhizome / Fresh / Dried; root collected in autumn / Fresh. **Geographic distribution:** North America (United States of America).
Reference(s): Bharatan *et al.* 2002; Dorta Soares, n.d.; Gotfredsen, 2009; Tiwari *et al.* 2013.

Verbascum thapsus

Scientific Name(s) / [Botanical Family]: *Verbascum thapsus* L. [Scrophulariaceae].
Common Name(s): Aaron's-rod, common mullein, flannelleave, flannelplant, great mullein, hag taper, mullein,

torches, velvet-dock, velvetplant [English]. Bouillon blanc, molène [French]. Barbasco, verbasco [Portuguese]. Gordolobo común, guardalobo [Spanish].
Life form: Herb. **Part(s) Used:** Flower, leaf / Fresh. **Geographic distribution:** Europe, Temperate-Asia & tropical. Naturalized in several places.
Reference(s): Bharatan *et al.* 2002; Dorta Soares, n.d.; Guermonprez *et al.* 1989; Tiwari *et al.* 2013; American Institute of Homeopathy, 1979.

Verbena officinalis

Scientific Name(s) / [Botanical Family]: *Verbena officinalis* L. = *Verbena setosa* Middle Martens & Galeotti [Verbenaceae].
Common Name(s): Ma bian cao [Chinese]. Common verbena, common vervain, vervain [English]. Véronique officinale [French]. Kumatsuzura [Japanese]. Erva-de-ferro, ferraria, planta-da-sorte [Portuguese].Girbao, verbena [Spanish].
Life form: Herb. **Part(s) Used:** Complete plant / Fresh; complete plant collected in bloom / Fresh. **Geographic distribution:** Asia. Africa. Europe. Madagascar. Mexico. Oceania. United States of America. Extensively naturalized in several temperate places.
Reference(s): Bharatan *et al.* 2002; Dorta Soares, n.d.; Provings, 2008-2009; Plants for a future, 2009; Tiwari *et al.* 2013; American Institute of Homeopathy, 1979.

Veronica beccabunga

Scientific Name(s) / [Botanical Family]: *Veronica beccabunga* L. [Scrophulariaceae].
Common Name(s): Brooklime, neckweed, speed-weell, water pimpernell [English]. Véronique [French]. Verónica acuatica, becabunga [Spanish].
Life form: Herb. **Part(s) Used:** Complete plant / Fresh. Complete plant collected in bloom / Fresh. **Geographic distribution:** Asia.

Europe. Cultivated in North America.

Reference(s): Bharatan *et al.* 2002; Dorta Soares, n.d.; Plants for a future, 2009; American Institute of Homeopathy, 1979.

Veronica officinalis

Scientific Name(s) / [Botanical Family]: *Veronica officinalis* L. [Scrophulariaceae].

Common Name(s): Common speed-weell, gypsyweed, heath speedwell [English]. Verónica-da-mata [Portuguese].

Life form: Herb. **Part(s) Used:** Complete plant / Fresh; complete plant collected in bloom / Fresh. **Geographic distribution:** Europe. Temperate-Asia.

Reference: Dorta Soares, n.d.

Vesca

Scientific Name(s) / [Botanical Family]: *Castanea vulgaris* var. *americana* (Michx.) A. DC. = *Castanea vesca* var. *americana* Michx. = *Castanea vulgaris* Lam. = *Castanea sativa* Mill. [Fagaceae].

Common Name(s): European chestnut, Spanish chestnut, sweet chestnut [English]. Châtaignier commun [French]. Castanheiro-comum [Portuguese]. Castaño común, regoldo [Spanish].

Life form: Tree. **Part(s) Used:** Leaf / Fresh. **Geographic distribution:** Europe. North United States of America. Extensively cultivated & naturalized in Eurasia.

Reference(s): Dorta Soares, n.d.; Plants for a future, 2009; Provings, 2008-2009; Tiwari *et al.* 2013.

Viburnum opulus

Scientific Name(s) / [Botanical Family]: *Viburnum opulus* L. = *Viburnum pauciflorum* Raf. [Caprifoliaceae].

Common Name(s): Crampbark, guelder rose, high cranberry, marsh snowball tree, water elder elder [English]. Boule de neige,

obier, viorne obier [French]. Viburno [Portuguese]. Bola de nieve, mundillo, rodela, rosa de Gueldres [Spanish].
Life form: Shrub. **Part(s) Used:** Bark, leaf, stem / Fresh.
Geographic distribution: East Asia (Russia). North & West Asia. Europe. East North America.
Reference(s): Bharatan *et al.* 2002; Clarke, 2008; Dorta Soares, n.d.; Tiwari *et al.* 2013.

Viburnum prunifolium

Scientific Name(s) / [Botanical Family]: *Viburnum prunifolium* L. [Caprifoliaceae].
Common Name(s): American sloe, stagbush [English]. Viorne [French]. Viburno, mundo, bolo de nieve [Spanish]. Acerola negra, espinheiro preto, viburno americano [Portuguese].
Life form: Shrub. **Part(s) Used:** Bark-stem, root-bark / Fresh.
Geographic distribution: North America (preferably in the East states).-
Reference(s): Bharatan *et al.* 2002; Bolte *et al.* 1997; Dorta Soares, n.d.; Hutchens, 1991; Plants for a future, 2009; Tiwari *et al.* 2013; American Institute of Homeopathy, 1979.

Viburnum tinus

Scientific Name(s) / [Botanical Family]: *Viburnum tinus* L. [Caprifoliaceae].
Common Name(s): Laurustinus [English]. Laurier tin [French].
Life form: Shrub. **Part(s) Used:** Root, root-bark? / Fresh.
Geographic distribution: Africa. Temperate-Asia. South Europe & cultivated.
Reference(s): Bharatan *et al.* 2002; Bolte *et al.* 1997; Hutchens, 1991; American Institute of Homeopathy, 1979.

Vicia faba

Scientific Name(s) / [Botanical Family]: *Vicia faba* L. = *Faba*

bona Medik. = *Faba vulgaris* Harz [Fabaceae, Leguminosae].
Common Name(s): Bell-bean, faba-bean, fava bean [English]. Fève, féverole [French]. Fava, fava comum, faveira do campo [Portuguese]. Doju, haba, veza [Spanish].
Life form: Herb. **Part(s) Used:** Complete plant, seeds, pod / Fresh.
Geographic distribution: cultivated in temperate regions.
Reference(s): Bharatan *et al.* 2002; Bolte *et al.* 1997; Dorta Soares, n.d.; Plants for a future, 2009.

Vinca

Scientific Name(s) / [Botanical Family]: *Vinca major* L. [Apocynaceae].
Common Name(s): Greater periwinkle, large periwinkle [English]. Pervenche majeure [French]. Pervinca-maior, vinca-pendente [Portuguese]. Vinca [Spanish].
Life form: Shrub. **Part(s) Used:** leaf / Fresh. **Geographic distribution:** Central & South Europe. North Africa. Naturalized in Great Britain. Cultivated in many places.
Reference(s): Fuentes, 1996; Plants for a future, 2009.

Vinca minor

Scientific Name(s) / [Botanical Family]: *Vinca minor* L. [Apocynaceae].
Common Name(s): Common Periwinkle, lesser periwinkle, running-myrtle [English]. Pervenche mineure [French]. Pervinca, pervinca pequena, vinca [Portuguese]. Cielo raso, Flor de paragûito, pervinca, vincapervinca [Spanish].
Life form: Shrub. **Part(s) Used:** leaf / Fresh; complete plant in bloom / Fresh; leaves collected during the bloom / Dried.
Geographic distribution: Europe. Extensively cultivated & naturalized.
Reference(s): Dorta Soares, n.d.; Plants for a future, 2009; Tiwari *et al.* 2013.

Vincetoxicum

Scientific Name(s) / [Botanical Family]: *Vincetoxicum hirundinaria* Medik = *Vincetoxicum officinale* Moench = *Asclepias vincetoxicum* L. = *Cynanchum laxum* Bartl. = *Cynanchum luteum* (Miller) Steudel = *Cynanchum vincetoxicum* (L.) Pers. [Asclepiadaceae].

Common Name(s): German ipecac, swallow wort, tame poison, white swallow-wort [English]. Dompte-venin [French]. Erva-contraveneno [Portuguese]. Centósigo, hierba contraveneno, hirundinaria, mataveneno, vencetósigo [Spanish].

Life form: Herb. **Part(s) Used:** Root / Fresh. **Geographic distribution:** Europe-Asia. Weed-invasive (United States of America).

Reference(s): Bharatan *et al.* 2002; Bolte *et al.* 1997; Dorta Soares, n.d.; Plants for a future, 2009; Tiwari *et al.* 2013.

Viola odorata

Scientific Name(s) / [Botanical Family]: *Viola odorata* L. [Violaceae].

Common Name(s): English violet, florist's violet, garden violet, sweet violet [English]. Violette odorante [French]. Violeta, violeta comum [Portuguese]. Violeta [Spanish].

Life form: Herb. **Part(s) Used:** Complete plant, flower, leaf / Fresh. **Geographic distribution:** Temperate-Asia. Europe. Cultivated & naturalized in several places.

Reference(s): Bolte *et al.* 1997; Bharatan *et al.* 2002; Dorta Soares, n.d.; Provings, 2008-2009; Tiwari *et al.* 2013.

Viola tricolor

Scientific Name(s) / [Botanical Family]: *Viola tricolor* L. [Violaceae].

Common Name(s): European wild pansy, field pansy, heart's-

ease, heart-sease, johnny-jump-up, love-in-idleness, miniature pansy [English]. Pensée sauvage [French]. Pensamento, violeta tricolor, amor perfeito [Portuguese]. Pensamiento [Spanish].
Life form: Herb. **Part(s) Used:** Complete plant in bloom / Fresh; Seeds / Dried. **Geographic distribution:** Europe, North de Asia. Cultivated & naturalized in several places.
Reference(s): Bharatan *et al.* 2002; Fuentes, 1996; Dorta Soares, n.d.; Plants for a future, 2009; Tiwari *et al.* 2013.

Viscum

Scientific Name(s) / [Botanical Family]: *Viscum album* L. [Viscaceae, Loranthaceae].
Common Name(s): European mistletoe [English]. Gui de chêne, gui du pommier [French]. Agárico, erva de passarinho, guirarepoti [Portuguese]. Muérdago europeo [Spanish].
Life form: Epiphyte, Shrub. **Part(s) Used:** Complete plant, fruit, leaf / Fresh; Mature fruits. **Geographic distribution:** Europe & Temperate-Asia. Living as parasit of several tree's species.
Reference(s): Bharatan *et al.* 2002; Dorta Soares, n.d.; Fuentes, 1996; Plants for a future, 2009; Tiwari *et al.* 2013.

Vitex

Scientific Name(s) / [Botanical Family]: *Vitex trifolia* L. [Verbenaceae].
Common Name(s): Man jing, san ye man jing [Chinese]. Hand-of-Mary, Indian privet, Indian three-leaf vitex, Indian wild pepper, simple-leaf chaste tree [English]. Árnica india [Spanish].
Life form: Herb. **Part(s) Used:** Complete plant. **Geographic distribution:** Temperate-Asia.
Reference(s): Bharatan *et al.* 2002; Clarke, 2008; Plants for a future, 2009.

Vitis

Scientific Name(s) / [Botanical Family]: *Vitis vinifera* L. [Vitaceae].

Common Name(s): Grapevine [English]. Vigne vinifère [French]. Parreira, videira, vinha [Portuguese]. Parra, pasa, pasas, uva, vid [Spanish].

Life form: Shrub. **Part(s) Used:** Fruit, leaf / Fresh. **Geographic distribution:** Western Asia. Extensively world cultivated.

Reference(s): Bharatan *et al.* 2002; Boericke, 1927, 1927b.; Dorta Soares, n.d.

Wyethia

Scientific Name(s) / [Botanical Family]: *Wyethia helenioides* (DC.) Nutt. = *Alarconia helenioides* DC. [Asteraceae, Compositae].

Common Name(s): Poison wed, whitehead mule-ears [English].

Life form: Herb. **Part(s) Used:** Root. **Geographic distribution:** North America (California, United States of America).

Reference(s): Bharatan *et al.* 2002; Dorta Soares, n.d.; Plants for a future, 2009; Provings, 2008-2009; Tiwari *et al.* 2013.

Xanthium

Scientific Name(s) / [Botanical Family]: *Xanthium spinosum* L. = *Xanthium ambrosioides* Hook. & Arn. = *Xanthium catharticum* Kunth = *Xanthium spinosum* var. *inerme* Bel = *Acanthoxanthium spinosum* (L.) Fourr. [Asteraceae, Compositae].

Common Name(s): Spiny cocklebur. [English]. Lampourde épineuse [French]. Amor de negro, carrapicho de Santa Helena, esoinho de carneiro [Portuguese].

Life form: Herb. **Part(s) Used:** Complete plant / Fresh.
Geographic distribution: North America (Canada, United States of America). South America (Argentine, Bolivia, Chile, Ecuador). South Africa.
Reference(s): Bharatan *et al.* 2002; Boericke, 1927, 1927b.; Clarke, 2008; Dorta Soares, n.d.; Tiwari *et al.* 2013.

Xanthium spinosum see *Xanthium*

Xanthorhiza apiifolia

Scientific Name(s) / [Botanical Family]: *Xanthorhiza apiifolia* (L'Her.) Guimpel, Otto. & Hage = *Xanthorhiza apifolia* L'Her. = *Xanthorhiza simplicissima* Marshall [Ranunculaceae].
Common Name(s): Shurb yellow root, yellowroot [English].
Life form: Shrub. **Part(s) Used:** Bark, Root. **Geographic distribution:** North America.
Reference(s): Bharatan *et al.* 2002; Boericke, 1927, 1927b.; Remedia/at, 2010.

Xanthorrhoea

Scientific Name(s) / [Botanical Family]: *Xanthorrhoea arborea* R. Br. [Xanthorrhoeaceae].
Common Name(s): Black boy, broad-leaf ed grass tree [English].
Life form: Shrub, Tree. **Part(s) Used:** Root's resin?. **Geographic distribution:** Australia.
Reference(s): Bolte *et al.* 1997; Plants for a future, 2009.

Xanthoxylon fraxineum see *Zanthoxylum*

Xerophyllum tenax

Scientific Name(s) / [Botanical Family]: *Xerophyllum tenax* (Pursh) Nutt. [Melanthiaceae, Liliaceae Xerophyllaceae].
Common Name(s): Bear-grass, bear-lily, elk-grass, fire-lily, Indian basket-grass, tamalpais lily, western turkey-beard

[English]. Hierba de oso, tamalpais [Spanish].
Life form: Herb. **Part(s) Used:** Root. **Geographic distribution:** North America (Canada, United States of America). Cultivated.
Reference: Remedia/at, 2010.

Xylosteum see *Lonicera xylosteum*

Zantedeschia aethiopica see *Calla*

Zanthoxylum

Scientific Name(s) / [Botanical Family]: *Zanthoxylum americanum* Mill. = *Zantoxylum fraxineum* Willd. [Rutaceae].
Common Name(s): Common prickly ash, northern prickly-ash, prickly-ash, toothachetree [English]. Clavalier.Frêne épineux [French]. Freixo espinhento da America, freixo espinhoso [Portuguese]. Fresno espinoso [Spanish].
Life form: Tree. **Part(s) Used:** Bark, fruit, root / Fresh.
Geographic distribution: North America (Canada-United States of America).
Reference(s): Bharatan *et al.* 2002; Dorta Soares, n.d.

Zea

Scientific Name(s) / [Botanical Family]: *Zea mays* L. [Gramineae, Poaceae].
Common Name(s): Corn, sweat corn [English]. Maïs [French]. Milho [Portuguese]. Cu, maíz, maíz oc, mojc, shobe, shuba, xoopa, yoobe [Spanish].
Life form: Herb. **Part(s) Used:** Flower, leaf, root, seeds; flower styles / Dried. **Geographic distribution:** cultivated in several world's places.
Reference(s): Boericke, 1927, 1927b.; Bharatan *et al.* 2002;

Dorta Soares, n.d.; Remedia/at, 2010;

Zea italica see *Zea mays*

Zizia aurea

Scientific Name(s) / [Botanical Family]: *Zizia aurea* (L.) W. D. J. Koch = *Smyrnium aureum* L. [Apiaceae, Umbelliferae].
Common Name(s): Golden alexanders, golden Alexanders, golden zizia [English].
Life form: Herb. **Part(s) Used:** Roots. **Geographic distribution:** Australia. North America (Canada. United States of America). Reference: Bharatan *et al.* 2002.

CHAPTER IV. Illustrations of some plants mentioned in the book.

The illustrations of: *Aesculus hippocastanum, Aethusa cynapium, Argemone mexicana, Caltha palustris, Cimifuga racemosa, Hydrastis canadensis, Podophyllum peltatum, Sambucus canadensis, Sinapis alba,* and *Viola tricolor,* was photographs taked by Mr. Alberto Waizel-Haiat from the book written and illustrated by Charles Frederick Millspaug: "American Medicinal Plants: An Illustrated and Descriptive Guide to the American Plants Used as Homeopathic Remedies. Their History, Preparation, Chemistry and Physiological Effects". Boericke & Taffel, Editor, USA. 1887. While the other photos: *Achillea millefolium, Ambrosia artemisiaefolia, Apium graveolens, Arnica montana, Asarum eropaeum, Artemisia absinthium, Petroselinum sativum, Pimpinella anisum, Raphanus raphanistrum, Rhus toxicodendron, Schinus molle & Vinca minor,* were taken by the book's author from specimens of the Herbarium of the Escuela Nacional de Medicina y Homeopatía in Mexico City. However the photos of *Myrtus communis,* & *Bougainvillea* sp. are from a private garden, and was taken by Jose Waizel-Bucay, and Alberto Waizel-Haiat respectively.

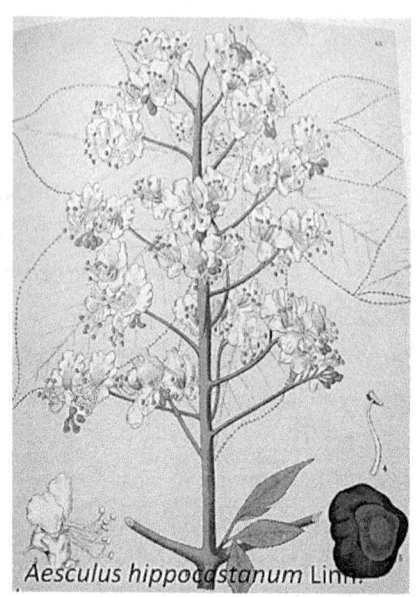

Aesculus hippocastanum Linn.

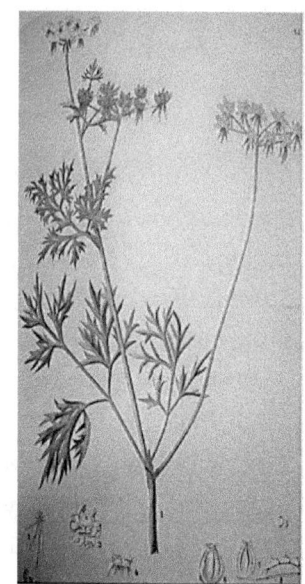

Aethusa cynapium L.

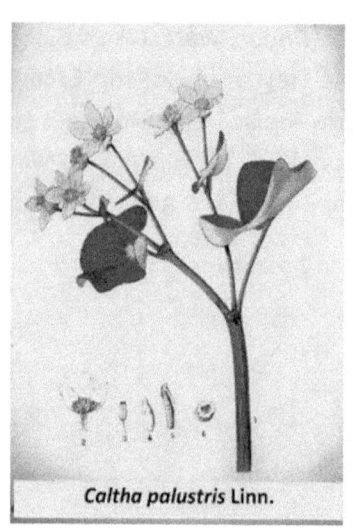

Caltha palustris Linn.

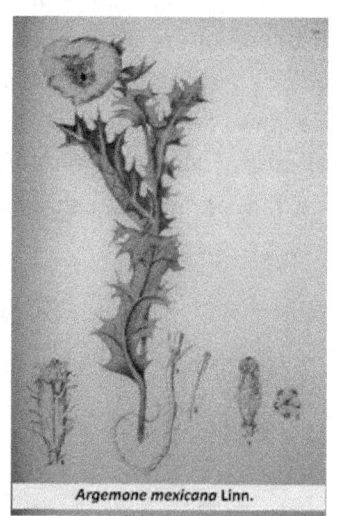

Argemone mexicana Linn.

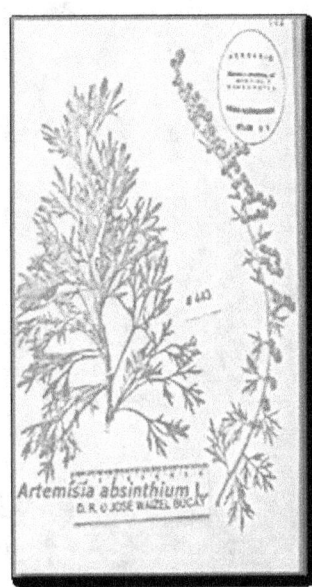
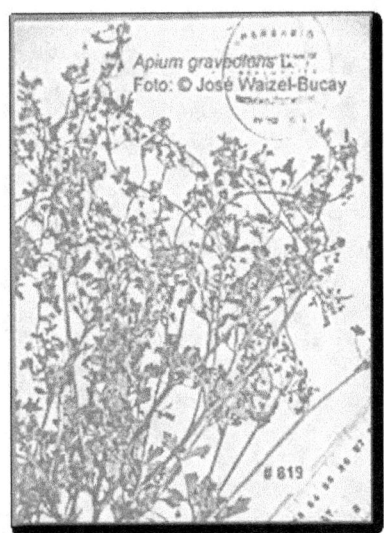
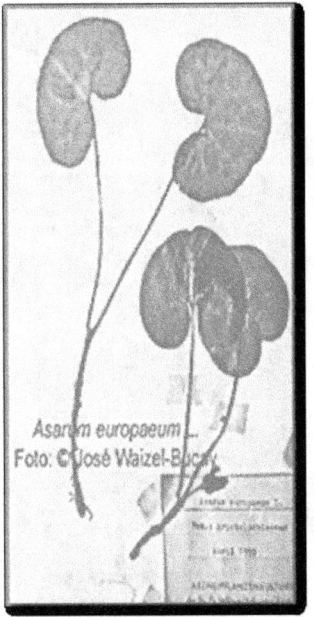

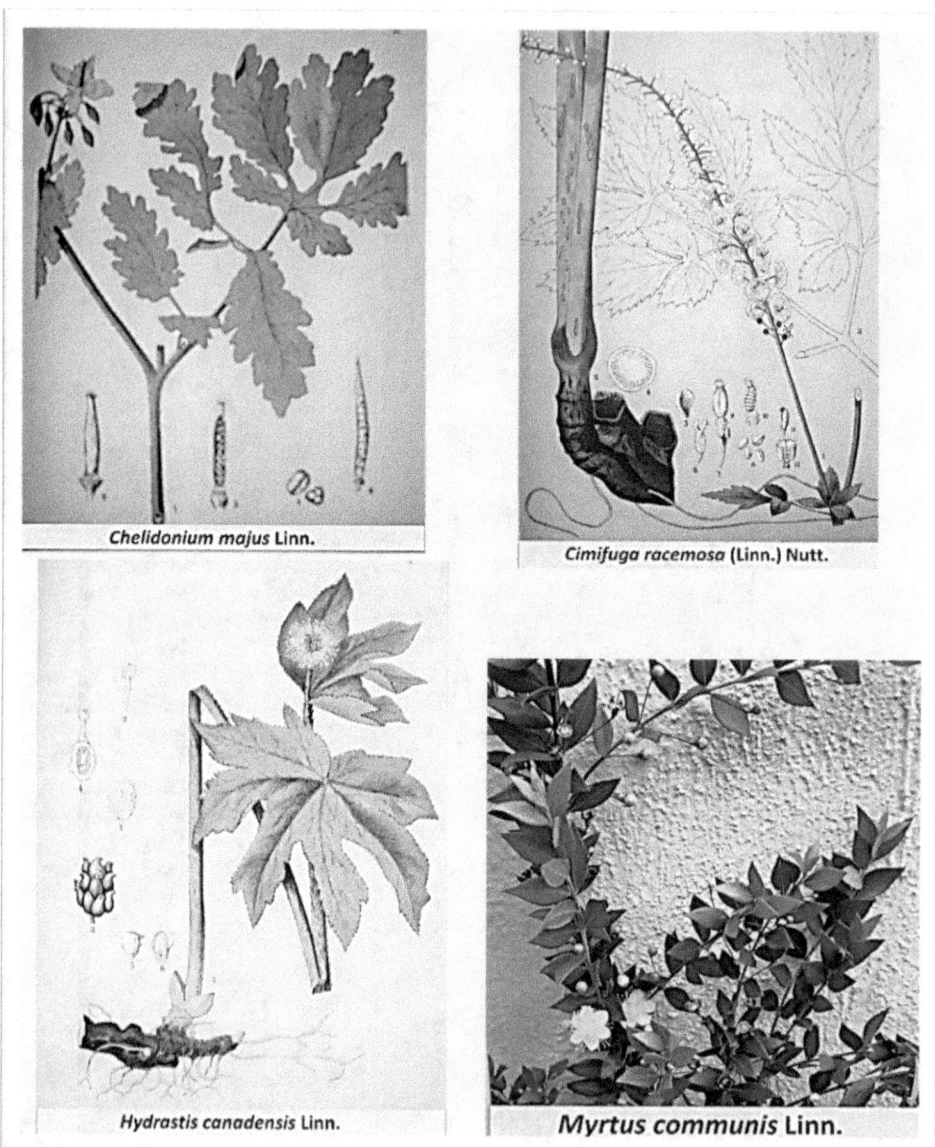

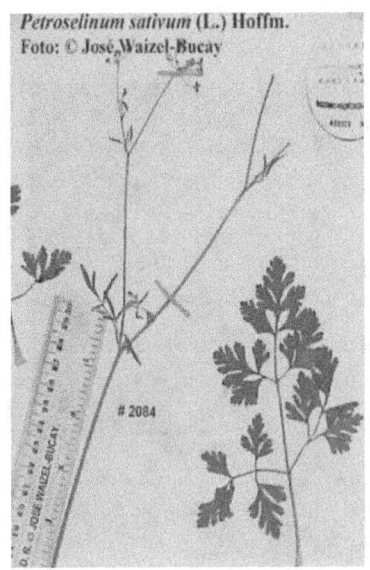

Petroselinum sativum (L.) Hoffm.
Foto: © José Waizel-Bucay

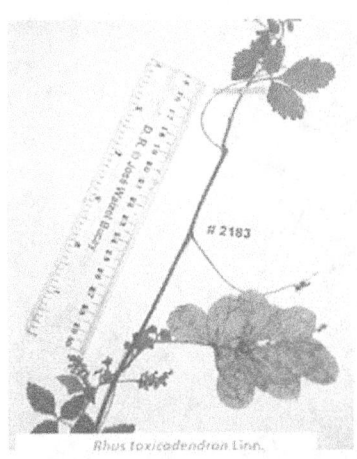

Rhus toxicodendron Linn.

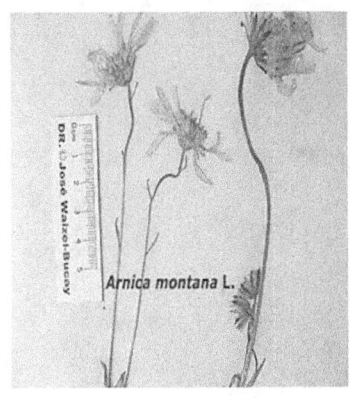

Arnica montana L.

Bougainvillea glabra Choisy
Photo: Alberto Waizel

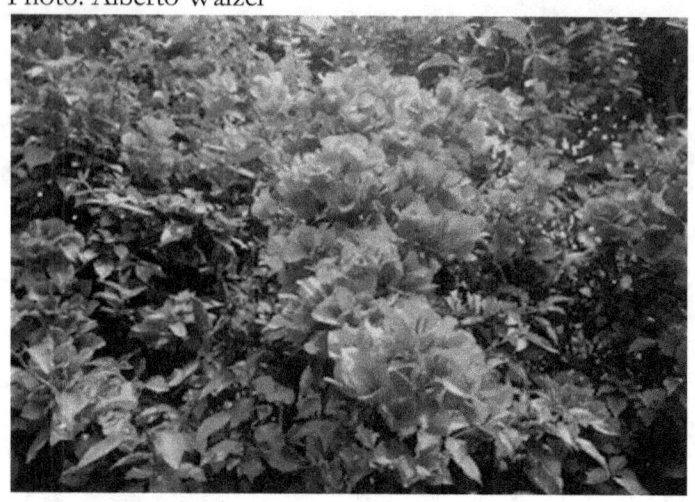

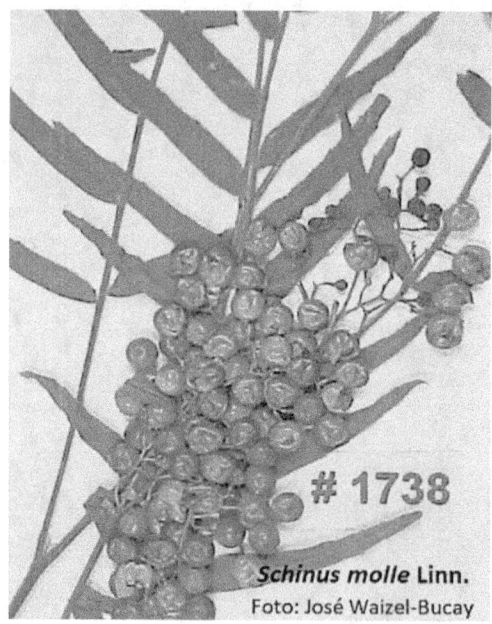

Schinus molle Linn.
Foto: José Waizel-Bucay

PLANTS FROM TEMPERATE ZONES

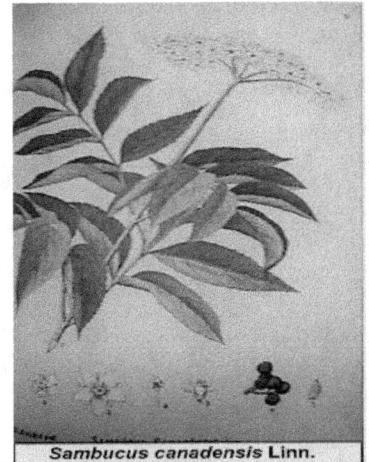
Sambucus canadensis Linn.

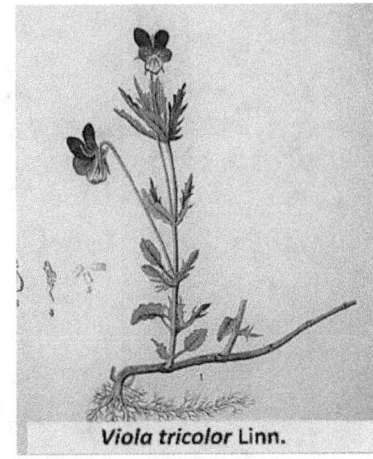
Viola tricolor Linn.

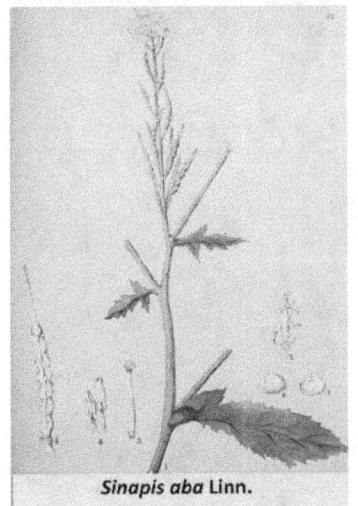
Sinapis aba Linn.

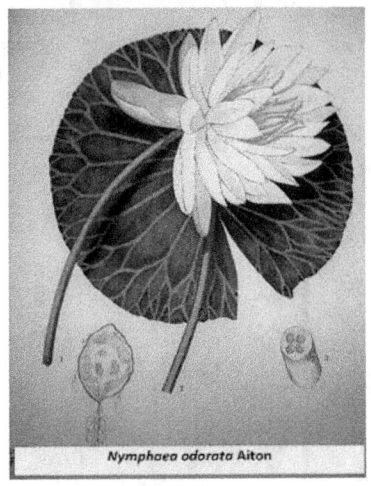
Nymphaea odorata Aiton

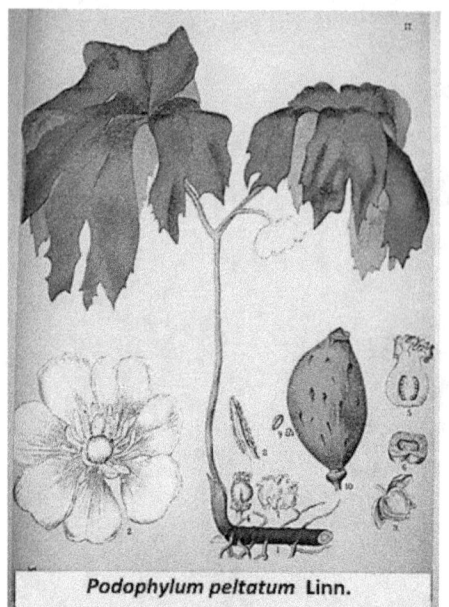

Podophylum peltatum Linn.

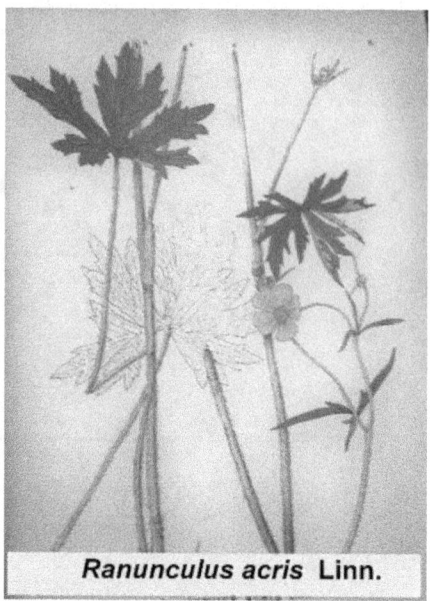

Ranunculus acris Linn.

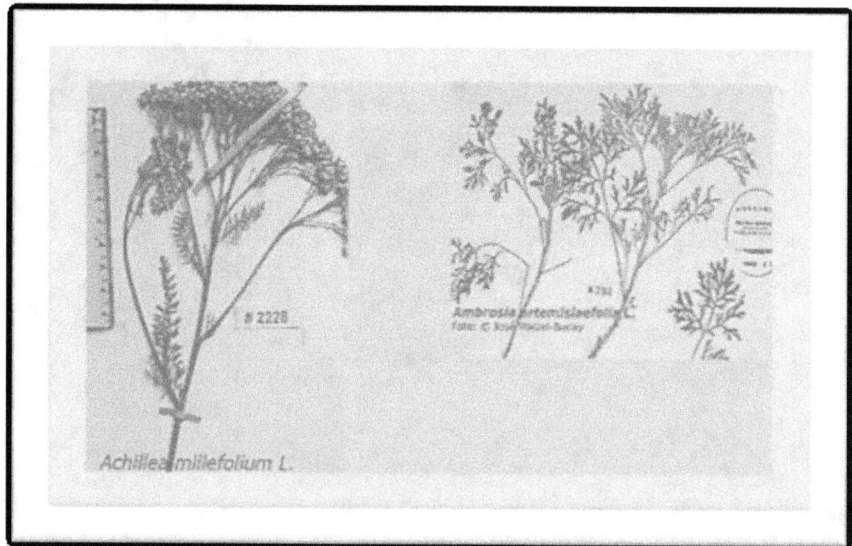

Achillea millefolium L.

Ambrosia artemisiaefolia L.

CHAPTER V. References

Allen, TF. 2006-2010. The Encyclopedia of Pure Materia Medica. [Available on line] http://homeoint.org/allen/a/agn.htm

American Institute of Homeopathy. 1979. The Homeopathic Pharmacopoeia of the United States of America. American Institute of Homeopathy. Fall Church's, Virginia, USA.

Anonymous. a. Sambong. *Blumea balsamifera* (L.) DC. In: Philippine Medicinal Plants. [Available on line] http://www.stuartxchange.org/Sambong.html <retrieved: August, 28 2008>.

Anshutz, PE. 2008. *Chionanthus virginica*. New, Old & Forgotten Remedies. In: Séror, R. Pathogénésies de l'an 1900. [Available on line] http://homeoint.org/seror/patho1900/chionant.htm <retrieved: November 28, 2008>.

Argimon, X. y MM. Trigo. n.d. Flora ornamental Española. In: Glosario de Botánica. http://www.arbolesornamentales.es/glosario.htm <retrieved: August 12, 2013>.

Bharatan, V. Humphries, JC. & RJ. Barnett. 2002. Plant Names in Homeopathy. The Natural History Museum. London. UK.

Boericke, W. 1927. Homoeophathic Materia Medica. [Available on line] http://www.homeoint.org/books/boericmm/index.htm

Boericke, W. 1927b. Una edición aumentada. Manual de Bolsillo de Matéria Médica Homeopática. B. Jain Publishers

PVT. LTD. India. [Available on line] http://books.google.com.mx/books?id=k_YLae-qEX0C&pg=RA1-PA116&lpg=RA1- <retrieved: January 1, 2009>.

Bolte, A. & I. Wichmann. 1997. The natural relationship of Remedies. Fagus-Verlag. [Available on line] http://www.homoeopathie-wichmann.de/heilmittel/order_of_remedies_intro.htm

Bruneton, J. 2001. Farmacognosia. Fitoquímica Plantas Medicinales. Editorial Acribia, S.A. Zaragoza, Spain.

Clarke, HJ. 2008. A Dictionary of Practical Materia Medica. [Available on line] http://homeoint.org/clarke/l/lact_vir.htm

Clarke, HJ. n.d. Un Diccionario de Materia Médica Práctica. Vol. I. [Available on line] http://books.google.com.mx/books?id=RnL--jMkG0sC&pg=PA623&lpg=PA623&dq=Armoracia+homeopatia&source=web&ots=uLQhBO3s23&sig=1y_N-7WSy9u-nWwXKIK9BJkq-YY&hl=es&sa=X&oi=book_result&resnum=3&ct=result#PPP1,M1 <retrieved: December 26, 2008>.

Comisión Editora de la Farmacopea Homeopática de los Estados Unidos Mexicanos. 1988. Farmacopea Homeopática de los Estados Unidos Mexicanos. Altres, Costa-Amic. México.

Cowperthwaith, CA. 2008. A Text-Book of Materia Medica. [Available on line] http://homeoint.org/seror/cowperthwaite/caulo.htm <retrieved: November 28, 2008>.

D'Ambrosio, S. n.d. El clima. [Available on line] http://www.monografias.com/trabajos4/elclima/elclima.shtml <retrieved: December 22, 2008>.

De Legarreta, L. 1961. M. M. Homéopathique des Plantes Mexicaines. In: Eliud Garcia-Trevino. 1966. Pathogénèses de quelques nouveaux remèdes Mexicains. *Journal of the American Institute of Homeopathy*. # 11/12. pp. 330-337. Cited by: Seror, R. 2000. Pathogénèses de l'an 2000. Agave Tequilana: [Available on line] http://homeoint.org/seror/pathog/agaveteq.htm

Domínguez, AX. 1979. Métodos de Investigación Fitoquímica. Limusa, S.A. México.

Dorta Soares, AA. n.d. Estudo comparativo das matérias-primas de origem vegetal utilizadas em Homeopatia em farmacopéias homeopáticas. [Available on line] http://lamasson.com.br/biblioteca/biblioteca/pesquisahomeopatica/artigogigio.htm <retrieved: March-April, 2013>.

Farias, DA. 2001. Repertório Homeopático Essencial. [Available on line] http://www.reocities.com/hotspring/spa/5086/prefacio.pdf <retrieved: April, 2011>.

Filipowicz, N. Piotrowski, A. Ochocka, JR. & M. Asztemborska. 2006. The phytochemical and genetic survey of common and dwarf juniper (*Juniperus communis* and *Juniperus depeana*) identifies chemical races and close taxonomic identity of the species. *Planta Medica*. 72(9):850-3.

François-Flores, DF. 2007. La Investigación Patogenética en México. (The Patogenetic Research in Mexico). [Available on line] http://www.homeopatia.com.mx/memorias2004/memorias/INVESTIGACION%20PATOGENETICA%20.doc <retrieved: February, 2007>.

Fuentes, FRV. 1996. Especies vegetales in Cuba empleadas en la preparación de medicamentos homeopáticos. *Revista*

Cubana de Plantas Medicinales. 1(3): 3-8.

Gotfredsen, E. 2009. Liber Herbarium II: The incomplete reference-guide to herbal medicine. [Available on line] http://www.liberherbarum.com/Pn1221.HTM <retrieved: 2008, 2013>.

Greuter, W. 2006. Compositae (pro parte majore). In: Euro+Med: Euro+Med PlantBase - the information resource for Euro-Mediterranean plant diversity. [Available on line] http://ww2.bgbm.org/EuroPlusMed, [01 November, 2013].

Guajardo, GB. 1988. El Estudio de la Farmacodinamia Homeopática. Instituto Politécnico Nacional. México.

Guermonprez, M. Pinkas M. *et* M.Torck. 1989. Matière Médicale Homéopathique. Editions Boiron. France.

Hering, C. 2006. The Guiding Symptoms of our Materia Medica. [Available on line] http://homeoint.org/hering/

Hutchens, RA. 1991. Indian Herbalogy of North America. Shambhala Publications Inc. Boston, USA.

International Plant Names (Database) 2004. [Available on line] http://www.ipni.org/index.html

Llorente-Bousquets, J., y S. Ocegueda. 2008. Estado del conocimiento de la biota. In: Capital Natural de México, vol. I: Conocimiento actual de la biodiversidad. CONABIO. México, pp. 283-322. [Available on line] http://www.biodiversidad.gob.mx/especies/cuantasesp.html <retrieved: July18, 2011>.

Materia Médica (*Ex libris*). 1999. Red-Radar Data Base. Assesse, Belgium: CD Edition by Red-Radar & Archibel S. A. Medical software.

Millspaugh, FC. 1974. American Medicinal Plants. Dover Publications. USA.

Missouri Botanical Garden. 2004. (Tropicos) Nomenclatural Data Base. [Available on line] http://mobot.mobot.org/cgi-bin/search_vast <retrieved: 2006, 2011, 2013 >.

Müntz, R. n.d. Remedia Homoopathie. [Available on line] http://www.remedia.at/homeopathy/Peganum%2Bharmala.html?arzneinr=3148&PHPSESSID=u002r8tqsn8ekuhn7m4cfmm7h1 <retrieved: January, 2009>.

Plants for a future. Species Database. [Available on line] http://www.pfaf.org/index.php <retrieved: January 1, 2009>.

Porcher, Michel H. *et al.* 1995. Sorting Medicinal Plant Names. Multilingual Multiscript Plant Name Database - A Work in Progress. Institute of Land & Food Resources. The University of Melbourne. Australia. [Available on line] http://www.plantnames.unimelb.edu.au/Sorting/Med_index.html < retrieved 2010-2011>.

Provings.info Systematics and Homeopathy Database. Fagus Publishing. [Available on line] http://www.provings.info/in/index.html <retrieved: 2008-2009>.

Remedia/at. 2010. [Available on line] http://www.remedia.at/homeopathy/index.html

Rosenberg, M. 1999. Temperate, Torrid & Frigid Zones. [Available on line] http://geography.about.com/library/weekly/aa011899.htm

Rosenberg, M. 2005. Köppen Climate Map. [Available on line] http://geography.about.com/library/weekly/aa011700a.htm

Ross, E. 1994. Climate and Biomes. Plant Physiology

Information Website. [Available on line] http://plantphys.info/principles/biomes.html. < retrieved: July 29, 2005>.

Rotblatt, M. & I. Ziment. 2002. Evidence-Based Herbal Medicine. Hanley & Belfus Inc. Philadelphia, USA.

Rowe, T. 2006. The Desert World. A Homeopathic Exploration. Desert Institute Publishing. USA.

Sachs, DJ. Mellinger, DA. & LJ. Gallup. 2000. The Geography of Poverty and Wealth. Center for international development. Harvard University. [Available on line] http://www.cid.harvard.edu/cidinthenews/articles/Sciam_03 01_article.html

Sandoval, GL. n.d. Farmacopea Homeopática Mexicana. B. Jain Publishers PVT. LTD. New Delhi, India.

Schumacher, H. 2007. Materia medica. [Available on line] http://openhomeo.org/openhomeopath/materia-medica.php?mittel=Malva-s.&lang=in <retrieved: April, 2011>.

Schwabe, W. 1929. Farmacopéa Homeopática. Willmar Schawe Ed. Leipzig.

Seror, R. 2000. Pathogénésies de l'an 2000. [Available on line] http://homeoint.org/seror/rp/rp014.htm

Sugden, A. 1997. Diccionario Ilustrado de la Botánica. Editorial Everest, S. A. Madrid, España (Spain).

Tiwari, L. Rai, N. & Kr R. Sharma. Regulatory Standards on Homoeophatic Drugs: Indian Perspective. *International Journal of Advanced Pharmaceutical Science and Technology*. 2013; 1(1):1-20. [Available on line] http://scientific.cloud-journals.com/index.php/IJAPST/article/view/Sci-72   <

retrieved: August 12, 2013>

USDA 2013. (United States of America Department of Agriculture) - Natural Resources Conservation Service (NRCS). Plants Database. [Available on line] http://plants.usda.gov/index.html <retrieved: January 5, 2009, November 2, 2013>.

USDA, ARS, National Genetic Resources Program. *Germplasm Resources Information Network - (GRIN)* [Online Database]. Species Nomenclature in GRIN taxonomy. National Germplasm Resources Laboratory, Beltsville, Maryland. [Available on line] http://www.ars-grin.gov/cgi-bin/npgs/html/taxgenform.pl?language=in <retrieved: March-December, 2008>.

Vithoulkas, G. n.d. Homeopathic Materia Medica. Online Materia Medica. [Available on line] http://www.vithoulkas.com/content/view/131/118/lang,in / <retrieved: December, 2008>.

Waizel, BJ. 1979. Cultivo, aislamiento y variación de principios activos de tres especies de plantas con propiedades anticancerígenas (Culture, isolation & variation of active principles of three species of plants with anticancer properties). Tesis Doctoral (Biología). (Ph D Thesis). Facultad de Ciencias. Universidad Nacional Autónoma de México. México. pp. 27-31.

Waizel, BJ. 2001. *Index Herbarium*, Índice de las plantas contenidas en el Herbario de la Escuela Nacional de Medicina & Homeopatía, con referencia a su uso en la terapéutica homeopática (Index of plants contained in the Herbarium of the National School of Medicine & Homeopathy, with reference to its use in homeopathic therapeutic) Instituto Politécnico Nacional. México.

Waizel, BJ. 2005. Some Plants from Arid Zones Used by Homeopathic Medicine. *American Journal of Homeopathic Medicine*. 98 (3): 179-206.

Waizel, BJ. 2006. La denominación de los seres vivos y la nomenclatura científica, su relevancia en los estudios científicos. In: Waizel, BJ. (Editor). Las Plantas Medicinales y las Ciencias. Una visión multidisciplinaria. Instituto Politécnico Nacional. México.

Waizel, BJ. (Editor). 2006. Las Plantas Medicinales y las Ciencias. Una visión multidisciplinaria (Sciences & medicinal plants. A multidisciplinary vision). Instituto Politécnico Nacional. México. Reprinted 2008.

Waizel, BJ. 2014. Plantas de Zona Templada Empleadas en Homeopatía. Aspectos Botánicos, Fitoquímicos y Farmacognósticos. Instituto Politécnico Nacional. México.

Waizel, BJ. & SH. Waizel. 2009. Antitussive plants used in Mexican traditional medicine. *Pharmacognosy Reviews*. 3(5): 22-36. [Available on line] http://phcogmag.com/antitussive-plants-used-mexican-traditional-medicine

Wang, Y. Sheir, W. & M. Ono. 2010. Ancient wisdom, modern kitchen: recipes from the East for Health, healing and long life. (Google eBook). De Capo Press.

Yépez, BM. Introducción a la Taxonomía Vegetal. In: Waizel, BJ. Las Plantas Medicinales y las Ciencias. Una visión multidisciplinaria. Instituto Politécnico Nacional. México. 2006, 2008.

Zandvoort, Van R. 2006. The Manual Complet Repertory 4.5 Ed. of the Institute for Research in Homeopathic Information and Symptomatology. Netherlands. [Available on line] http://www.mac-repertory.com/45.pdf <retrieved: July 13, 2006>.

ZOO Brno, Czechoslovakia, 1998. [Available on line] ZOO Brno, &

PLANTS FROM TEMPERATE ZONES

Koning.

CHAPTER VI. Index of Homeopathic Remedies

A
Abies canadensis: 17
Abies nigra: 17
Abrotanum: 18
Abrus: 18
Absinthium: 18
Acanthus mollis: 19
Achyrantes calea: 19
Aconitum anthora: 20
Aconitum cammarum: 20
Aconitum e radice: 21
Aconitum ferox: 21
Aconitum lycoctonum: 21
Aconitum napellus: 22
Aconitum septentrionale: 22
Acorus calamus: 22
Actaea racemosa: 23
Actaea spicata: 23
Actinidia chinensis e flores femineibus: 23
Adlumia fungosa: 24
Adonis vernalis: 24
Adoxa: 25
Aesculus glabra: 25
Aesculus hippocastanum: 25
Aethusa: 26
Agaricus: 26
Agaricus citrina: 27
Agaricus emeticus: 27
Agaricus pantherina: 27
Agaricus phalloides: 28
Agaricus procera: 28
Agave americana: 28
Agnus castus: 29
Agraphis nutans: 29
Agrimonia: 30

Agrostema githago: 30
Ailanthus glandulosus: 30
Ajuga reptans: 31
Aletris: 31
Alkekengi officinarum: 32
Alfalfa: 32
Allium cepa: 32
Allium sativum: 32
Allium ursinum: 33
Alnus: 33
Alnus serrulata: 34
Aloe: 34
Alpinia officinarum: 35
Althaea officinalis: 35
Ambrosia artemisiaefolia: 35
Ampelopsis quincefolia: 36
Amygdala amara: 36
Amygdalus dulcis: 36
Amygdalus persica: 37
Anacardium orientale: 37
Anagallis arvensis: 37
Anantherum muricatum: 37
Anchusa officinalis: 38
Anemone nemorosa: 38
Anethum: 39
Anisum stellatum: 39
Anthemis: 39
Anthoxanthum odoratum: 40
Apium graveolens: 40
Apocynum androsaemifolium: 40
Apocynum cannabinum: 41
Aquilegia vulgaris: 41
Aragallus lambertii: 42
Aralia: 42
Aralia hispida: 42
Aralia racemosa: 42
Arbutus andrachne: 43
Arbutus menziesii: 43
Argemone mexicana: 43

Argemone ochroleuca: 44
Argemone pleicantha: 44
Aristolochia clematitis: 45
Arnica montana: 45
Artemisia abrotanum: 46
Artemisia absinthum: 47
Artemisia dracunculus: 47
Artemisia vulgaris: 47
Arum dracontium: 48
Arum maculatum: 48
Arum triphyllum: 48
Asarum canadense: 49
Asarum europaeum: 49
Asclepias cornuti: 49
Asclepias incarnata: 50
Asclepias syriaca: 50
Asclepias tuberosa: 51
Asimina triloba: 51
Asparagus officinalis: 51
Assa-foetida: 52
Astragallus lamberti: 52
Astragalus campestris: 53
Astragalus exscapus: 53
Astragalus menziesii: 53
Astragalus mollisimus: 53
Athamanta oreoselinum: 54
Avena sativa: 54

B
Baptisia confusa: 55
Baptisia tinctoria: 55
Belladona: 55
Bellis perennis: 56
Benzoin: 56
Berberis: 56
Berberis aquifolium: 57
Berberis vulgaris: 57
B etula alba: 58

Blumea balsamifera: 58
Blumea odorata: 59
Boerhavia diffusa: 59
Boletus: 59
Borago officinalis: 59
Bougainvillea: 60
Bovista: 60
Branca ursina: 60
Brassica napus: 61
Brassica oleracea: 61
Brucea: 62
Bryonia: 62
Bunias orientalis: 63
Buxus: 63

C
Cainca (cahinca): 64
Cajuputum: 64
Calabar: 64
Caladium seguinum: 65
Calea: 65
Calendula: 66
Calendula arvensis: 66
Calla aethiopica: 67
Calotropis: 67
Caltha palustris: 67
Calystegia sepium: 68
Camphora: 68
Canchalagua: 69
Cannabis indica: 69
Cannabis sativa: 70
Capsicum: 70
Capsicum frutescens: 71
Carduus benedictus: 71
Carduus marianus: 71
Carissa schimperi: 72
Carpinus betulus: 72
Carya alba: 72
Cascara sagrada: 73

Castanea sativa: 73
Castanea vesca: 74
Catalpa: 74
Cataria nepeta: 74
Caulophyllum: 74
Ceanothus: 75
Ceanothus thyrisiflorus: 75
Celtis: 76
Centaurea tagana: 76
Centaurium umbellatum: 76
Cephalanthus: 77
Ceratonia siliqua: 268
Cetraria: 77
Chamomilla: 78
Chelidonium: 78
Chenopodium ambrosioides: 79
Chenopodium vulvaria: 79
Chimaphila: 80
Chionanthus: 80
Chrysanthemum: 81
Cichorium: 81
Cicuta maculata: 82
Cimifuga racemosa: 82
Cina: 83
Cineraria: 83
Cirsium arvense: 84
Cistus: 84
Citrus aurantium: 85
Citrus decumana: 85
Citrus limonum: 86
Citrus sinensis: 86
Citrus vulgaris: 86
Claviceps purpurea: 86
Clematis: 86
Clematis erecta: 86
Clematis vitalba: 87
Cocculus indicus: 88
Cochlearia armoracia: 88
Colchicum: 89

Colocynthis: 89
Conium: 90
Convolvulus stans: 90
Coriaria ruscifolia: 91
Corn-smut: 91
Corydalis: 91
Corydalis cava: 92
Corylus avellana: 92
Crataegus oxyacantha: 93
Crocus: 93
Cucurbita citrullus: 94
Cucurbita pepo: 94
Cundurango: 95
Cuphea viscosissima: 95
Cupressus australis: 96
Cupressus lawsoniana: 96
Cuscuta: 96
Cyclamen europaeum: 97
Cydonia vulgaris: 97
Cynara scolymus: 98
Cynoglossum officinale: 98
Cypripedium pubescens: 98
Cytisus scoparius: 99

D
Daphne indica: 99
Datura arborea: 100
Datura candida: 100
Datura ferox: 101
Datura inoxia: 101
Datura metel: 101
Datura sanguinea: 102
Desmodium gangeticum: 102
Dictamnus albus: 102
Digitalis lutea: 103
Digitalis purpurea: 103
Dioscorea villosa: 104
Dipsacus sylveaster: 104
Dirca palustris: 104

Draconitum foetidum: 105
Drosera rotundifolia: 105
Dulcamara: 105

E
Echinacea angustifolia: 106
Echinacea purpurea: 106
Elaeagnus: 107
Elaterium: 107
Eleutherococcus senticosus: 107
Ephedra: 108
Ephedra vulgaris: 108
Equisetum arvense: 108
Equisetum hyemale: 109
Equisetum limosum: 109
Erechites: 109
Erigeron: 110
Eriodictyon californicum: 110
Eryngium maritimum: 111
Eucalyptus globulus: 111
Euonymus atropurpurea: 111
Euonymus europaea: 112
Eupatorium aromaticum: 112
Eupatorium cannabinum: 112
Eupatorium perfoliatum: 113
Eupatorium purpureum: 113
Euphorbia corollata: 113
Euphorbia cyparissias: 114
Euphorbia esula: 114
Euphorbia helioscopia: 115
Euphorbia pilosa: 115
Euphorbia prostrata: 115
Euphorbia pulcherrima: 116
Euphrasia officinalis: 116
Eysenhardtia polystachya: 117

F
Fabiana: 117
Fagopyrum esculentum: 117

Fagus: 118
Ferula communis: 118
Filix: 118
Foeniculum anethum: 119
Foenum-graecum: 119
Fragaria: 120
Fraxinus: 120
Fraxinus excelsior: 120
Fumaria officinalis: 121

G
Galega: 121
Galium aparine: 122
Galium odoratum: 122
Galium verum: 123
Ganoderma lucidum: 123
Gaultheria: 123
Gelsemium: 124
Genista tinctoria: 124
Gentiana cruciata: 125
Gentiana lutea: 125
Gentiana quinquefolia: 126
Geranium: 126
Geranium robertianum: 127
Ginseng: 127
Gnaphalium: 127
Gnaphalium arenarium: 128
Gnaphalium polycephalum: 128
Granatum: 129
Gratiola officinalis 129
Grindelia robusta: 129
Grindelia squarrosa: 130
Gymnocladus canadensis: 130

H
Hamamelis: 131
Helianthus: 131
Heliotropium: 132
Helleborus: 132

Helleborus foetidus: 132
Helleborus orientalis: 133
Helleborus viridis: 133
Helonias dioica: 134
Hepatica: 134
Heracleum: 134
Hoitzia coccinea: 134
Hoya carnosa: 135
Humulus lupulus: 135
Hydrangea: 135
Hydrastis: 136
Hydrophyllum virginicum: 136
Hydropiper: 137
Hyoscyamus: 137
Hypericum: 137
Hyssopus officinalis: 138

I
Iberis amara: 138
Ictodes foetida: 138
Ignatia: 139
Ilex aquifolium: 139
Illicium anisatum: 139
Illicium verum: 140
Imperatoria: 140
Inula helenium: 140
Ipomoea: 141
Ipomoea stans: 141
Iris: 142
Iris florentina: 142
Iris germanica: 142
Iris versicolor: 143

J
Jacaranda mimosifolia: 143
Jalapa: 144
Jequirity: 144
Juglans cinerea: 144
Juglans nigra: 145

Juglans regia: 145
Juncus effusus: 145
Juniperus communis: 146
Juniperus oxycedrus: 146
Juniperus sabina: 147
Juniperus virginiana: 147
Justicia adhatoda: 148

K
Kalmia latifolia: 148
Karwinskia humboldtiana: 149

L
Laburnum anagyroides: 149
Lachnanthes tinctoria: 150
Lactuca: 150
Lactuca virosa: 150
Lamium: 151
Lamium laevigarum: 151
Lamium maculatum: 151
Lapathum acutum: 151
Lappa major: 152
Lariciformes officinalis: 152
Lathyrus: 153
Laurocerasus officinalis: 153
Laurus nobilis: 154
Lavandula angustifolia: 154
Leccinum testaceoscabrum: 154
Ledum palustre: 155
Lemna: 155
Lentinula edodes: 155
Lentinus edodes: 156
Leontopodium alpinum: 156
Leonurus: 156
Leptandra virginica: 157
Lespedeza capitata: 157
Liatris: 157
Lilium tigrinum: 158
Linaria vulgaris: 158

Linum catharticum: 158
Linum usitatissimum: 159
Lippia mexicana: 159
Lithospermum officinale: 160
Lobelia: 160
Lobelia cardinalis: 161
Lobelia dortmanna: 161
Lobelia erinus: 161
Lobelia purpurascens: 162
Lobelia siphilitica: 162
Lobelia syphilitica: 162
Lolium: 162
Lonicera: 163
Lonicera caprifolium: 163
Lupulina: 164
Lupulinum: 164
Lupulus humulus: 164
Lycium berberis: 164
Lycopersicum: 164
Lycopodium: 165
Lycopodium clavatum: 165
Lycopus: 165, 166
Lysimachia: 166

M
Macrozamia spiralis: 167
Magnolia glauca: 167
Magnolia grandiflora: 167
Magnolia virginiana: 168
Mahonia aquifolium: 168
Malva silvestris: 168
Mandragora: 168
Manzanita: 168
Marrubium vulgare: 169
Mate: 169
Mathiola: 170
Matricaria maritima: 170
Matricaria parthenium: 170
Melaleuca alternifolia: 170

PLANTS FROM TEMPERATE ZONES

Melilotus: 171
Melilotus alba: 171
Melissa: 171
Menispermum: 172
Mentha: 172
Mentha piperita: 173
Mentha pulegium: 173
Mentha viridis: 173
Menyanthes: 174
Mercurialis: 174
Mercurialis perennis: 174
Mezereum: 175
Millefolium: 175
Mimosa humilis: 176
Mimosa pudica: 176
Mitchella: 176
Momordica charantia: 177
Monotropa uniflora: 177
Morus nigra: 177
Myosotis arvensis: 178
Myosotis symphytifolia: 178
Myrica cerifera: 179
Myrtus communis: 179

N
Nabalus: 180
Nabalus albus: 180
Nabalus serpentaria: 180
Narcissus poeticus: 180
Narcissus pseudonarcissus: 181
Nasturtium: 182
Nelumbo nucifera: 182
Nepeta: 183
Nigella sativa: 183
Nolana paradoxa: 183
Nuphar: 184
Nuphar luteum: 184
Nymphaea: 184
Nymphaea alba: 185

O

Ocimum: 186
Oenanthe aquatica: 186
Oenanthe crocata: 186
Oenothera: 187
Oleander: 187
Oleum cajeputum: 188
Oleum cajuputi: 188
Oleum europaeum: 188
Ononis: 188
Onosmodium: 189
Opium: 189
Opuntia alba spina: 189
Opuntia ficus-indica: 190
Opuntia microdasys: 190
Opuntia vulgaris: 190
Orchis mascula: 190
Oreodaphne california: 191
Oreodaphne californica: 191
Origanum: 191
Origanum vulgare: 192
Ornithogalum umbellatum: 192
Orthosiphon stamineus: 192
Ostrya: 193
Ostrya virginica: 193
Oxalis acetosa: 193
Oxydendrum arboreum: 194
Oxytropis: 194
Oxytropis campestris: 195
Oxytropis lambertii: 195
Ozothamnus diosmifolius: 195

P

Padus avium: 195
Paeonia officinalis: 195
Papaver orientale: 195
Papaver rhoeas: 196
Parietaria: 196

Paris: 196
Paronichia illecebrum (Paronychia): 197
Parthenium: 197
Passiflora incarnata: 198
Pastinaca sativa: 198
Peganum harmala: 199
Pelargonium odoratissimum: 199
Penthorum sedoides: 200
Perilla frutescens: 200
Periploca graeca: 200
Persea americana: 201
Petiveria: 201
Petroselinum: 202
Petroselinum sativum: 202
Peumus boldus: 202
Phaseolus: 202
Phaseolus lunatus: 203
Phaseolus nanus: 203
Phellandrium: 203
Philadelphus coronarius: 204
Phleum: 204
Phragmites vulgaris: 204
Phyla scaberrima: 205
Phyllitis scolopendrium: 205
Physalis: 205
Physalis peruviana: 206
Phytolacca decandra: 206
Pichi pichi: 207
Pimpinella anisum: 207
Pimpinella saxifraga: 207
Pinguicula vulgaris: 208
Pinus abies: 208
Pinus cembra: 208
Pinus lambertiana: 208
Pinus palustres: 209
Pinus pumillionis: 209
Pinus silvestris: 209
Pinus teocote: 210
Pistacia lentiscus: 210

Plantago lanceolata: 210
Plantago major: 211
Plantago minor: 211
Platanus acerifolia: 212
Platanus occidentalis: 212
Platanus orientalis: 213
Platycerium bifurcatum: 213
Plumbago capensis: 213
Plumeria celinus: 213
Podophyllum peltatum: 214
Poinsettia: 214
Polei: 214
Polygala amara: 214
Polygala senega: 215
Polygonatum officinale: 215
Polygonum aviculare: 215
Polygonum hydropiperoides: 216
Polygonum persicaria: 216
Polygonum sagittatum: 216
Polygonum viviparum: 217
Polymnia: 217
Polyporus pinicola: 217
Polyporus pinicolus: 217
Populus alba: 218
Populus balsamifera: 218
Populus candicans: 218
Populus gileadensis: 219
Populus tremula: 219
Populus tremuloides: 219
Portulaca grandiflora: 220
Potentilla anserina: 220
Potentilla erecta: 221
Potentilla tomentilla: 221
Pothos foetidus: 221
Primula farinosa: 221
Primula obconca: 222
Primula obconica: 222
Primula veris: 222
Primula vulgaris: 223

Prunus armeniaca: 223
Prunus cerasifera: 223
Prunus cerasus: 223
Prunus domestica: 224
Prunus mahaleb: 224
Prunus padus: 224
Prunus persica: 225
Prunus spinosa: 225
Prunus virginiana: 225
Pseudotsuga menziesii: 226
Psilocybe: 226
Psoralea: 226
Psoralea corylifolia: 227
Ptelea trifoliata: 227
Pulmonaria officinalis: 228
Pulsatilla: 228
Pulsatilla nuttalliana: 228
Pulsatilla vulgaris: 229
Punica granatum: 229
Pyracantha coccinea: 229
Pyrethrum: 230
Pyrethrum parthenium: 230
Pyrola rotundifolia: 230
Pyrus americana: 231
Pyrus communis: 231
Pyrus malus: 231

Q
Quebracho: 232
Quercus: 232
Quercus robur: 233
Quillaia (Quillaja) saponaria: 233
Quillaja: 234
Quillaya saponaria: 234

R
Rajania subsamarata: 234
Ranunculus acris: 234
Ranunculus bulbosus: 235

Ranunculus ficaria: 235
Ranunculus flammula: 236
Ranunculus glacialis: 236
Ranunculus repens: 236
Ranunculus sceleratus: 237
Raphanistrum arvense: 237
Raphanus sativus: 237
Ratanhia: 238
Ratanhia peruviana: 238
Rauwolfia: 238
Rhamnus californica: 239
Rhamnus cathartica: 239
Rhamnus frangula: 240
Rheum: 240, 241
Rhododendron: 241
Rhododendron campylocarpum: 242
Rhododendron chrysanthemum: 242
Rhododendron chrysanthum: 242
Rhododendron ferrugineum: 242
Rhus aromatica: 242
Rhus coriaria: 242
Rhus diversiloba: 242
Rhus diversilobum: 242
Rhus glabra: 243
Rhus lentii: 243
Rhus ovata: 244
Rhus radicans: 244
Rhus toxicodendron: 244
Rhus typhina: 245
Rhus venenata: 245
Rhus vernix: 245
Ribes nigrum: 246
Ribes rubrum: 246
Ribes uva-crispa: 247
Ricinus communis: 247
Robinia: 247
Robinia bessoniana: 248
Robinia pseudoacacia: 248
Rosa canina: 248

Rosa centifolia: 248
Rosa damascena: 249
Rosmarinus: 249
Rubia tinctorum: 250
Rubus fruticosus: 250
Rubus idaeus: 250
Rumex: 251
Rumex acetosa: 251
Ruscus aculeatus: 252
Russula: 252
Ruta chalepensis: 252

S
Sabina: 253
Salix alba: 253
Salix fragilis: 254
Salix mollissima: 254
Salix nigra: 254
Salix purpurea: 255
Salvia: 255
Salvia sclarea: 255
Sambucus canadensis: 256
Sambucus ebulus: 256
Sambucus nigra: 257
Sanguinaria canadensis: 257
Sanguisorba officinalis: 258
Sanicula europaea: 258
Saponaria: 258
Sarracenia purpurea: 259
Sarsaparilla: 259
Sassafras: 259
Satureja: 260
Saxifraga granulata: 260
Scabiosa arvensis: 261
Scabiosa succisa: 261
Scammonium: 262
Schinus: 262
Scilla: 262
Scleranthus annus: 262

Scolopendrium: 263
Scorzonera hispanica: 263
Scrofularia nodosa: 263
Scutellaria: 264
Scutellaria galericulata: 264
Scutellaria laterifolia: 264
Secale cornutum: 264
Selaginella lepidophylla: 264
Semecarpus anacardium: 265
Senecio aureus: 265
Senecio hieracifolia: 266
Senecio jacobaea: 266
Senecio vulgaris: 266
Senega: 266
Sequoiadendron giganteum: 267
Serpentaria: 267
Siegesbeckia: 267
Siegesbeckia orientalis: 268
Sigesbeckia: 268
Siliqua dulcis: 268
Silphion: 268
Sinapis alba: 268
Sinapis nigra: 269
Smilax cordifolia: 269
Solanum carolinense: 269
Solanum malacoxylon: 270
Solanum mammosum: 270
Solanum nigrescens: 271
Solanum nigrum: 271
Solanum oleraceum: 272
Solanum pseudocapsicum: 272
Solanum tuberosum: 272
Solanum xanthocarpum: 273
Solanum xanthocarpus: 273
Solidago: 273
Sophora japonica: 274
Sorbus aucuparia: 274
Soya blüte: 274
Soya fluor: 275

PLANTS FROM TEMPERATE ZONES

Spartium scoparium: 275
Spigelia: 275
Spigelia marilandica: 275
Spilanthes acmella: 276
Spiraea: 276
Spiranthes: 277
Spiranthes autumnalis: 277
Spiritus glandium Quercus: 277
Squilla: 277
Stachys betonica: 278
Staphisagria: 278
Staphysagria: 279
Sticta pulmonaria: 279
Stillingia: 279
Stramonium: 280
Sumbul: 280
Sumbul plant: 281
Symphoricarpos albus: 281
Symphoricarpos racemosus: 281
Symphytum: 281
Syringa vulgaris: 282

T
Tabacum: 282
Tagetes: 283
Talauma mexicana: 283
Tanacetum: 283
Tanacetum parthenium: 284
Tanacetum vulgare: 284
Taraxacum officinale: 284
Taxus baccata: 284
Taxus brevifolia: 285
Telopea speciosissima: 285
Teucrium: 285
Teucrium scorodonia: 286
Thea: 286
Thea chinensis: 286
Thlaspi: 286
Thuja: 287

Thuja lobbii: 287
Thuya: 288
Thymus: 288
Tilia cordata: 288
Tilia europaea: 288
Tomentilla: 289
Torula: 289
Trifolium pratense: 289
Trillium: 290
Trillium cernuum: 290
Triosteum perfoliatum: 290
Triticum aestivum: 290
Tropaeolum: 291
Tussilago: 291
Tussilago fragans: 292
Tussilago petasites: 292

U
Ulex europaeus: 292
Ulmus: 293
Urtica: 293
Urtica dioica: 294
Urtica urens: 294
Uva-ursi: 294

V
Valeriana officinalis: 295
Veratrum: 295
Veratrum nigrum: 296
Veratrum viride: 296
Verbascum thapsus: 296
Verbena officinalis: 297
Veronica beccabunga: 297
Veronica officinalis: 298
Vesca: 298
Viburnum opulus: 298
Viburnum prunifolium: 299
Viburnum tinus: 299
Vicia faba: 299

Vinca: 300
Vinca: minor: 300
Vincetoxicum: 301
Viola odorata: 301
Viola tricolor: 301
Viscum: 302
Vitex: 302
Vitis: 303

W
Wyethia: 303

X
Xanthium: 303
Xanthium spinosum: 304
Xanthorhiza apiifolia: 304
Xanthorrhoea: 304
Xanthoxylon fraxineum: 304
Xerophyllum tenax: 304
Xylosteum: 305

Z
Zantedeschia aethiopica: 305
Zanthoxylum: 305
Zea: 305
Zea italica: 306
Zizia aurea: 306

CHAPTER VII. About the Author

José Waizel-Bucay, Biologist (B. Sc., M. Sc. & Dr. Sc.), was Professor and Senior Researcher in the Escuela Nacional de Medicina y Homeopatía (National Medicine & Homeopathy School) dependent of the Instituto Politécnico Nacional (IPN) or National Polytechnic Institute, in Mexico City, where 36 years ago, he worked in Medical Botany area, also was the founder of the Medicinal Plants Scholar Herbarium.

He had published articles and several lectures. Also is author and co-author (editor) of six books, one of them (his Doctoral Thesis) published by UNAM (1979) and the other five by IPN, three of which already have been reprinted (In one of them was a coauthor-editor, and in the other was a single creator). All are about medicinal plants (cancer, asthma, Homeopathy, and general medicinal plants history).

He was also the Coordinator and coauthor of the book: 1) "Las Plantas Medicinales y las Ciencias, una visión multidisciplinaria" (2006), 587 pp. ISBN: 970-36-0025-5. [The Medicinal plants and the sciences, a multidisciplinary vision].

He also wrote (as single author):

2) "La Medicina por Medio de las Plantas. Su recorrido a través de las culturas y la Historia" (2011), 120 pp. ISBN: 978-607-414-232-7. [Medicine across Plants. His journey throughout the cultures & history].

3) "Las Plantas y su Uso Antitumoral. Un Conocimiento Ancestral con Futuro Prometedor" (2012), 495 pp. ISBN: 978-607-414-298-3. [Plants and their antitumor use. An ancestral knowledge with promising future],

4) "Plantas de Zona Templada empleadas por la Homeopatía. Aspectos Botánicos, Fitoquímicos y

Farmacognósticos". (2014), 268 pp. ISBN: 978-607-414-443-7.
And,

5) "Plantas empleadas en el tratamiento del asma, Botánica, Fitoquímica, Etnofarmacología" (2016), 495 pp. ISBN: 978-607-414-556-4. [Plants used in asthma treatment. Botany, phytochemistry & ethnopharmacology].

The five books were printed in Spanish language, by Instituto Politécnico Nacional (IPN), in Mexico City.

6) e-Book "Plants from Temperate zones used in Homeopathic Medicine, Botanical, Ecological & Pharmacognostc Features" available as kindle e-book in amazon.com until september 8, 2019.

I. Articles from José Waizel-Bucay in English:

1. **Waizel, B.J.** "A chapter in therapeutics history. The affinity principles". Homoeopathic Links. [International Journal for Classical Homoeopathy]. Winter 2001; 14(1):199-201.
2. **Waizel, B.J.** "Atropa belladonna. Plants with relevance to medicine". Homoeopathic Links [International Journal for Classical Homoeopathy]. Vol. 15 (3):157-160. Autumn 2002.
3. **Waizel, B.J.** "Some Plants from Arid Zones Used by Homeopathic Medicine". American Journal of Homeopathic Medicine. Autumn, 2005; 98(3).
4. **Waizel, B.J.** "Some Cactaceous and Succulent Plants Used in Homeopathic Therapy" Homoeopathic Links [International Journal for Classical Homoeopathy]. Vol. 19(2), pp. 92-96, Summer 2006.
5. **Waizel, B.J.**, Waizel, H.S. "Antitussive plants used in Mexican traditional medicine". Pharmacognosy Reviews. 5 – January-June, 2009. http://phcogmag.com/antitussive-plants-used-mexican-traditional-medicine
6. De la Peña, SS., Sothern, RB., López, FS., Lujambio, IM., **Waizel-Bucay, J.**, Sánchez, CO., Pérez MC., Tena, BE. "Circadian aspects of hyperthermia in mice induced

by *Aconitum napellus*". Pharmacognosy Magazine. 2011:7(27); 234-242.
7. **Waizel-Bucay, J.**, Cruz-Juárez, Ma.L. "*Arnica montana* L., relevant European medicinal plant". (*Arnica montana* L. Planta medicinal europea con relevancia). Revista Mexicana de Ciencias Forestales. 2014; 5(25): 99-109. (Bilingual Edition; Spanish & English).

II. Research articles published in spanish in Mexican or International Scientific Journals (some available on the internet, Academia. edu; ResearchGate, & others pages)

1) **Waizel, B.J.** "Cultivo y aislamiento de principios activos anticancerosos en tres especies de plantas". Revista de la Sociedad Mexicana de Historia Natural. 1988; XXXVIII: 47 - 65.
2) Pulido A. M. E., G.A Ciurlizza, **Waizel B.J.** *et al.* "Yumel un medicamento homeopático verdadero" Revista de Homeopatía (Brasil). 1989; 54 (2): 47-56.
3) **Waizel, B.J.** "La colección de plantas medicinales de la Esc. Nal. de Medicina y Homeopatía del I.P.N." Rev. Mex. de Ciencias Farmacéuticas. 1991; 22(3):72.
4) **Waizel, B.J.**, Herrera Santoyo, J., Alonso Cortés D., Villarreal Ortega ML. Estudios preliminares de la actividad citotóxica de muérdagos mexicanos: *Cladocolea grahami, Phoradendron reichenbachianum* y *Phoradendron galeottii* (Loranthaceae). Revista del Instituto Nacional de Cancerología (Méx.). 1994; 40(3): 133-137.
5) **Waizel, B.J.** "Algunas notas sobre la planta medicinal *Arnica montana* L". Revista Médica del Instituto Mexicano del Seguro Social .1995; 33 (3): 306, 312, 326.
6) Serrano Nafate, José E. y **Waizel B.J.** "El cultivo de vegetales de utilidad medicinal". VIII Congreso Nacional Estudiantil de Investigación en el área de la Salud. Escuela Médico Militar. México, D. F. 25-27 mayo de l995. En: Gaceta Médica de México. l995; 131 (Supl.1).
7) **Waizel, B.J.** "Ecología y Salud: Experiencia de la Enseñanza de temas Ecológicos en una Escuela de Medicina." Salud en el trabajo (Rev. de la Soc. Mex. de Med. del Trabajo, A. C.). 1996; I(3): 9-13.
8) **Waizel, B.J.** y A. Salas C. "Situación actual del Jardín Botánico de Plantas Medicinales de la Escuela Nacional de Medicina y Homeopatía". Amaranto (Rev. de la Soc. Mex. de

Jardines Botánicos, A. C.) Vol. 9 # 1, pp. 18-28. (1996, 1997?).
9) **Waizel, B.J.** "Las Plantas y dermatitis por contacto ocupacional, una contribución a su conocimiento y estudio. Salud en el Trabajo (Soc. Mex. de Med. del Trabajo, A. C.). 1997. Vol. 2 # 4, pp.32-36.
10) **Waizel, B.J.** "Plantas con relevancia en la Medicina. I. La digital (*Digitalis* spp.).Revista Médica del Instituto Mexicano del Seguro Social. marzo-abril-1999; 37(2): 147-154.
11) **Waizel, B.J.**, Torres-Cabrera, M.L. Uso Tradicional e investigación científica de *Talauma mexicana* (D.C.) Don, "Yoloxóchitl o flor-corazón" (Magnoliaceae), Revista Mexicana de Cardiología. 2002. Vol. 12 # 4:31-38.
12) **Waizel, B.J.**, Martínez-Porcayo, G., Villarreal-Ortega, Ma. L., Alonso-Cortés, D., Pliego-Castañeda, A "Estudio preliminar etnobotánico, fitoquímico, de la actividad citotóxica y antimicrobiana de *Cuphea aequipetala* Cav. (Lythraceae)", Polibotánica (Editada por el Instituto Politécnico Nacional, México). 2003; #15: 99-108.
13) **Waizel, B.J.** y Waizel, H. S. "Algunas plantas empleadas popularmente en el tratamiento de enfermedades respiratorias. Parte I". Anales de Otorrinolaringología Mexicana. 2005; 50(4): 76-87.
14) Marines M. E., Torres, M. J., Hernández, H, F., Salas, B. SJ.y **Waizel, B.J.** Efecto del *Eupatorium perfoliatum* en la parasitemia de ratones BALB/c infectados con Plasmodium berghei. Revista De Fitoterapia (España) 2006; 6 (Supl. 1): P08.
15) **Waizel-Bucay, J.**, Martínez RIM. "Plantas empleadas en odontalgias I" Revista ADM (Asociación Dental Mexicana) 2007; 64 (5): 173-186.
16) **Waizel-Bucay, J.** "Plantas empleadas popularmente en el tratamiento de verrugas". Revista de Fitoterapia (España) 2007; 7(2): 153-170.
17) **Waizel, B.J.**, Waizel, HS. "Algunas plantas empleadas en México en el tratamiento del asma". *Revista Latinoamericana de Química*. 2008; (Suplemento especial).
18) **Waizel, B.J.** "El uso tradicional de las especies del género Dioscorea". Revista de Fitoterapia (España). 2009; 9(1): 63-67.

19) Waizel, H.S., **Waizel, B.J.** "Algunas plantas utilizadas en México para el tratamiento del asma". Anales de Otorrinolaringología Mexicana. 2009; 54(4): 145-171.
20) **Waizel-Bucay, J.**, Martínez RIM. "Algunas Plantas usadas en México en padecimientos periodontales" Revista ADM (Asociación Dental Mexicana) 2011; 68(2): 73-88.
21) **Waizel-Bucay, J.**, Camacho, MR. "El género Capsicum spp. ("chile"). Una versión panorámica". Revista Alephzero (Univ. de las Américas, Puebla, Méx.) 2011; 16(60): 67-79. En Internet: http://hosting.udlap.mx/profesores/miguela.mendez/alephzero/archivo/historico/az60/capsicum60.html
22) **Waizel-Bucay, J.** "Plantas y compuestos importantes para la medicina: Los sauces, los salicilatos y la aspirina". *Revista de Fitoterapia* (España). 2011: 11(1); 61-75.
23) López-González, SK., **Waizel-Bucay, J.**, Ríos-Guerra, H., Querejeta-Villagómez, E., Araujo-Álvarez, JM. "Prevalencia de molestias musculoesqueléticas en violinistas de una orquesta sinfónica". Revista Mexicana de Salud en el Trabajo. 2011; 1(8): 4-9.
24) Waizel-Haiat, S. **Waizel-Bucay, J.** "Cacao y chocolate: Seducción y terapéutica". Anales Médicos (México). 2012; 57(3): 236-245.
25) **Waizel-Bucay, J.**, Waizel-Haiat, S. "El estornudo. Fisiología, mitos, tradiciones, etnomedicina y plantas con propiedades estornutatorias". Anales de Otorrinolaringología Mexicana. 2015; 60(3): 179-193.
26) **Waizel-Bucay, J.**, Waizel-Haiat, S. "Las especias o condimentos vegetales. ¿Sólo saborizantes o también remedios medicinales?" Anales de Otorrinolaringología Mexicana. 2016; 61(3): 208-230.
27) **Waizel-Bucay, J.**, Waizel-Haiat, S., Revilla-Peñaloza, F. "Los productos herbolarios, la coagulación sanguínea y la cirugía otorrinolaringológica". Anales de Otorrinolaringología Mexicana. 2017; 62(2): 115-142.
28) **Waizel-Bucay, J.** "Perspectivas de las plantas medicinales". Revista digital Enosi (Escuela Nacional de Medicina y Homeopatía, IPN), México. 2019; junio-agosto

www.ingramcontent.com/pod-product-compliance
Lightning Source LLC
Chambersburg PA
CBHW072027230526
45466CB00020B/943